McMinn's Color Atlas of
Human Anatomy

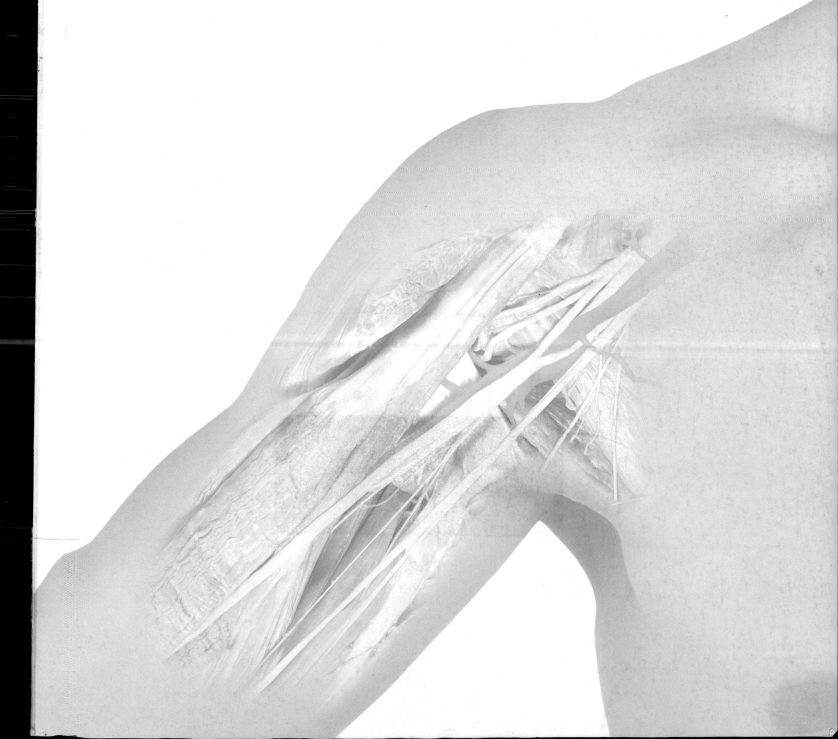

Dedicated to the memory of Peter Wolfe

Publisher: Richard Furn
Project Development Manager: Sarah Keer-Keer
Project Controller: Frances Affleck
Designer: George Ajayi
Page Makeup: Kate Walshaw
Illustration Manager: Bruce Hogarth

McMinn's Color Atlas of
Human Anatomy

Peter H. Abrahams MB BS, FRCS (Ed), FRCR
Professor of Clinical Anatomy
Kigezi International School of Medicine, Cambridge, UK
St. George's University, Grenada, West Indies

Fellow, Girton College, Cambridge, UK

Examiner to the Royal College of Surgeons of Edinburgh, UK

Family Practitioner, London, UK

Sandy C. Marks Jr BS, DDS, PhD FACD
Professor of Cell Biology, Radiology and Surgery,
University of Massachusetts Medical School,
Worcester, Massachusetts, USA

Ralph Hutchings
Photographer for Imagingbody.com

Formerly Chief Medical Laboratory Scientific Officer,
Royal College of Surgeons of England, London, UK

New dissections prepared by
Lynette Nearn Hardwick
Ross University School of Medicine, Dominica, West Indies

Radiological Adviser
Dr J Spratt MA (Cantab) FRCS (Eng) FRCS (Glas) FRCR
Honorary Lecturer in Anatomy, University of Durham, UK

Consultant Clinical Radiologist, University Hospital of North Durham, UK

Examiner in Anatomy, Royal College of Surgeons of England, UK

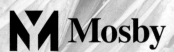

EDINBURGH LONDON NEW YORK PHILADELPHIA ST LOUIS SYDNEY TORONTO 2003

MOSBY
An imprint of Elsevier Science Limited

First edition published	1977 by Wolfe Publishing
Second edition published	1988 by Wolfe Publishing
Third edition published	1993 by Mosby-Wolfe, an imprint of Times Mirror International Publishers Ltd
Fourth edition published	1998 by Mosby, an imprint of Mosby International Ltd
This edition published	2003 by Elsevier Science Limited

Main edition ISBN 0723432120
International edition ISBN 0723432139

British Library Cataloguing in Publication Data
A catalogue record for this book is available from the British Library

Library of Congress Cataloging in Publication Data
A catalog record for this book is available from the Library of Congress

Note
Medical knowledge is constantly changing. As new information becomes available, changes in treatment, procedures, equipment and the use of drugs become necessary. The authors and the publishers have taken care to ensure that the information given in this text is accurate and up to date. However, readers are strongly advised to confirm that the information, especially with regard to drug usage, complies with the latest legislation and standards of practice.

The
publisher's
policy is to use
**paper manufactured
from sustainable forests**

Printed in China

Contents

Thorax 5

Abdomen and pelvis 6

Lower Limb 7

Appendices

Preface

In preparing the fifth edition of McMinn's Color Atlas of Human Anatomy, we have concentrated on making its use as intuitive as possible to the wide audience that the book enjoys, particularly to students of medicine, physical and occupational therapy, radiography, surgery, and dentistry. Towards that end we have:

- Prepared 50 new 'big picture' dissections that help provide an improved view of the anatomy of each region;
- Added an introductory page at the beginning of each chapter to provide a 'macro' view of the region;
- Adopted a completely redesigned, integrated page layout to make the book more intuitively user-friendly;
- Increased the use of orientation diagrams by including more than 90 surface anatomy 'locators' that place the region dissected on a live model;
- Used sequential dissections of the same specimen (for example, see infratemporal fossa, popliteal fossa, and sole of foot) to enhance the presentation of spatial relationships;
- Improved the clarity of each page by reducing the amount of text – citing the popular clinical correlations at the foot of the page but moving their explanation to the end of each chapter;
- Moved the Systemic Review to the front of the book and expanded it to include dermatome maps and cross sections from the Visible Human Project.

Another unique educational feature of this edition is the inclusion of a CD-ROM developed by Primal Pictures that contains stunning 3D anatomical models that illustrate the following regions; the Head, Vertebral Column, Thorax, Hand, Pelvis, Knee and Leg.

The functionality of the CD-ROM includes the ability to:

- Add and remove layers of muscle, etc. from the models;
- Rotate models completely for views from all angles;
- Activate labels on or off to test recognition skills;
- Export images to a hard drive;
- Self-test by means of an image-related multi-choice question format and quiz function.

Given the increasing significance of 3-dimensional data in medical education and clinical practice, use of this CD-ROM will provide the student with the earliest possible experience of multimodality learning of spatial data. Note that the most suitable 'jumping off points' from the book to the CD-ROM are indicated by the use of the CD icon thus:

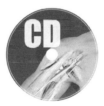

The general order of presentation in the Fifth Edition follows that used in the Fourth, except that (as noted above) the Systemic Review has been moved to the front of the book and each region is introduced by an overview. Our aim has been to make each page as self-explanatory as possible with respect to location and orientation. There are 50 new full-color plates in this edition. Most of these replace previous images, thus improving the overall quality of the presentations. We have also added 70 new radiographic and laparoscopic images to illustrate the anatomical foundation of contemporary health sciences.

P H Abrahams, S C Marks Jr. and R Hutchings
2003

Users Guide

This book is arranged in the general order 'head to toe'. The Head and Neck section (including the brain) is followed by the Vertebral Column and Spinal Cord, then Thorax, Upper Limb, Abdomen and Pelvis and finally the Lower Extremity. In each section skeletal elements are shown first followed by dissections, with surface views included for orientation. All structures are labelled by numbers, and these are identified in lists beside each image. An arrowhead at the end of a leader indicates that the structure labelled is just out of view beyond the tip of the arrow. Text has been limited to that needed to understand how the preparation was made, and is not intended to be comprehensive. The most suitable 'jumping off points' from the book to the CD-ROM are indicated by the use of the CD icon thus:

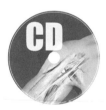

Acknowledgements

The sources for each of the new, updated images and laparoscopic photographs are acknowledged individually in the text. From the fourth edition of this book we have reused images from Prof. A. Darzi, Imperial College, London, UK, on pages 206, 228 and 243.

All the new dissections were produced at the University of Massachusetts Medical School by Lynette Nearn Hardwick (Ross University School of Medicine, Commonwealth of Dominica, West Indies). To add these new preparations to the 5th edition we are indebted to her special skills in the art and science of dissection and to the meticulous photographic expertise of Charlene Baron and Marie Craig. These new photographs augment the original ones taken by Ralph Hutchings, an author of every edition of this Atlas.

For assistance in proof reading we acknowledge the work of numerous colleagues:
David Choi MA (hons) MB ChB FRCS
Roy Choudhury PhD FRCS
Elanor Clarke BSc MBChB MD
John Cooke PhD
Andrew Fletcher PhD
Anne Gilroy MA
Vishy Mahadevan PhD FRCS
J D Spratt MA FRCS FRCR
T Welch FRCS
R Whitaker MS FRCS

Finally, it has been our pleasure to work closely with Sarah Keer-Keer and Richard Furn at Elsevier throughout the preparation of this edition.

Orientation

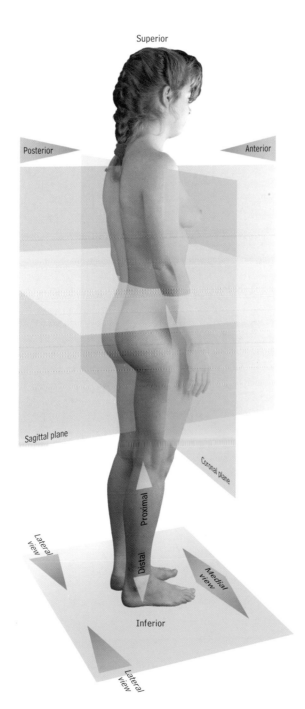

Superior

Posterior

Anterior

Transverse plane

Sagittal plane

Coronal plane

Proximal

Distal

Lateral view

Medial view

Inferior

Lateral view

Systemic review

Skeleton

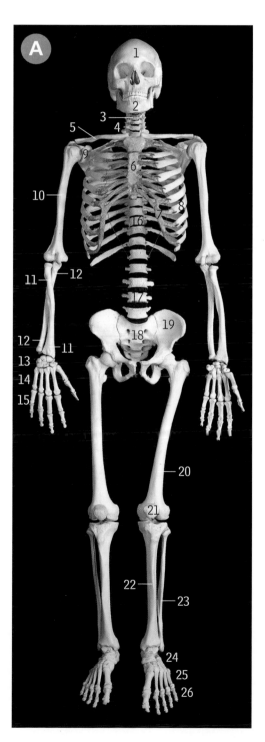

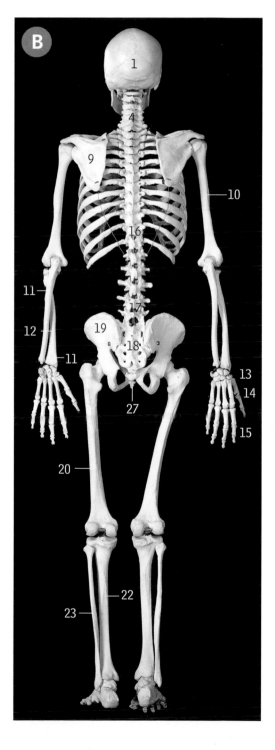

Ⓐ *from the front*
Ⓑ *from behind*

The left forearm is in the position of supination, the right in pronation.

1 Skull
2 Mandible
3 Hyoid bone
4 Cervical vertebrae
5 Clavicle
6 Sternum
7 Costal cartilages
8 Ribs
9 Scapula
10 Humerus
11 Radius
12 Ulna
13 Carpal bones
14 Metacarpal bones
15 Phalanges of thumb and fingers
16 Thoracic vertebrae
17 Lumbar vertebrae
18 Sacrum
19 Hip bone
20 Femur
21 Patella
22 Tibia
23 Fibula
24 Tarsal bones
25 Metatarsal bones
26 Phalanges of toes
27 Coccyx

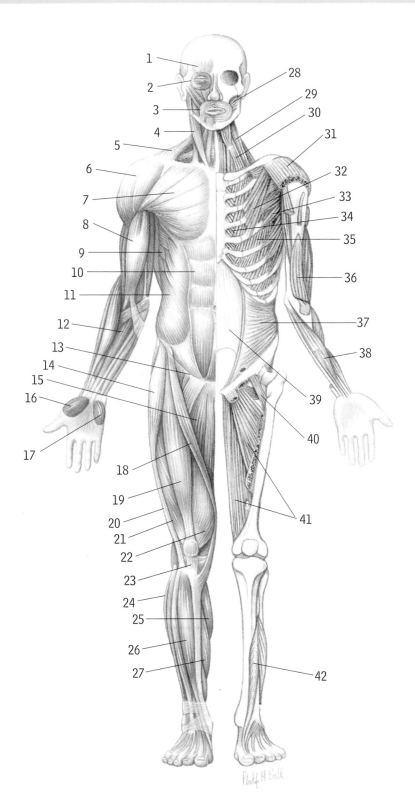

Muscles *from the front*

Superficial muscles on the right side of the body, deep muscles on the left side.

1 Frontalis part of occipitofrontalis
2 Orbicularis oculi
3 Orbicularis oris
4 Sternocleidomastoid
5 Trapezius
6 Deltoid
7 Pectoralis major
8 Biceps brachii
9 Serratus anterior
10 Rectus abdominis
11 External oblique
12 Superficial flexor muscles of forearm
13 Inguinal ligament
14 Tensor fasciae latae
15 Adductor muscles
16 Thenar muscles
17 Hypothenar muscles
18 Sartorius
19 Rectus femoris
20 Iliotibial tract
21 Vastus lateralis
22 Vastus medialis
23 Patellar ligament
24 Peroneal (fibular) muscles
25 Gastrocnemius
26 Extensor muscles of leg
27 Soleus
28 Buccinator
29 Levator scapulae
30 Scalenus anterior
31 Deltoid
32 Pectoralis minor
33 Serratus anterior
34 Internal intercostal
35 External intercostal
36 Brachialis
37 Internal oblique
38 Deep flexor muscles of forearm
39 Rectus sheath (posterior wall)
40 Psoas major and iliacus
41 Adductor magnus
42 Extensor hallucis longus

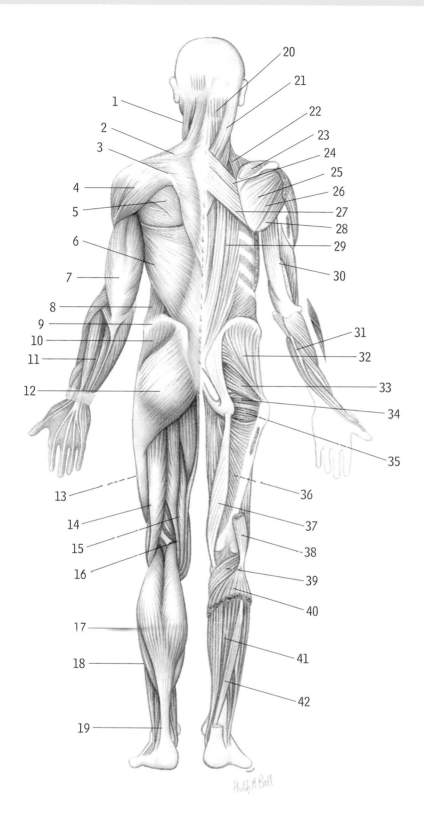

Muscles *from behind*

Superficial muscles on the left side of the body, deep muscles on the right side.

1 Sternocleidomastoid
2 Trapezius
3 Spine of scapula
4 Deltoid
5 Infraspinatus
6 Latissimus dorsi
7 Triceps
8 External oblique
9 Iliac crest
10 Gluteus medius
11 Superficial extensor muscles of forearm
12 Gluteus maximus
13 Iliotibial tract
14 Biceps femoris
15 Semimembranosus
16 Semitendinosus
17 Gastrocnemius
18 Soleus
19 Tendo calcaneus (Achilles tendon)
20 Semispinalis capitis
21 Splenius
22 Levator scapulae
23 Supraspinatus
24 Rhomboid minor
25 Infraspinatus
26 Teres minor
27 Rhomboid major
28 Teres major
29 Erector spinae
30 Triceps
31 Deep extensor muscles of forearm
32 Gluteus medius
33 Piriformis
34 Obturator internus
35 Quadratus femoris
36 Adductor magnus
37 Semimembranosus
38 Biceps femoris
39 Popliteus
40 Soleus
41 Deep flexor muscles of leg
42 Flexor hallucis longus

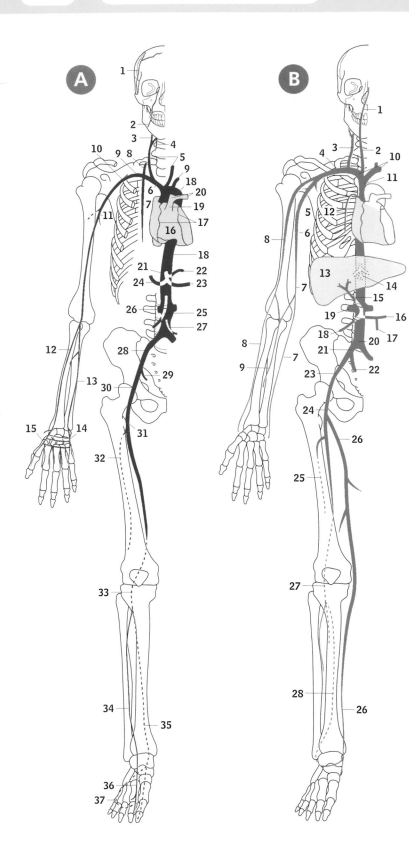

Ⓐ Arteries

major arteries, from the front

1	Superficial temporal a.	**20**	Pulmonary a.
2	Facial a.	**21**	Coeliac trunk
3	Internal carotid a.	**22**	Left gastric a.
4	External carotid a.	**23**	Splenic a.
5	Common carotid a.	**24**	Common hepatic a.
6	Brachiocephalic trunk	**25**	Superior mesenteric a.
7	Internal thoracic a.	**26**	Renal a.
8	Vertebral a.	**27**	Inferior mesenteric a.
9	Subclavian a.	**28**	Common iliac a.
10	Axillary a.	**29**	Internal iliac a.
11	Brachial a.	**30**	External iliac a.
12	Radial a.	**31**	Femoral a.
13	Ulnar a.	**32**	Profunda femoris a.
14	Deep palmar arch	**33**	Popliteal a.
15	Superficial palmar arch	**34**	Anterior tibial a.
16	Heart	**35**	Posterior tibial a.
17	Coronary a.	**36**	Dorsalis pedis a.
18	Aorta	**37**	Plantar arch
19	Pulmonary trunk		

Ⓑ Veins

major veins, from the front

(The pulmonary veins enter the left atrium at the back of the heart and are not shown)

1	Facial v.	**15**	Portal v.
2	Internal jugular v.	**16**	Splenic v.
3	External jugular v.	**17**	Inferior mesenteric v.
4	Subclavian v.	**18**	Superior mesenteric v.
5	Axillary v.	**19**	Renal v.
6	Brachial v.	**20**	Inferior vena cava
7	Basilic v.	**21**	Common iliac v.
8	Cephalic v.	**22**	Internal iliac v.
9	Median forearm v.	**23**	External iliac v.
10	Brachiocephalic v.	**24**	Femoral v.
11	Superior vena cava	**25**	Profunda femoris v.
12	Azygos v.	**26**	Great saphenous v.
13	Liver	**27**	Popliteal v.
14	Hepatic v.	**28**	Small saphenous v.

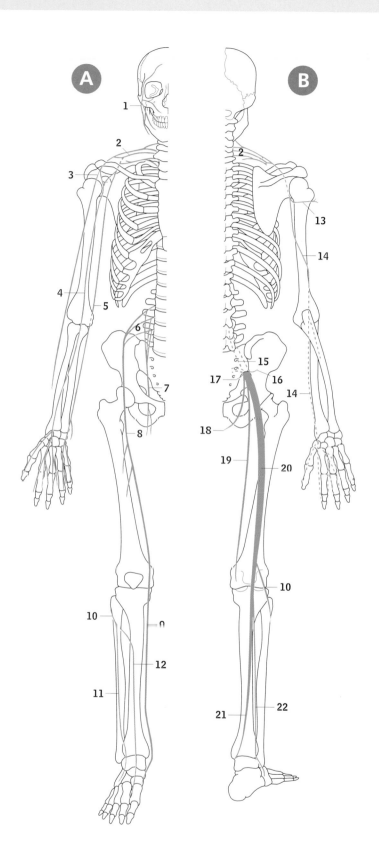

Nerves
the facial nerve and major branches of the brachial, lumbar and sacral plexuses

A from the front

B from the back

1 Facial n.
2 Brachial plexus
3 Musculocutaneous n.
4 Median n.
5 Ulnar n.
6 Lumbar plexus
7 Obturator n.
8 Femoral n.
9 Saphenous n.
10 Common peroneal (fibular) n.
11 Superficial peroneal (fibular) n.
12 Deep peroneal (fibular) n.
13 Axillary n.
14 Radial n.
15 Sacral plexus
16 Superior gluteal n.
17 Inferior gluteal n.
18 Pudendal n.
19 Posterior femoral cutaneous n.
20 Sciatic n.
21 Tibial n.
22 Sural n.

Spinal dermatomes and peripheral nerves

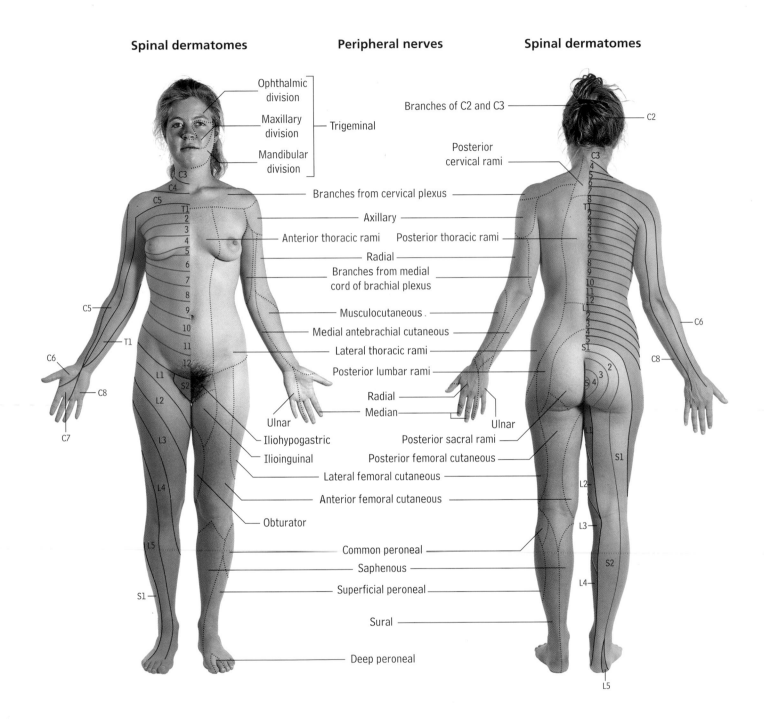

Spinal dermatomes   Peripheral nerves   Spinal dermatomes

Ophthalmic division
Maxillary division — Trigeminal
Mandibular division

Branches of C2 and C3

Posterior cervical rami

Branches from cervical plexus

Axillary

Anterior thoracic rami   Posterior thoracic rami

Radial

Branches from medial cord of brachial plexus

Musculocutaneous

Medial antebrachial cutaneous

Lateral thoracic rami

Posterior lumbar rami

Radial
Median
Ulnar
Iliohypogastric
Ilioinguinal
Ulnar
Posterior sacral rami
Posterior femoral cutaneous
Lateral femoral cutaneous
Anterior femoral cutaneous
Obturator
Common peroneal
Saphenous
Superficial peroneal
Sural
Deep peroneal

After Keegan et al, Anatomical Record 102, 1948. There is great personal variation, see Foerster, Brain 56, 1933.
Overlap of dermatomes occurs over 2–3 spinal root levels.

Cross-sections of the human body

Head and neck *cross-sections*

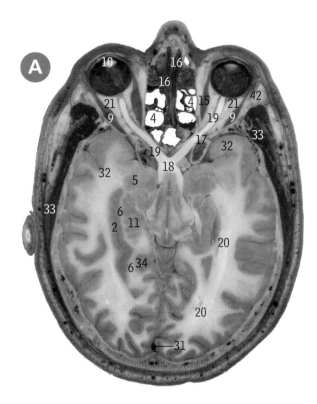

A section at level of optic chiasma

B section at level of vocal cords

1 Arytenoid cartilage
2 Claustrum
3 Common carotid artery
4 Ethmoidal air cells
5 Head of caudate nucleus
6 Internal capsule of cerebrum
7 Internal jugular vein
8 Lamina of vertebra
9 Lateral rectus muscle
10 Lens
11 Lentiform nucleus
12 Levator scapulae muscle
13 Ligamentum nuchae
14 Longus colli muscle
15 Medial rectus muscle
16 Nasal cavity
17 Optic canal
18 Optic chiasma
19 Optic nerve
20 Optic radiation
21 Orbital fat
22 Piriform fossa, pharynx
23 Platysma muscle
24 Scalenus anterior muscle
25 Scalenus medius and scalenus posterior
26 Semispinalis capitis muscle
27 Spinal cord
28 Spinalis muscle
29 Splenius capitis muscle
30 Sternocleidomastoid muscle
31 Superior sagittal sinus
32 Temporal lobe, cerebrum
33 Temporalis muscle
34 Thalamus
35 Thyroid cartilage
36 Thyroid gland, lateral lobe
37 Trapezius muscle
38 Vertebral artery in transverse foramen
39 Vertebral body
40 Vertebral canal
41 Vocal cord
42 Zygomatic bone

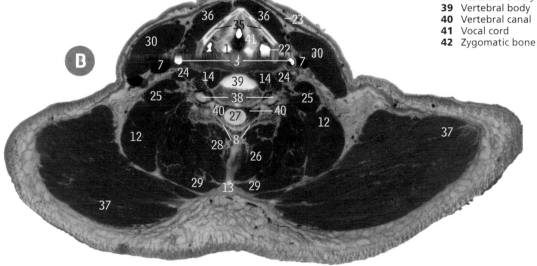

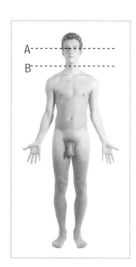

Images on pages 7–10 inclusive are from the National Library of Medicine (USA), Visible Human Data Set.

Thorax *cross-sections*

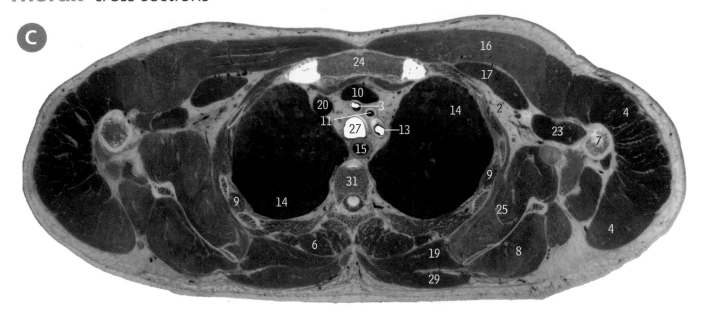

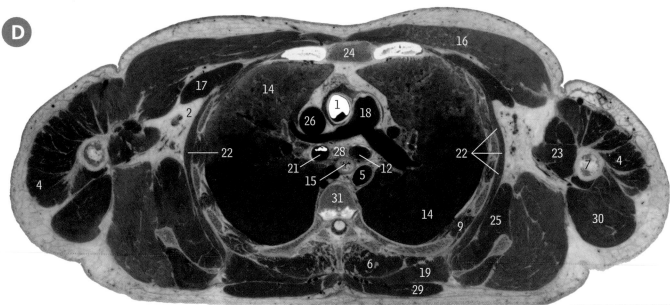

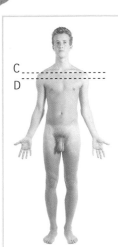

| C | section at T2 vertebral level |
| D | section at T4 vertebral level |

9 Intercostal muscles
10 Left brachiocephalic vein
11 Left common carotid artery
12 Left main bronchus
13 Left subclavian artery
14 Lung
15 Oesophagus
16 Pectoralis major muscle
17 Pectoralis minor muscle
18 Pulmonary trunk
19 Rhomboid major muscle
20 Right brachiocephalic vein
21 Right main bronchus

22 Serratus anterior muscle
23 Short head of biceps brachii
   and coracobrachialis muscles
24 Sternal marrow
25 Subscapularis muscle
26 Superior vena cava
27 Trachea
28 Tracheobronchial lymph
   nodes (carinal nodes)
29 Trapezius muscle
30 Triceps muscle
31 Vertebral body

1 Ascending aorta
2 Axillary fat with brachial plexus
3 Brachiocephalic artery
4 Deltoid muscle
5 Descending aorta
6 Erector spinae muscle
7 Humerus
8 Infraspinatus muscle

Abdomen *cross-sections*

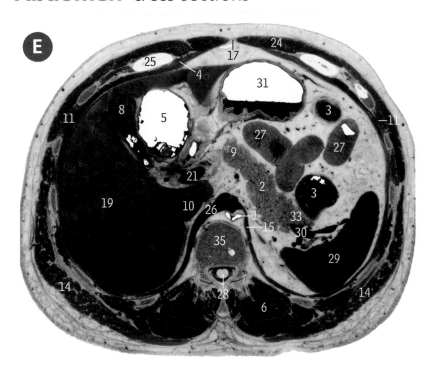

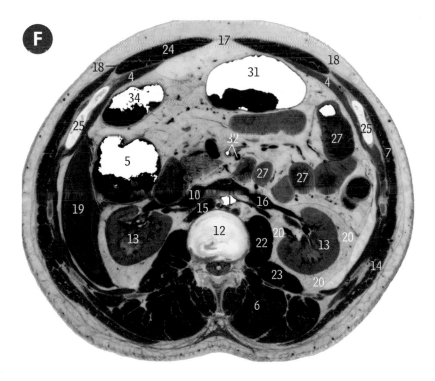

E section at L1 vertebral level

F section at L2 vertebral level

1 Aorta
2 Body of pancreas
3 Descending colon
4 Diaphragm
5 Duodenum
6 Erector spinae muscle
7 External oblique muscle
8 Gall bladder
9 Head of pancreas
10 Inferior vena cava
11 Intercostal muscle
12 Intervertebral disc
13 Kidney
14 Latissimus dorsi muscle
15 Left crus of diaphragm
16 Left renal vein
17 Linea alba
18 Linea semilunaris
19 Liver
20 Perirenal fat
21 Portal vein
22 Psoas muscle
23 Quadratus lumborum muscle
24 Rectus abdominis muscle
25 Rib
26 Right crus of diaphragm
27 Small intestine
28 Spinal cord
29 Spleen
30 Splenic artery and vein
31 Stomach
32 Superior mesenteric vessels
33 Tail of pancreas
34 Transverse colon
35 Vertebral body

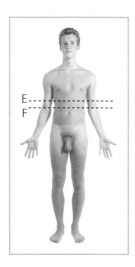

Pelvic region *cross-sections*

G

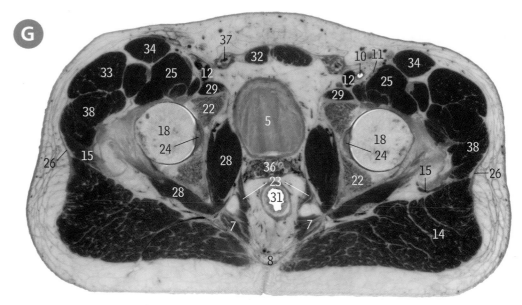

H

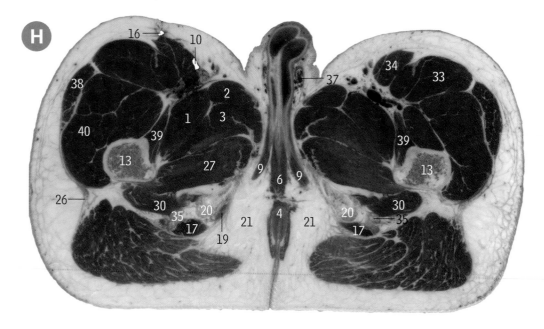

G section at level of the
hip joint in a male pelvis

H section at level of the
upper thigh in a male pelvis

1 Adductor brevis muscle
2 Adductor longus muscle
3 Adductor magnus muscle
4 Anal canal
5 Bladder
6 Bulb of penis
7 Coccygeus part of levator ani muscle
8 Coccyx

9 Crus of penis
10 Femoral artery
11 Femoral nerve
12 Femoral vein
13 Femur
14 Gluteus maximus muscle
15 Gluteus minimus muscle
16 Great saphenous vein
17 Hamstring origin
18 Head of femur
19 Ischiocavernosus
20 Ischial tuberosity
21 Ischioanal fossa
22 Ischium
23 Levator ani muscle
24 Ligament of head of femur

25 Iliopsoas muscle
26 Iliotibial tract
27 Obturator externus muscle
28 Obturator internus muscle
29 Pectineus muscle
30 Quadratus femoris muscle
31 Rectum
32 Rectus abdominis muscle
33 Rectus femoris muscle
34 Sartorius muscle
35 Sciatic nerve
36 Seminal vesicles
37 Spermatic cord
38 Tensor fasciae latae muscle
39 Vastus intermedius muscle
40 Vastus lateralis muscle

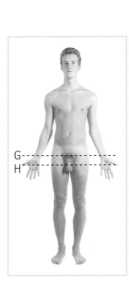

Head, neck and brain

Skull *from the front*

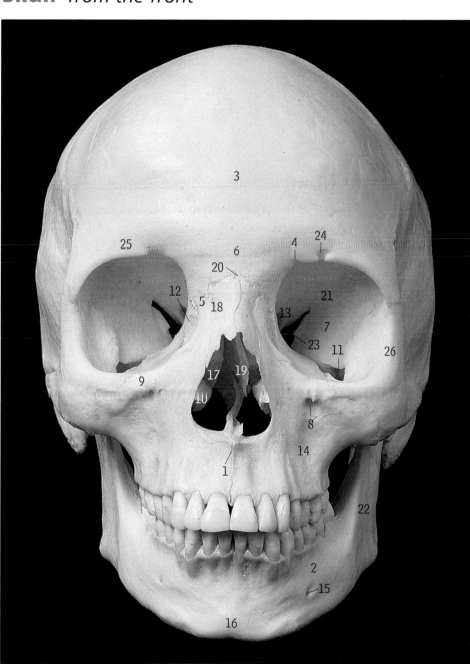

1 Anterior nasal spine
2 Body of mandible
3 Frontal bone
4 Frontal notch
5 Frontal process of maxilla
6 Glabella
7 Greater wing of sphenoid bone
8 Infra-orbital foramen
9 Infra-orbital margin
10 Inferior nasal concha
11 Inferior orbital fissure
12 Lacrimal bone
13 Lesser wing of sphenoid bone
14 Maxilla
15 Mental foramen
16 Mental protuberance
17 Middle nasal concha
18 Nasal bone
19 Nasal septum
20 Nasion
21 Orbit (orbital cavity)
22 Ramus of mandible
23 Superior orbital fissure
24 Supra-orbital foramen
25 Supra-orbital margin
26 Zygomatic bone

The term 'skull' includes the mandible, and 'cranium' refers to the skull without the mandible.

The calvaria is the vault of the skull (cranial vault or skull-cap) and is the upper part of the cranium that encloses the brain.

The front part of the skull forms the facial skeleton.

The supra-orbital, infra-orbital and mental foramina (24, 8 and 15) lie in approximately the same vertical plane.

Details of individual skull bones are given on pages 30 to 37, of the bones of the orbit and nose on page 22, and of the teeth on page 23.

Skull *muscle attachments, from the front*

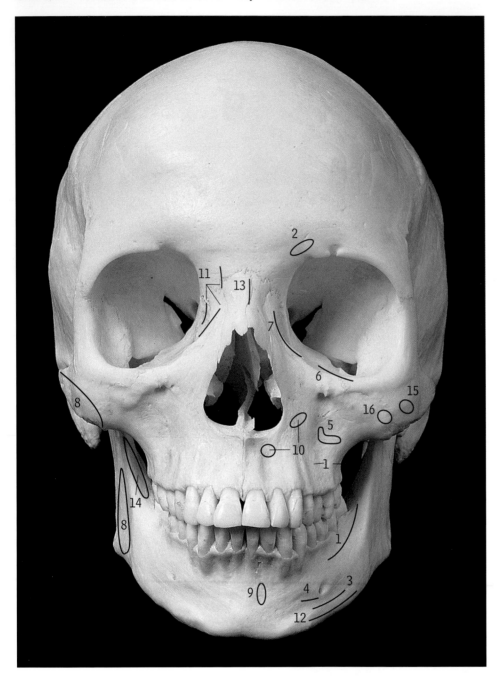

1   Buccinator
2   Corrugator supercilii
3   Depressor anguli oris
4   Depressor labii inferioris
5   Levator anguli oris
6   Levator labii superioris
7   Levator labii superioris alaeque nasi
8   Masseter
9   Mentalis
10 Nasalis
11 Orbicularis oculi
12 Platysma
13 Procerus
14 Temporalis
15 Zygomaticus major
16 Zygomaticus minor

Skull *radiograph, occipitofrontal 15° projection*

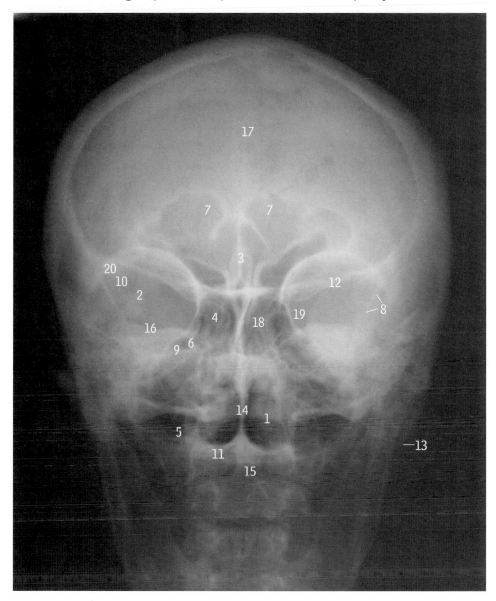

1 Basi-occiput
2 Body of sphenoid
3 Crista galli
4 Ethmoidal air cells
5 Floor of maxillary sinus (antrum)
6 Foramen rotundum
7 Frontal sinus
8 Greater wing of sphenoid
9 Internal acoustic meatus
10 Lambdoid suture
11 Lateral mass of atlas
   (first cervical vertebra)
12 Lesser wing of sphenoid
13 Mastoid process
14 Nasal septum
15 Odontoid process (dens) of axis
   (second cervical vertebra)
16 Petrous part of temporal bone
17 Sagittal suture
18 Sella turcica
19 Superior orbital fissure
20 Temporal surface of greater wing
   of sphenoid

Skull *from the right*

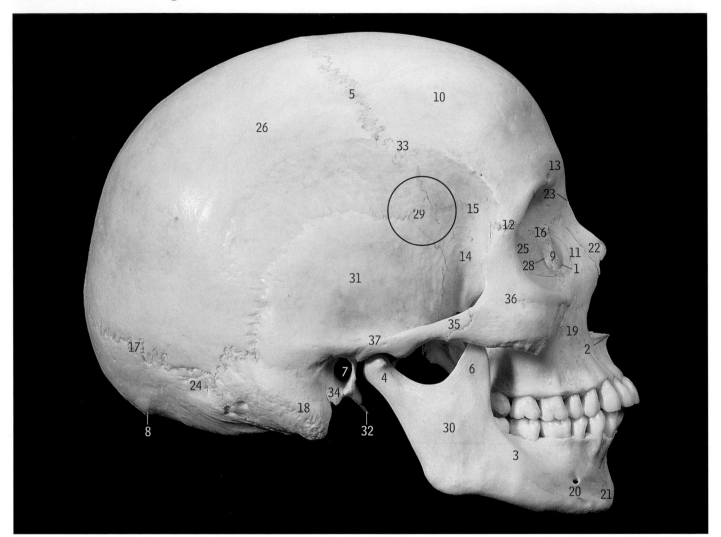

1 Anterior lacrimal crest	**11** Frontal process of maxilla	**21** Mental protuberance	**32** Styloid process of
2 Anterior nasal spine	**12** Frontozygomatic suture	**22** Nasal bone	temporal bone
3 Body of mandible	**13** Glabella	**23** Nasion	**33** Superior temporal line
4 Condyle of mandible	**14** Greater wing of	**24** Occipital bone	**34** Tympanic part of
5 Coronal suture	sphenoid bone	**25** Orbital part of ethmoid bone	temporal bone
6 Coronoid process of mandible	**15** Inferior temporal line	**26** Parietal bone	**35** Zygomatic arch
7 External acoustic meatus of	**16** Lacrimal bone	**27** Pituitary fossa (sella turcica)	**36** Zygomatic bone
temporal bone	**17** Lambdoid suture	**28** Posterior lacrimal crest	**37** Zygomatic process of
8 External occipital	**18** Mastoid process of	**29** Pterion (encircled)	temporal bone
protuberance (inion)	temporal bone	**30** Ramus of mandible	
9 Fossa for lacrimal sac	**19** Maxilla	**31** Squamous part of	
10 Frontal bone	**20** Mental foramen	temporal bone	

Pterion (29) is not a single point but an area where the frontal (10), parietal (26), squamous part of the temporal (31) and greater wing of the sphenoid bone (14) adjoin one another.

It is an important landmark for the anterior branch of the middle meningeal artery which underlies this area on the inside of the skull (page 27).

 Extradural haemorrhage, see page 90.

Skull *radiograph, lateral projection*

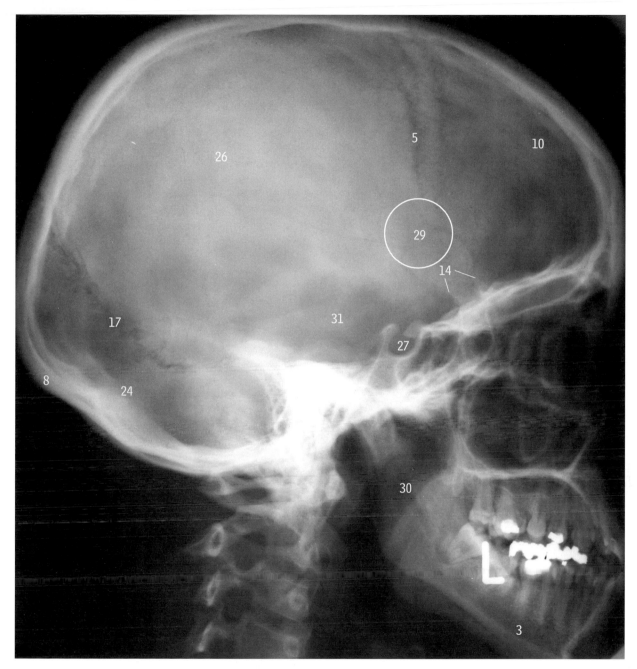

The position of mandibular ramus (30) is superimposed by air shadow in the nasopharynx.

Skull *muscle attachments, from the right*

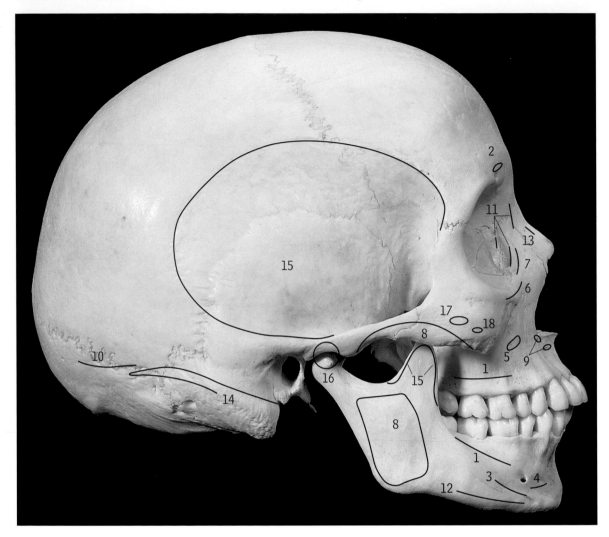

1   Buccinator
2   Corrugator supercilii
3   Depressor anguli oris
4   Depressor labii inferioris
5   Levator anguli oris
6   Levator labii superioris
7   Levator labii superioris alaeque nasi
8   Masseter
9   Nasalis
10 Occipital part of occipitofrontalis
11 Orbicularis oculi
12 Platysma
13 Procerus
14 Sternocleidomastoid
15 Temporalis
16 Temporomandibular joint
17 Zygomaticus major
18 Zygomaticus minor

The bony attachments of the buccinator muscle (1) are to the upper and lower jaws (maxilla and mandible) opposite the three molar teeth. (The teeth are identified on page 23, C.)

The upper attachment of temporalis (upper 15) occupies the temporal fossa (the narrow space above the zygomatic arch at the side of the skull). The lower attachment of temporalis (lower 15) extends from the lowest part of the mandibular notch of the mandible, over the coronoid process and down the front of the ramus almost as far as the last molar tooth.

Masseter (8) extends from the zygomatic arch to the lateral side of the ramus of the mandible.

Temporomandibular joint (TMJ) reduction, see page 91.

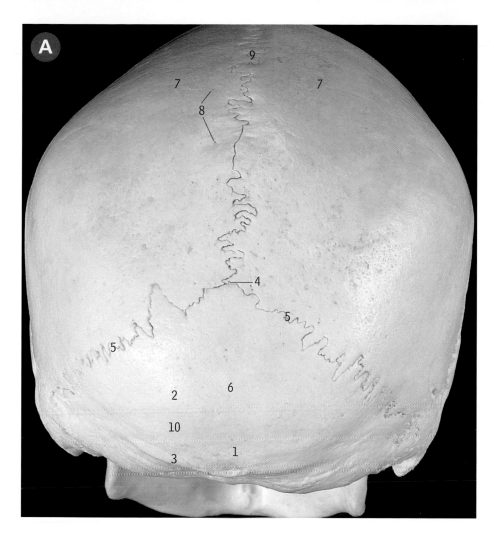

A Skull *from behind*

1 External occipital protuberance (inion)
2 Highest nuchal line
3 Inferior nuchal line
4 Lambda
5 Lambdoid suture
6 Occipital bone
7 Parietal bone
8 Parietal foramen
9 Sagittal suture
10 Superior nuchal line

B Skull *right infratemporal region, obliquely from below*

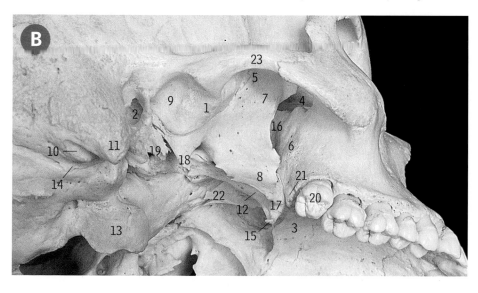

1 Articular tubercle
2 External acoustic meatus
3 Horizontal plate of palatine bone
4 Inferior orbital fissure
5 Infratemporal crest
6 Infratemporal (posterior) surface of maxilla
7 Infratemporal surface of greater wing
   of sphenoid bone
8 Lateral pterygoid plate
9 Mandibular fossa
10 Mastoid notch
11 Mastoid process
12 Medial pterygoid plate
13 Occipital condyle
14 Occipital groove
15 Pterygoid hamulus
16 Pterygomaxillary fissure and
   pterygopalatine fossa
17 Pyramidal process of palatine bone
18 Spine of sphenoid bone
19 Styloid process and sheath
20 Third molar tooth
21 Tuberosity of maxilla
22 Vomer
23 Zygomatic arch

 Burr holes, see page 89.

Skull *from above*

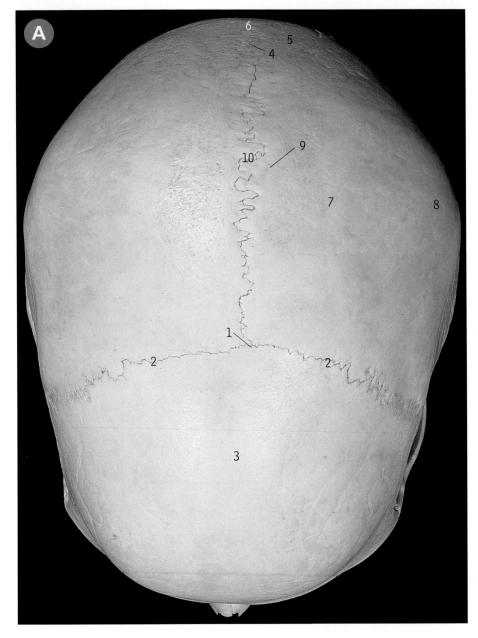

Skull
internal surface of the cranial vault, central part

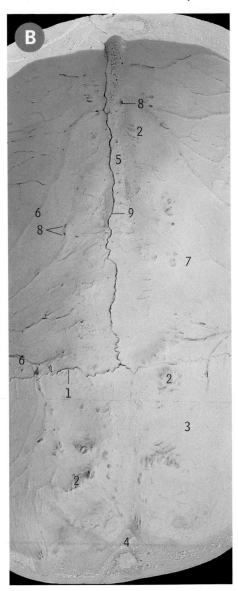

1	Bregma
2	Coronal suture
3	Frontal bone
4	Lambda
5	Lambdoid suture
6	Occipital bone
7	Parietal bone
8	Parietal eminence
9	Parietal foramen
10	Sagittal suture

In this skull the parietal eminences are prominent (A8).

The point where the sagittal suture (A10) meets the coronal suture (A2) is the bregma (A1). At birth the unossified parts of the frontal and parietal bones in this region form the membranous anterior fontanelle (page 24, D1).

The point where the sagittal suture (A10) meets the lambdoid suture (A5) is the lambda (A4). At birth the unossified parts of the parietal and occipital bones in this region form the membranous posterior fontanelle (page 24, C13).

The label 3 in the centre of the frontal bone indicates the line of the frontal suture in the fetal skull (page 24, A5). The suture may persist in the adult skull and is sometimes known as the metopic suture.

The arachnoid granulations (page 72, B1), through which cerebrospinal fluid drains into the superior sagittal sinus, cause the irregular depressions (B2) on the parts of the frontal and parietal bones (B3 and 7) that overlie the sinus.

1	Coronal suture
2	Depressions for arachnoid granulations
3	Frontal bone
4	Frontal crest
5	Groove for superior sagittal sinus
6	Grooves for middle meningeal vessels
7	Parietal bone
8	Parietal foramen
9	Sagittal suture

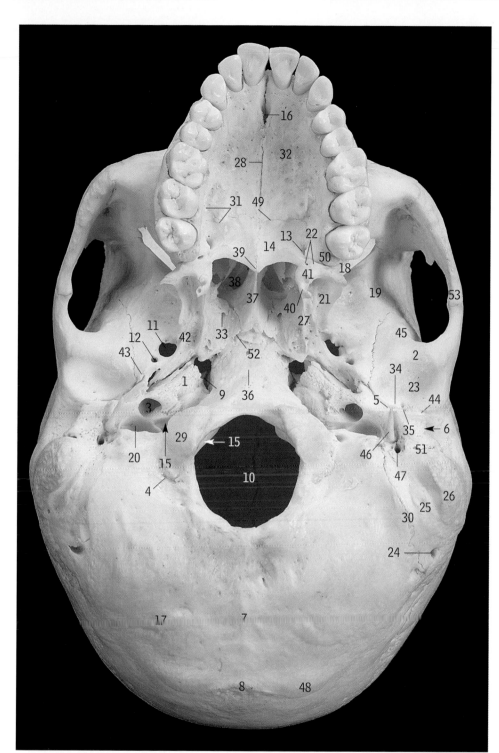

Skull

external surface of the base

1 Apex of petrous part of temporal bone
2 Articular tubercle
3 Carotid canal
4 Condylar canal (posterior)
5 Edge of tegmen tympani
6 External acoustic meatus
7 External occipital crest
8 External occipital protuberance
9 Foramen lacerum
10 Foramen magnum
11 Foramen ovale
12 Foramen spinosum
13 Greater palatine foramen
14 Horizontal plate of palatine bone
15 Hypoglossal (anterior condylar) canal
16 Incisive fossa
17 Inferior nuchal line
18 Inferior orbital fissure
19 Infratemporal crest of greater wing
    of sphenoid bone
20 Jugular foramen
21 Lateral pterygoid plate
22 Lesser palatine foramina
23 Mandibular fossa
24 Mastoid foramen
25 Mastoid notch
26 Mastoid process
27 Medial pterygoid plate
28 Median palatine (intermaxillary) suture
29 Occipital condyle
30 Occipital groove
31 Palatine grooves and spines
32 Palatine process of maxilla
33 Palatinovaginal canal
34 Petrosquamous fissure
35 Petrotympanic fissure
36 Pharyngeal tubercle
37 Posterior border of vomer
38 Posterior nasal aperture (choana)
39 Posterior nasal spine
40 Pterygoid hamulus
41 Pyramidal process of palatine bone
42 Scaphoid fossa
43 Spine of sphenoid bone
44 Squamotympanic fissure
45 Squamous part of temporal bone
46 Styloid process
47 Stylomastoid foramen
48 Superior nuchal line
49 Transverse palatine
    (palatomaxillary) suture
50 Tuberosity of maxilla
51 Tympanic part of temporal bone
52 Vomerovaginal canal
53 Zygomatic arch

The palatine process of the maxilla (32) and the horizontal plate of the palatine bone (14) form the hard palate (roof of the mouth and floor of the nose).

The carotid canal (3), recognized by its round shape on the inferior surface of the petrous part of the temporal bone, does not pass straight upwards to open into the inside of the skull but takes a right-angled turn forwards and medially within the petrous temporal to open into the back of the foramen lacerum (9).

Intracranial spread of infections, see p. 90.

Skull *muscle attachments, external surface of the base*

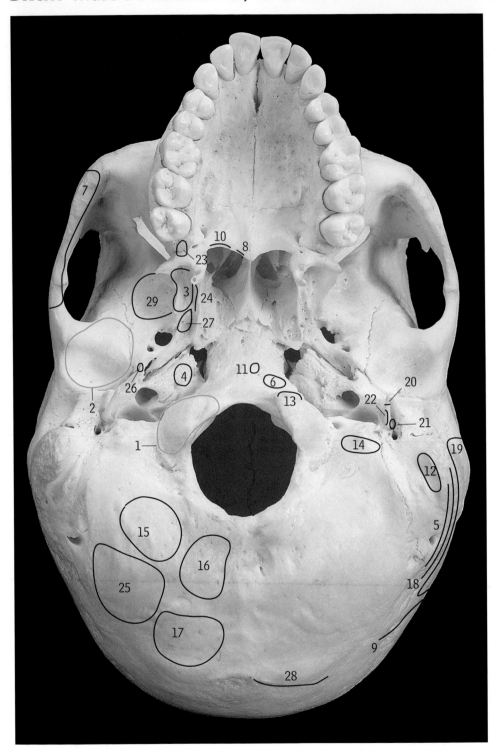

Green line = capsule attachments of atlanto-occipital and temporomandibular joints

1 Capsule attachment of atlanto-occipital joint
2 Capsule attachment of temporomandibular joint
3 Deep head of medial pterygoid
4 Levator veli palatini
5 Longissimus capitis
6 Longus capitis
7 Masseter
8 Musculus uvulae
9 Occipital part of occipitofrontalis
10 Palatopharyngeus
11 Pharyngeal raphe
12 Posterior belly of digastric
13 Rectus capitis anterior
14 Rectus capitis lateralis
15 Rectus capitis posterior major
16 Rectus capitis posterior minor
17 Semispinalis capitis
18 Splenius capitis
19 Sternocleidomastoid
20 Styloglossus
21 Stylohyoid
22 Stylopharyngeus
23 Superficial head of medial pterygoid
24 Superior constrictor
25 Superior oblique
26 Tensor tympani
27 Tensor veli palatini
28 Trapezius
29 Upper head of lateral pterygoid

The medial pterygoid plate has no pterygoid muscles attached to it. It passes straight backwards, giving origin at its lower end to part of the superior constrictor of the pharynx (24).

The lateral pterygoid plate has both pterygoid muscles attached to it: medial and lateral muscles from the medial and lateral surfaces, respectively (3 and 29). The plate becomes twisted slightly laterally because of the constant pull of these muscles which pass backwards and laterally to their attachments to the mandible (page 29).

Skull *internal surface of the base (cranial fossae)*

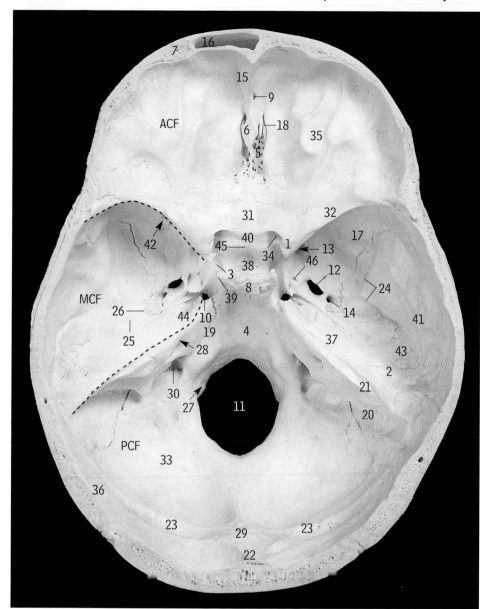

1 Anterior clinoid process
2 Arcuate eminence
3 Carotid groove
4 Clivus
5 Cribriform plate of ethmoid bone
6 Crista galli
7 Diploë
8 Dorsum sellae
9 Foramen caecum
10 Foramen lacerum
11 Foramen magnum
12 Foramen ovale
13 Foramen rotundum
14 Foramen spinosum
15 Frontal crest
16 Frontal sinus
17 Greater wing of sphenoid bone
18 Groove for anterior ethmoidal nerve and vessels
19 Groove for inferior petrosal sinus
20 Groove for sigmoid sinus
21 Groove for superior petrosal sinus
22 Groove for superior sagittal sinus
23 Groove for transverse sinus
24 Grooves for middle meningeal vessels
25 Hiatus and groove for greater petrosal nerve
26 Hiatus and groove for lesser petrosal nerve
27 Hypoglossal canal
28 Internal acoustic meatus
29 Internal occipital protuberance
30 Jugular foramen
31 Jugum of sphenoid bone
32 Lesser wing of sphenoid bone
33 Occipital bone
34 Optic canal
35 Orbital part of frontal bone
36 Parietal bone (postero-inferior angle only)
37 Petrous part of temporal bone
38 Pituitary fossa (sella turcica)
39 Posterior clinoid process
40 Prechiasmatic groove
41 Squamous part of temporal bone
42 Superior orbital fissure
43 Tegmen tympani
44 Trigeminal impression
45 Tuberculum sellae
46 Venous foramen

The anterior cranial fossa (ACF) is limited posteriorly on each side by the free margin of the lesser wing of the sphenoid (32) with its anterior clinoid process (1), and centrally by the anterior margin of the prechiasmatic groove (40).

The middle cranial fossa (MCF) is butterfly-shaped and consists of a central or median part and right and left lateral parts. The central part includes the pituitary fossa (38) on the upper surface of the body of the sphenoid, with the prechiasmatic groove (40) in front and the dorsum sellae (8) with its posterior clinoid processes (39) behind. Each lateral part extends from the posterior border of the lesser wing of the sphenoid (32) to the groove for the superior petrosal sinus (21) on the upper edge of the petrous part of the temporal bone.

The posterior cranial fossa (PCF), whose most obvious feature is the foramen magnum (11), is behind the dorsum sellae (8) and the grooves for the superior petrosal sinuses (21).

For cranial dural attachments and reflections see pages 61 and 63.

 Anosmia, see p. 89.

Skull *bones of the left orbit*

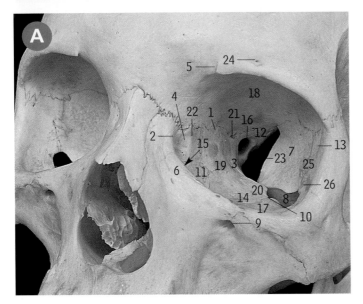

Nasal cavity *lateral wall*

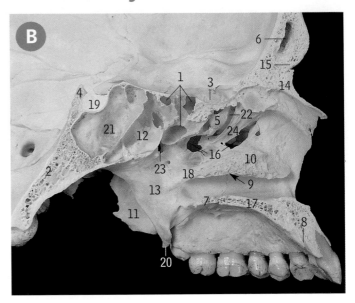

1 Anterior ethmoidal foramen	**14** Maxilla, forming floor
2 Anterior lacrimal crest	**15** Nasolacrimal canal
3 Body of sphenoid bone, forming medial wall	**16** Optic canal
4 Fossa for lacrimal sac	**17** Orbital border of zygomatic bone, forming floor
5 Frontal notch	**18** Orbital part of frontal bone, forming roof
6 Frontal process of maxilla, forming medial wall	**19** Orbital plate of ethmoid bone, forming medial wall
7 Greater wing of sphenoid bone, forming lateral wall	**20** Orbital process of palatine bone, forming floor
8 Inferior orbital fissure	**21** Posterior ethmoidal foramen
9 Infra-orbital foramen	**22** Posterior lacrimal crest
10 Infra-orbital groove	**23** Superior orbital fissure
11 Lacrimal bone, forming medial wall	**24** Supra-orbital foramen
12 Lesser wing of sphenoid bone, forming roof	**25** Zygomatic bone forming lateral wall
13 Marginal tubercle	**26** Zygomatico-orbital foramen

The fossa for the lacrimal sac (A4) is formed partly by the lacrimal groove of the frontal process of the maxilla (A6) and partly by the similar groove on the lacrimal bone (A11).

In this midline sagittal section of the skull, with the nasal septum removed, the superior and middle nasal conchae have been dissected away to reveal the air cells of the ethmoidal sinus, in particular the ethmoidal bulla (5).

1 Air cells of ethmoidal sinus	**13** Medial pterygoid plate
2 Clivus	**14** Nasal bone
3 Cribriform plate of ethmoid bone	**15** Nasal spine of frontal bone
4 Dorsum sellae	**16** Opening of maxillary sinus
5 Ethmoidal bulla	**17** Palatine process of maxilla
6 Frontal sinus	**18** Perpendicular plate of palatine bone
7 Horizontal plate of palatine bone	**19** Pituitary fossa (sella turcica)
8 Incisive canal	**20** Pterygoid hamulus
9 Inferior meatus	**21** Right sphenoidal sinus
10 Inferior nasal concha	**22** Semilunar hiatus
11 Lateral pterygoid plate	**23** Sphenopalatine foramen
12 Left sphenoidal sinus	**24** Uncinate process of ethmoid bone

The roof of the nasal cavity consists mainly of the cribriform plate of the ethmoid bone (B3) with the body of the sphenoid containing the sphenoidal sinuses (B21 and 12) behind, and the nasal bone (B14) and the nasal spine of the frontal bone (B15) at the front.

The floor of the cavity consists of the palatine process of the maxilla (B17) and the horizontal plate of the palatine bone (B7).

The medial wall is the nasal septum (page 67) which is formed mainly by two bones – the perpendicular plate of the ethmoid and the vomer – and the septal cartilage.

The lateral wall consists of the medial surface of the maxilla with its large opening (B16), overlapped from above by parts of the ethmoid (B1, 5 and 24) and lacrimal bones, from behind by the perpendicular plate of the palatine (B18), and below by the inferior concha (B10).

When covered by mucous membrane, the ethmoidal bulla (B5) and the uncinate process of the ethmoid (B24) form the upper and lower boundaries, respectively, of the semilunar hiatus (page 68, D15).

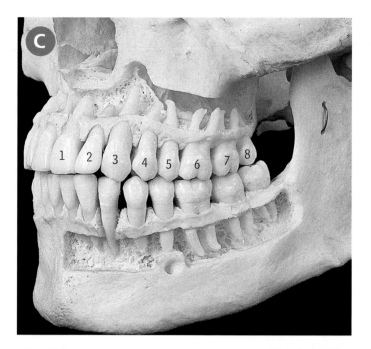

● Permanent teeth
from the left and in front

1	First (central) incisor	**5**	Second premolar
2	Second (lateral) incisor	**6**	First molar
3	Canine	**7**	Second molar
4	First premolar	**8**	Third molar

The corresponding teeth of the upper and lower jaws have similar names. In clinical dentistry the teeth are often identified by the numbers 1 to 8 (as listed here) rather than by name.

The third molar is sometimes called the wisdom tooth.

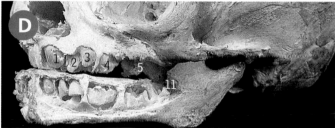

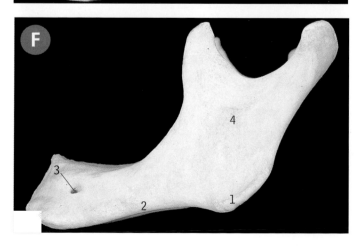

Upper and lower jaws
from the left and in front

D in the newborn with unerupted deciduous teeth

E in a four-year-old child with erupted deciduous teeth and unerupted permanent teeth

1	First (central) incisor of deciduous dentition	**7**	Second (lateral) incisor of permanent dentition
2	Second (lateral) incisor of deciduous dentition	**8**	Canine of permanent dentition
3	Canine of deciduous dentition	**9**	First premolar of permanent dentition
4	First molar of deciduous dentition	**10**	Second premolar of permanent dentition
5	Second molar of deciduous dentition	**11**	First molar of permanent dentition
6	First (central) incisor of permanent dentition	**12**	Second molar of permanent dentition

The deciduous molars occupy the positions of the premolars of the permanent dentition.

● Edentulous mandible
in old age, from the left

1	Angle	**3**	Mental foramen
2	Body	**4**	Ramus

With the loss of teeth the alveolar bone becomes absorbed, so that the mental foramen (3) and mandibular canal lie near the upper margin of the bone.

The angle (1) between the ramus (4) and body (2) becomes more obtuse, resembling the infantile angle (as in D and E, above).

Skull of a full-term fetus

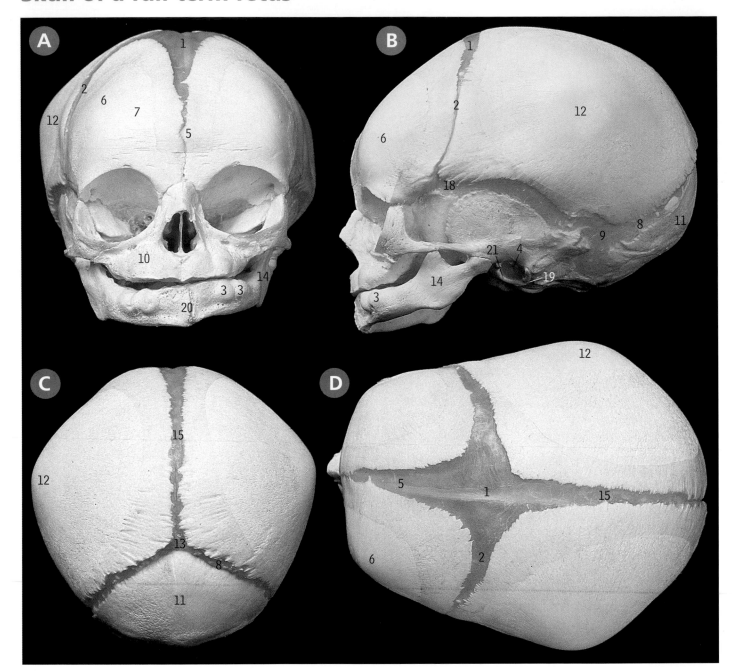

A　from the front

B　from the left and slightly below

C　from behind

D　from above

1	Anterior fontanelle	**11**	Occipital bone
2	Coronal suture	**12**	Parietal tuberosity
3	Elevations over deciduous teeth in body of mandible	**13**	Posterior fontanelle
		14	Ramus of mandible
4	External acoustic meatus	**15**	Sagittal suture
5	Frontal suture	**16**	Sella turcica
6	Frontal tuberosity	**17**	Semicircular canals
7	Half of frontal bone	**18**	Sphenoidal fontanelle
8	Lambdoid suture	**19**	Stylomastoid foramen
9	Mastoid fontanelle	**20**	Symphysis menti
10	Maxilla	**21**	Tympanic ring

Fetal skull radiographs **E** *frontal projection* **F** *lateral projection*

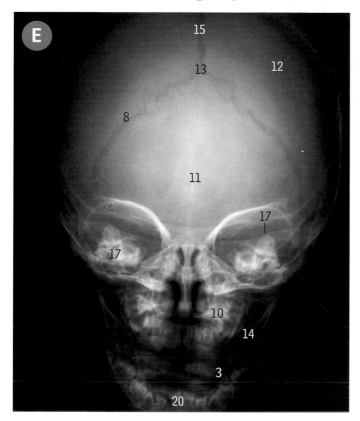

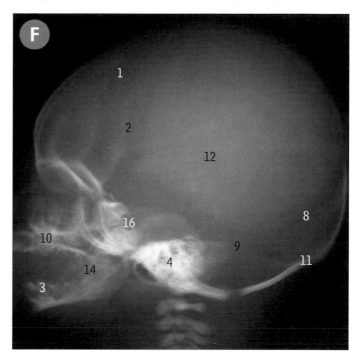

The face at birth forms a relatively smaller proportion of the cranium than in the adult (about one eighth compared with one half) because of the small size of the nasal cavity and maxillary sinuses and the lack of erupted teeth.

The posterior fontanelle (C13, E13) closes about two months after birth, the anterior fontanelle (A1, D1, F1) in the second year.

Owing to the lack of the mastoid process (which does not develop until the second year) the stylomastoid foramen (B19) and the emerging facial nerve are relatively near the surface and unprotected.

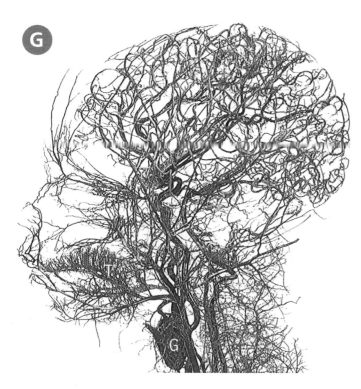

G Resin cast of head and neck arteries *full-term fetus, from the left*

In this cast of fetal arteries, note in the front of the neck the dense arterial pattern indicating the thyroid gland (G), and above and in front of it the fine vessels outlining the tongue (T).

Hydrocephalus, scalp wounds, see pp 90–91.

Skull Ⓐ cleared specimen from the front, illuminated from behind
Ⓑ radiograph of facial bones, occipitofrontal view

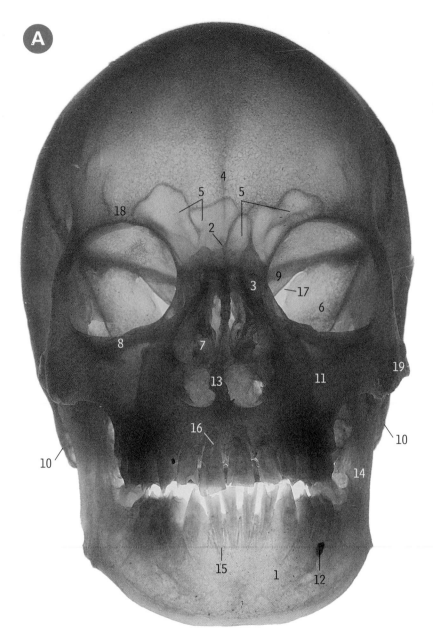

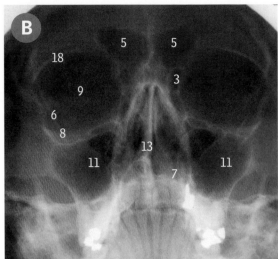

Compare with the skull on page 11.

1 Body of mandible
2 Crista galli
3 Ethmoidal sinus
4 Frontal crest
5 Frontal sinus
6 Greater wing of sphenoid bone
7 Inferior nasal concha
8 Infra-orbital margin
9 Lesser wing of sphenoid bone
10 Mastoid process
11 Maxillary sinus
12 Mental foramen
13 Nasal septum
14 Ramus of mandible
15 Root of lower lateral incisor
16 Root of upper central incisor
17 Superior orbital fissure
18 Supra-orbital margin
19 Zygomatic arch

Blow-out fractures, mastoiditis, see pp 89, 90.

Skull *left half of the skull in sagittal section*

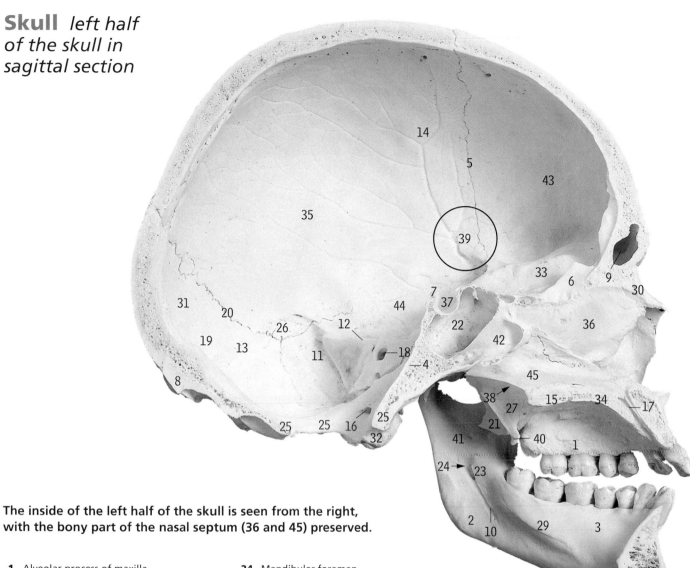

The inside of the left half of the skull is seen from the right, with the bony part of the nasal septum (36 and 45) preserved.

1 Alveolar process of maxilla	**24** Mandibular foramen
2 Angle of mandible	**25** Margin of foramen magnum
3 Body of mandible	**26** Mastoid (posterior inferior)
4 Clivus	angle of parietal bone
5 Coronal suture	**27** Medial pterygoid plate
6 Crista galli of ethmoid bone	**28** Mental protuberance
7 Dorsum sellae	**29** Mylohyoid line
8 External occipital protuberance	**30** Nasal bone
9 Frontal sinus	**31** Occipital bone
10 Groove for mylohyoid nerve	**32** Occipital condyle
11 Groove for sigmoid sinus	**33** Orbital part of frontal bone
12 Groove for superior petrosal sinus	**34** Palatine process of maxilla
13 Groove for transverse sinus	**35** Parietal bone
14 Grooves for middle meningeal vessels	**36** Perpendicular plate of ethmoid bone
(anterior division)	**37** Pituitary fossa (sella turcica)
15 Horizontal plate of palatine bone	**38** Posterior nasal aperture (choana)
16 Hypoglossal canal	**39** Pterion (encircled)
17 Incisive canal	**40** Pterygoid hamulus of medial
18 Internal acoustic meatus in petrous	pterygoid plate
part of temporal bone	**41** Ramus of mandible
19 Internal occipital protuberance	**42** Right sphenoidal sinus
20 Lambdoid suture	**43** Squamous part of frontal bone
21 Lateral pterygoid plate	**44** Squamous part of temporal bone
22 Left sphenoidal sinus	**45** Vomer
23 Lingula	

The bony part of the nasal septum consists of the vomer (45) and the perpendicular plate of the ethmoid bone (36). The anterior part of the septum consists of the septal cartilage (page 67, A6).

In this skull the sphenoidal sinuses (42 and 22) are large, and the right one (42) has extended to the left of the midline. The pituitary fossa (37) projects down into the left sinus (22).

The grooves for the middle meningeal vessels (14) pass upwards and backwards. The circle (39) marks the region of the pterion, and corresponds to the position shown on the outside of the skull on page 14, 29.

 Extradural haemorrhage, pituitary tumour, see pp 90, 91.

Mandible

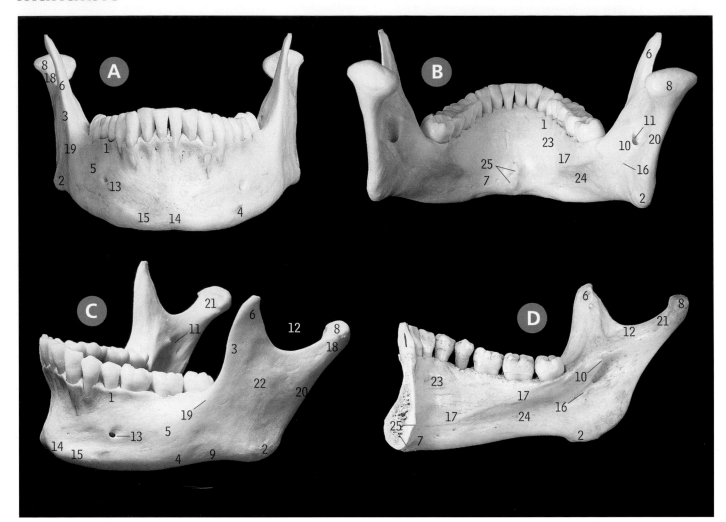

A from the front

B from behind and above

C from the left and front

D internal view from the left

1 Alveolar part
2 Angle
3 Anterior border of ramus
4 Base
5 Body
6 Coronoid process
7 Digastric fossa
8 Head
9 Inferior border of ramus
10 Lingula
11 Mandibular foramen
12 Mandibular notch
13 Mental foramen
14 Mental protuberance
15 Mental tubercle
16 Mylohyoid groove
17 Mylohyoid line
18 Neck
19 Oblique line
20 Posterior border of ramus
21 Pterygoid fovea
22 Ramus
23 Sublingual fossa
24 Submandibular fossa
25 Superior and inferior mental spines (genial tubercles)

The head (8) and the neck (18, including the pterygoid fovea, 21) constitute the condyle.

The alveolar part (1) contains the sockets for the roots of the teeth.

The base (4) is the inferior border of the body (5), and becomes continuous with the inferior border (9) of the ramus (22).

Mandible *muscle attachments*

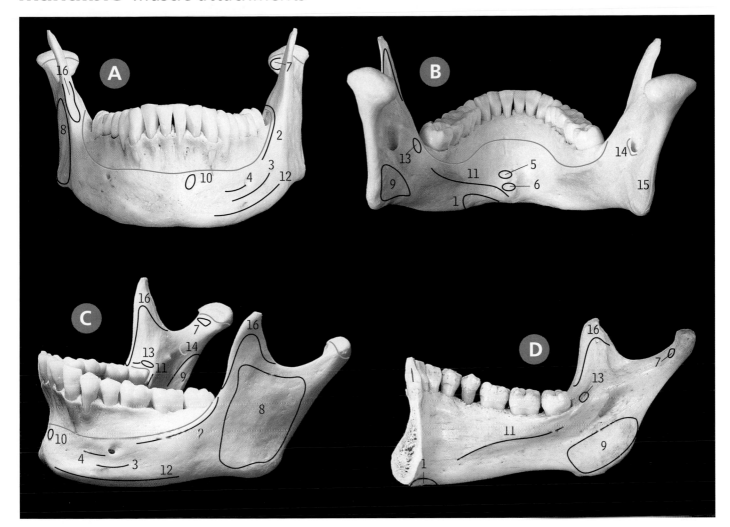

A from the front

B from behind and above

C from the left and front

D internal view from the left

Green line = capsular attachment of temporomandibular joint;
blue line = limit of attachment of the oral mucous membrane;
pale green line = ligament attachment

1	Anterior belly of digastric	**10**	Mentalis
2	Buccinator	**11**	Mylohyoid
3	Depressor anguli oris	**12**	Platysma
4	Depressor labii inferioris	**13**	Pterygomandibular raphe
5	Genioglossus		and superior constrictor
6	Geniohyoid	**14**	Sphenomandibular ligament
7	Lateral pterygoid	**15**	Stylomandibular ligament
8	Masseter	**16**	Temporalis
9	Medial pterygoid		

The lateral pterygoid (A7) is attached to the pterygoid fovea on the neck of the mandible (and also to the capsule of the temporomandibular joint and the articular disc – see page 52, A27, A28).

The medial pterygoid (B9, C9) is attached to the medial surface of the angle of the mandible, below the groove for the mylohyoid nerve.

Masseter (C8) is attached to the lateral surface of the ramus.

Temporalis (C16) is attached over the coronoid process, extending back as far as the deepest part of the mandibular notch and downwards over the front of the ramus almost as far as the last molar tooth.

Buccinator (C2) is attached opposite the three molar teeth, at the back reaching the pterygomandibular raphe (C13).

Genioglossus (B5) is attached to the upper mental spine and geniohyoid (B6) to the lower.

Mylohyoid (11) is attached to the mylohyoid line.

The attachment of the lateral temporomandibular ligament to the lateral aspect of the neck of the condyle is not shown.

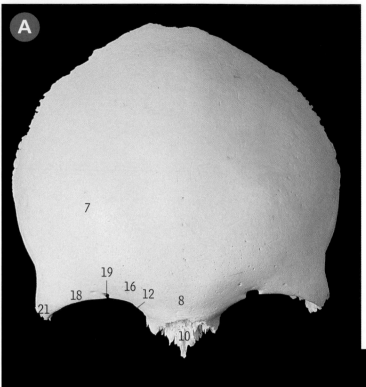

Frontal bone

A external surface from the front

B external surface from the left

C from below

D internal surface from above and behind
(right half removed; ethmoidal notch is inferior)

1	Anterior ethmoidal canal (position of groove)	**13**	Posterior ethmoidal canal (position of groove)
2	Ethmoidal notch	**14**	Roof of ethmoidal air cells
3	Foramen caecum	**15**	Sagittal crest
4	Fossa for lacrimal gland	**16**	Superciliary arch
5	Frontal crest	**17**	Superior temporal line
6	Frontal sinus	**18**	Supra-orbital margin
7	Frontal tuberosity	**19**	Supra-orbital notch or
8	Glabella		foramen
9	Inferior temporal line	**20**	Trochlear fovea
10	Nasal spine		(or tubercle)
11	Orbital part	**21**	Zygomatic process
12	Position of frontal notch or foramen		

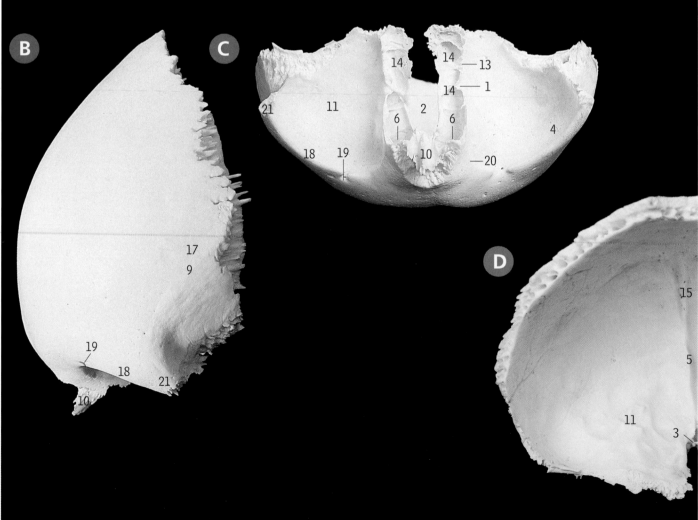

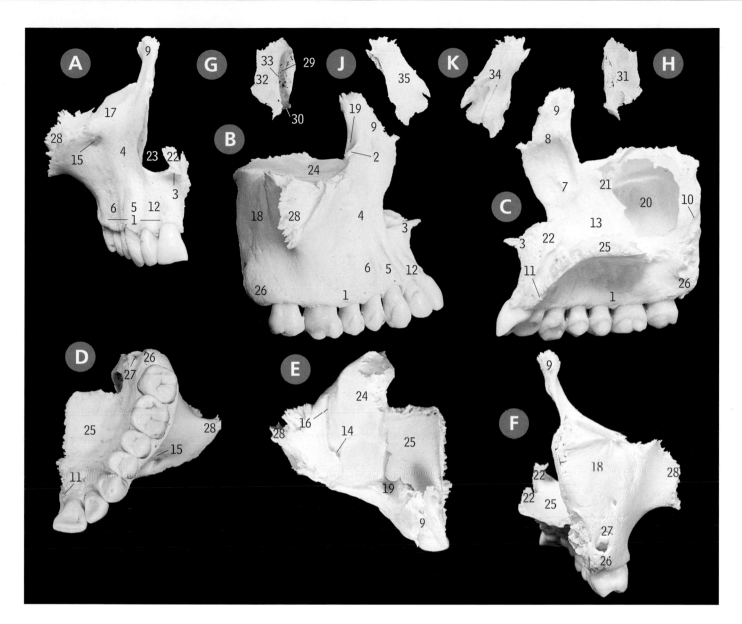

Right maxilla

A from the front

B from the lateral side

C from the medial side

D from below

E from above

F from behind

1 Alveolar process
2 Anterior lacrimal crest
3 Anterior nasal spine
4 Anterior surface
5 Canine eminence
6 Canine fossa
7 Conchal crest
8 Ethmoidal crest
9 Frontal process
10 Greater palatine canal
   (position of groove)
11 Incisive canal
12 Incisive fossa
13 Inferior meatus
14 Infra-orbital canal

15 Infra-orbital foramen
16 Infra-orbital groove
17 Infra-orbital margin
18 Infratemporal surface
19 Lacrimal groove
20 Maxillary hiatus and sinus
21 Middle meatus
22 Nasal crest
23 Nasal notch
24 Orbital surface
25 Palatine process
26 Tuberosity
27 Unerupted third molar tooth
28 Zygomatic process

Right lacrimal bone

G from the lateral (orbital) side

H from the medial (nasal) side

29 Lacrimal groove
30 Lacrimal hamulus
31 Nasal surface
32 Orbital surface
33 Posterior lacrimal crest

Right nasal bone

J from the lateral side

K from the medial side

34 Internal surface and groove for
   anterior ethmoidal nerve
35 Lateral surface

Right palatine bone

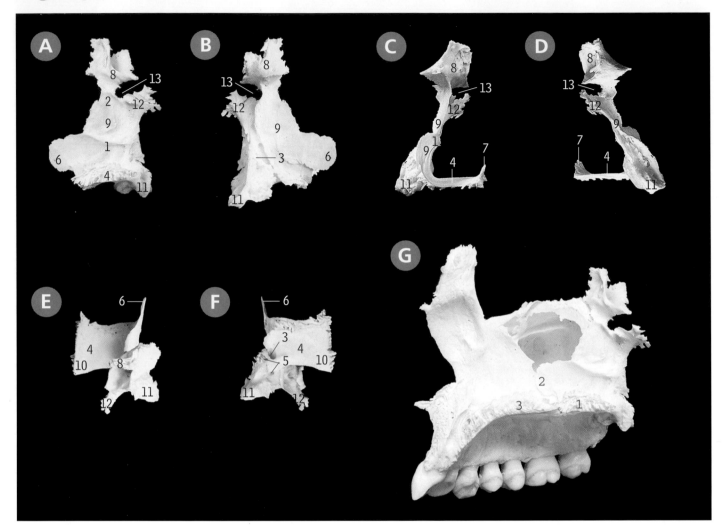

A from the medial side	**D** from behind	**G** Articulation of the right maxilla and the palatine bone, from the medial side.	
B from the lateral side	**E** from above		
C from the front	**F** from below	**1** Horizontal plate of palatine	
		2 Maxillary process of palatine	
		3 Palatine process of maxilla	

1 Conchal crest
2 Ethmoidal crest
3 Greater palatine groove
4 Horizontal plate
5 Lesser palatine canals
6 Maxillary process
7 Nasal crest

8 Orbital process
9 Perpendicular plate
10 Posterior nasal spine
11 Pyramidal process
12 Sphenoidal process
13 Sphenopalatine notch

Right temporal bone

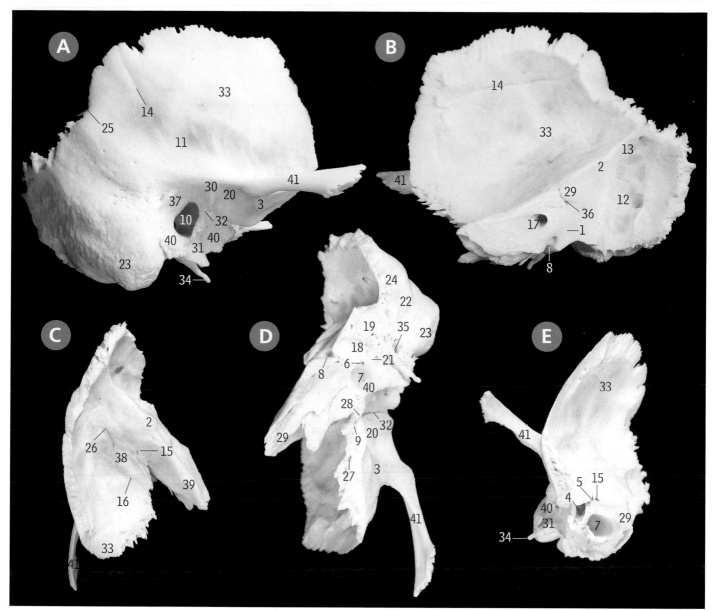

A external aspect

B internal aspect

C from above

D from below

E from the front

1 Aqueduct of vestibule
2 Arcuate eminence
3 Articular tubercle
4 Auditory tube
5 Canal for tensor tympani
6 Canaliculus for tympanic branch of glossopharyngeal nerve
7 Carotid canal
8 Cochlear canaliculus
9 Edge of tegmen tympani
10 External acoustic meatus
11 Groove for middle temporal artery
12 Groove for sigmoid sinus
13 Groove for superior petrosal sinus
14 Grooves for branches of middle meningeal vessels

15 Hiatus and groove for greater petrosal nerve
16 Hiatus and groove for lesser petrosal nerve
17 Internal acoustic meatus
18 Jugular fossa
19 Jugular surface
20 Mandibular fossa
21 Mastoid canaliculus for auricular branch of vagus nerve
22 Mastoid notch
23 Mastoid process
24 Occipital groove
25 Parietal notch
26 Petrosquamous fissure (from above)
27 Petrosquamous fissure (from below)

28 Petrotympanic fissure
29 Petrous part
30 Postglenoid tubercle
31 Sheath of styloid process
32 Squamotympanic fissure
33 Squamous part
34 Styloid process
35 Stylomastoid foramen
36 Subarcuate fossa
37 Suprameatal triangle
38 Tegmen tympani
39 Trigeminal impression on apex of petrous part
40 Tympanic part
41 Zygomatic process

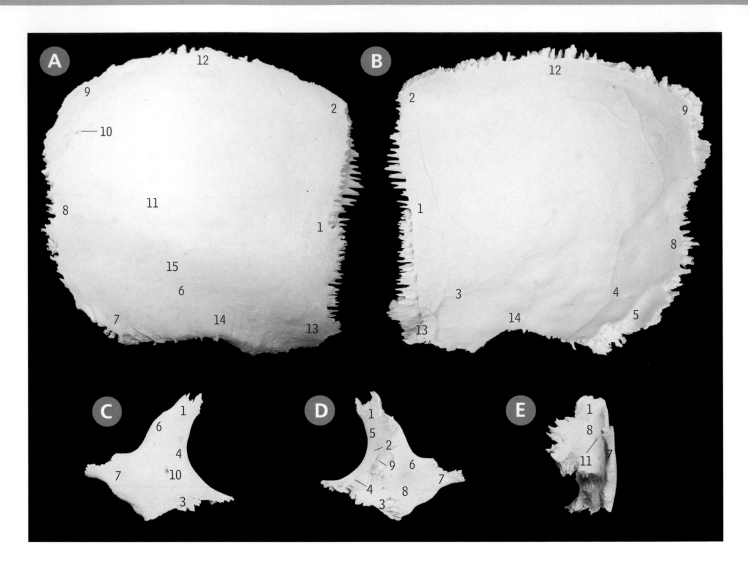

Right parietal bone

Ⓐ external surface

Ⓑ internal surface

1 Frontal (anterior) border
2 Frontal (anterosuperior) angle
3 Furrows for frontal branch of middle meningeal vessels (anterior division)
4 Furrows for parietal branch of middle meningeal vessels (posterior division)
5 Groove for sigmoid sinus at mastoid angle
6 Inferior temporal line
7 Mastoid (postero-inferior) angle
8 Occipital (posterior) border
9 Occipital (posterosuperior) angle
10 Parietal foramen
11 Parietal tuberosity
12 Sagittal (superior) border
13 Sphenoidal (antero-inferior) angle
14 Squamosal (inferior) border
15 Superior temporal line

Right zygomatic bone

Ⓒ lateral surface

Ⓓ from the medial side

Ⓔ from behind

1 Frontal process
2 Marginal tubercle
3 Maxillary border
4 Orbital border
5 Orbital surface
6 Temporal border
7 Temporal process
8 Temporal surface
9 Zygomatico-orbital foramen
10 Zygomaticofacial foramen
11 Zygomaticotemporal foramen

The zygomatic process of the temporal bone (page 33, 39) and the temporal process of the zygomatic bone (C7, D7) form the zygomatic arch (page 14, 35).

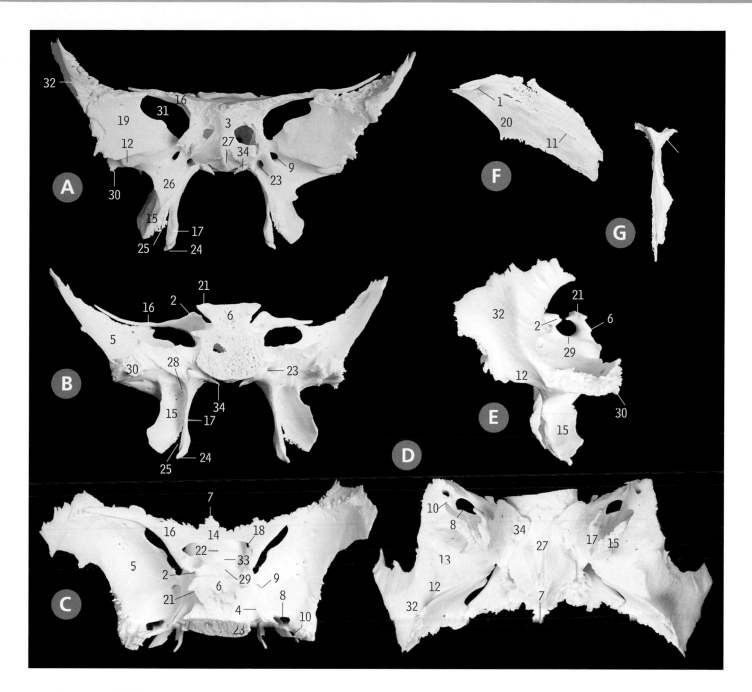

Sphenoid bone

A from the front   **D** from below
B from behind   **E** from the left
C from above and behind

Vomer

F from the right
G from behind

1 Ala
2 Anterior clinoid process
3 Body with openings of sphenoidal sinuses
4 Carotid groove
5 Cerebral surface of greater wing
6 Dorsum sellae
7 Ethmoidal spine
8 Foramen ovale
9 Foramen rotundum
10 Foramen spinosum
11 Groove for nasopalatine nerve and vessels
12 Infratemporal crest of greater wing
13 Infratemporal surface of greater wing
14 Jugum
15 Lateral pterygoid plate
16 Lesser wing
17 Medial pterygoid plate
18 Optic canal
19 Orbital surface of greater wing
20 Posterior border
21 Posterior clinoid process
22 Prechiasmatic groove
23 Pterygoid canal
24 Pterygoid hamulus
25 Pterygoid notch
26 Pterygoid process
27 Rostrum
28 Scaphoid fossa
29 Sella turcica (pituitary fossa)
30 Spine
31 Superior orbital fissure
32 Temporal surface of greater wing
33 Tuberculum sellae
34 Vaginal process

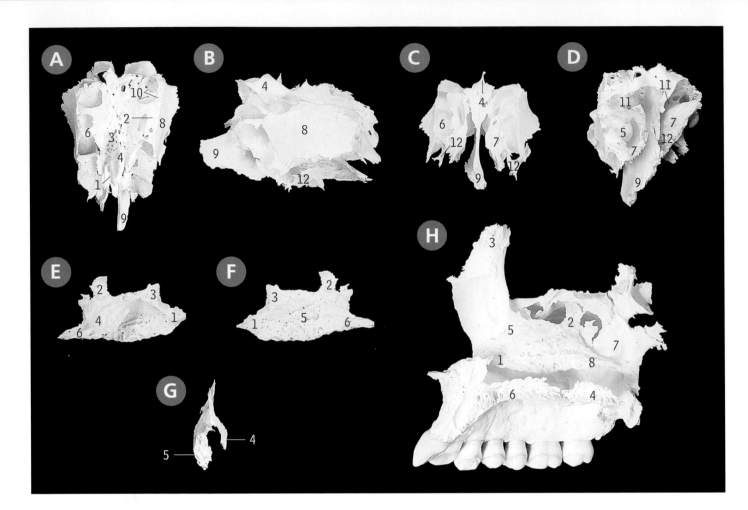

Ethmoid bone

A from above

B from the left

C from the front

D from the left, below and behind

1 Ala of crista galli
2 Anterior ethmoidal groove
3 Cribriform plate
4 Crista galli
5 Ethmoidal bulla
6 Ethmoidal labyrinth
   (containing ethmoidal air cells)
7 Middle nasal concha
8 Orbital plate
9 Perpendicular plate
10 Posterior ethmoidal groove
11 Superior nasal concha (meatus)
12 Uncinate process

Right inferior nasal concha

E from the lateral side

F from the medial side

G from behind

1 Anterior end
2 Ethmoidal process
3 Lacrimal process
4 Maxillary process
5 Medial surface
6 Posterior end

Maxilla

H Articulation of right maxilla, palatine bone and inferior nasal concha, from the medial side.

1 Anterior end of inferior nasal concha
2 Ethmoidal process of inferior nasal concha
3 Frontal process of maxilla
4 Horizontal plate of palatine
5 Lacrimal process of inferior nasal concha
6 Palatine process of maxilla
7 Perpendicular plate of palatine
8 Posterior end of inferior nasal concha

Occipital bone

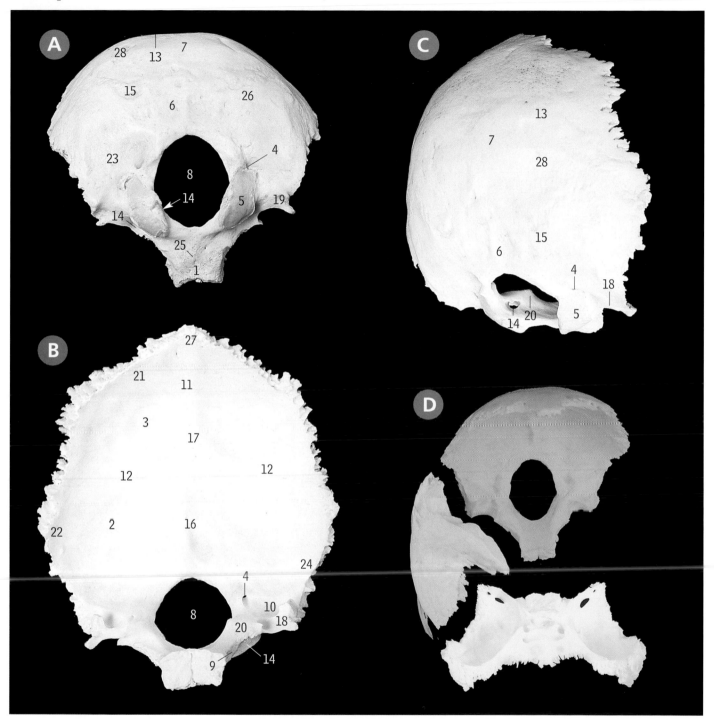

1 Basilar part
2 Cerebellar fossa
3 Cerebral fossa
4 Condylar fossa (and
   condylar canal in B and C)
5 Condyle
6 External occipital crest
7 External occipital
   protuberance
8 Foramen magnum
9 Groove for inferior
   petrosal sinus
10 Groove for sigmoid sinus
11 Groove for superior
    sagittal sinus
12 Groove for transverse
    sinus
13 Highest nuchal line
14 Hypoglossal canal
15 Inferior nuchal line
16 Internal occipital crest
17 Internal occipital
    protuberance
18 Jugular notch
19 Jugular process
20 Jugular tubercle
21 Lambdoid margin
22 Lateral angle
23 Lateral part
24 Mastoid margin
25 Pharyngeal tubercle
26 Squamous part
27 Superior angle
28 Superior nuchal line

Neck *surface markings of the front and right side*

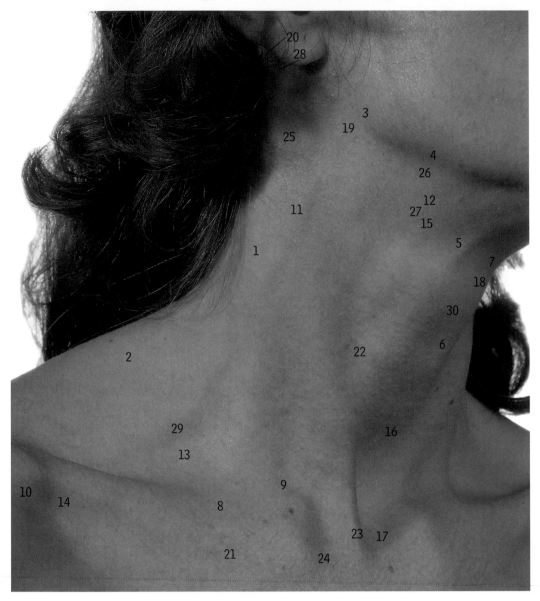

The pulsation of the common carotid artery (22, opposite page, 8) can be felt by backward pressure in the angle between the lower anterior border of sternocleidomastoid and the side of the larynx and trachea.

The cricoid cartilage (6) is about 5 cm (2 in) above the jugular notch of the manubrium of the sternum (17).

The lower end of the internal jugular vein lies behind the interval between the sternal (23) and clavicular (9) heads of sternocleidomastoid (when viewed from the front), just above the point where it joins the subclavian vein to form the brachiocephalic vein (24).

The uppermost part of the brachial plexus (29) can be felt as a cord-like structure in the lower part of the posterior triangle.

1 Accessory nerve emerging from sternocleidomastoid
2 Accessory nerve passing under anterior border of trapezius
3 Angle of mandible
4 Anterior border of masseter and facial artery
5 Anterior jugular vein
6 Arch of cricoid cartilage
7 Body of hyoid bone
8 Clavicle
9 Clavicular head of sternocleidomastoid
10 Deltoid
11 External jugular vein
12 Hypoglossal nerve
13 Inferior belly of omohyoid
14 Infraclavicular fossa and cephalic vein
15 Internal laryngeal nerve
16 Isthmus of thyroid gland
17 Jugular notch and trachea
18 Laryngeal prominence (Adam's apple)
19 Lowest part of parotid gland
20 Mastoid process
21 Pectoralis major
22 Site for palpation of common carotid artery
23 Sternal head of sternocleidomastoid
24 Sternoclavicular joint and union of internal jugular and subclavian veins to form brachiocephalic vein
25 Sternocleidomastoid
26 Submandibular gland
27 Tip of greater horn of hyoid bone
28 Tip of transverse process of atlas
29 Upper trunk of brachial plexus
30 Vocal fold

Torticollis, see p. 91.

Side of the neck *right side, deep dissection*

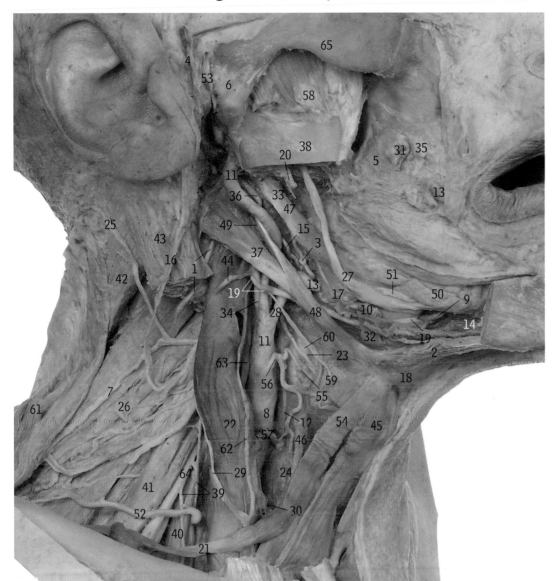

The lingual nerve (27) lies superficial to hyoglossus (17) and at this level is a flattened band rather than a typical round nerve, with the deep part of the submandibular gland (10) below it. The nerve crosses underneath the submandibular duct (51), lying first lateral to the duct and then medial to it.

The thyrohyoid membrane (60) is pierced by the internal laryngeal nerve (23) and the superior laryngeal artery (55).

Apart from supplying muscles of the tongue, the hypoglossal nerve (19) gives branches to geniohyoid (14) and thyrohyoid (59) and forms the upper root of the ansa cervicalis (62). These three branches consist of the fibres from the first cervical nerve that have joined the hypoglossal nerve higher in the neck; they are not derived from the hypoglossal nucleus. The C1 fibres in the upper root of the ansa contribute to the supply of sternohyoid (45) and omohyoid (21, 54).

1 Accessory nerve	**19** Hypoglossal nerve	**39** Roots of phrenic nerve	**59** Thyrohyoid and nerve
2 Anterior belly of digastric and nerve	**20** Inferior alveolar nerve	**40** Scalenus anterior	**60** Thyrohyoid membrane
3 Ascending palatine artery	**21** Inferior belly of omohyoid	**41** Scalenus medius	**61** Trapezius
4 Auriculotemporal nerve	**22** Internal jugular vein	**42** Splenius capitis	**62** Upper root of ansa cervicalis
5 Buccinator	**23** Internal laryngeal nerve	**43** Sternocleidomastoid	**63** Vagus nerve
6 Capsule of temporomandibular joint	**24** Lateral lobe of thyroid gland	**44** Sternocleidomastoid branch of occipital artery	**64** Ventral ramus of fifth cervical nerve
7 Cervical nerves to trapezius	**25** Lesser occipital nerve	**45** Sternohyoid	**65** Zygomatic arch
8 Common carotid artery	**26** Levator scapulae	**46** Sternothyroid	
9 Deep lingual artery	**27** Lingual nerve	**47** Styloglossus	
10 Deep part of submandibular gland	**28** Linguofacial trunk	**48** Stylohyoid	
11 External carotid artery	**29** Lower root of ansa cervicalis	**49** Stylohyoid ligament	
12 External laryngeal nerve	**30** Middle thyroid vein	**50** Sublingual gland	
13 Facial artery	**31** Molar glands	**51** Submandibular duct	
14 Geniohyoid	**32** Mylohyoid and nerve	**52** Superficial cervical artery	
15 Glossopharyngeal nerve	**33** Nerve to mylohyoid	**53** Superficial temporal artery	
16 Great auricular nerve	**34** Occipital artery	**54** Superior belly of omohyoid	
17 Hyoglossus	**35** Parotid duct	**55** Superior laryngeal artery	
18 Hyoid bone	**36** Posterior auricular artery	**56** Superior thyroid artery	
	37 Posterior belly of digastric	**57** Superior thyroid vein	
	38 Ramus of mandible	**58** Temporalis	

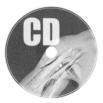

Front of the neck *superficial dissection*

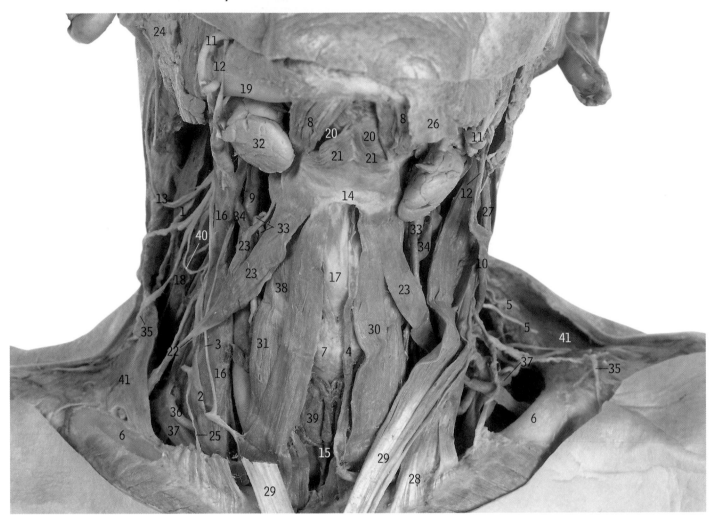

1 Accessory nerve	**16** Internal jugular vein
2 Ansa cervicalis, lower root	**17** Laryngeal prominence
3 Ansa cervicalis, upper root	**18** Levator scapulae
4 Anterior jugular vein	**19** Mandible
5 Cervical nerves to trapezius	**20** Mylohyoid
6 Clavicle	**21** Mylohyoid, anomalous fibres
7 Cricoid cartilage	**22** Omohyoid, intermediate
8 Digastric, anterior belly	tendon
9 External carotid artery	**23** Omohyoid, superior belly
10 External jugular vein	**24** Parotid gland
11 Facial artery	**25** Phrenic nerve
12 Facial vein	**26** Platysma
13 Great auricular nerve	**27** Retromandibular vein
14 Hyoid bone, body	**28** Sternocleidomastoid,
15 Inferior thyroid vein	clavicular head

29 Sternocleidomastoid, sternal head	**35** Supraclavicular nerve
30 Sternohyoid	**36** Suprascapular artery
31 Sternothyroid	**37** Suprascapular vein
32 Submandibular gland	**38** Thyrohyoid
33 Superior thyroid artery	**39** Thyroid gland, isthmus
34 Superior thyroid vein	**40** Transverse cervical nerve
	41 Trapezius

Midline landmarks in the neck include the body of the hyoid bone (14), the laryngeal prominence (Adam's apple, 17) and the arch of the cricoid cartilage (7).

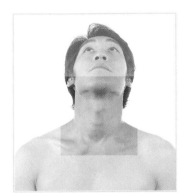

 Tracheostomy, see p. 92.

Front of the neck *deeper dissection*

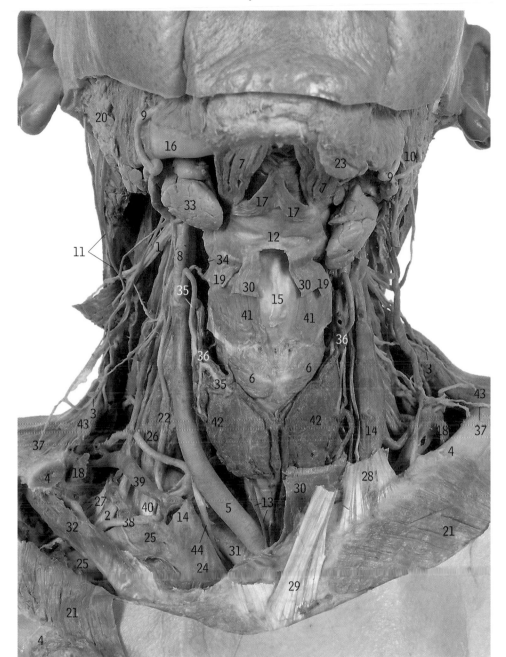

1 Accessory nerve
2 Brachial plexus (roots)
3 Cervical nerves to trapezius
4 Clavicle
5 Common carotid artery
6 Cricothyroid
7 Digastric, anterior belly
8 External carotid artery
9 Facial artery
10 Facial vein
11 Great auricular nerve
12 Hyoid bone, body
13 Inferior thyroid vein
14 Internal jugular vein
15 Laryngeal prominence
16 Mandible
17 Mylohyoid, anomalous fibres
18 Omohyoid, inferior belly
19 Omohyoid, superior belly
20 Parotid gland
21 Pectoralis major
22 Phrenic nerve
23 Platysma
24 Right brachiocephalic vein
25 Right subclavian vein
26 Scalenus anterior
27 Scalenus medius
28 Sternocleidomastoid, clavicular head
29 Sternocleidomastoid, sternal head
30 Sternohyoid
31 Subclavian artery
32 Subclavius
33 Submandibular gland
34 Superior laryngeal artery
35 Superior thyroid artery
36 Superior thyroid vein
37 Supraclavicular nerve
38 Suprascapular artery
39 Suprascapular vein
40 Tendon of scalenus anterior
41 Thyrohyoid
42 Thyroid gland, lateral lobe
43 Trapezius
44 Vagus nerve

On the right hand side the clavicle
(4) has been cut and retracted
forwards to reveal the underlying
subclavius (32).

Accessory nerve paralysis, goitre, sialolithiasis, see pp 89, 90, 91.

Right side of the neck Ⓐ *superficial* Ⓑ *deep*

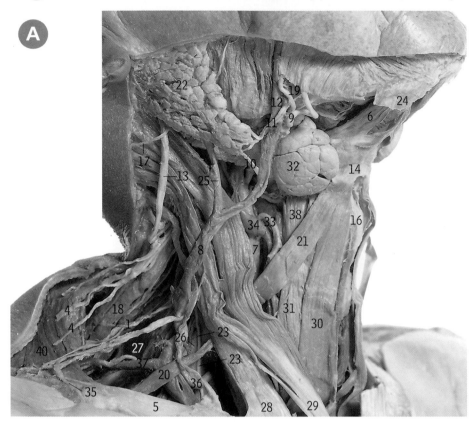

1	Accessory nerve
2	Ansa cervicalis, upper root
3	Brachial plexus (roots)
4	Cervical nerves to trapezius
5	Clavicle
6	Digastric, anterior belly
7	External carotid artery
8	External jugular vein
9	Facial artery
10	Facial nerve, cervical branch
11	Facial nerve, marginal mandibular branch
12	Facial vein
13	Great auricular nerve
14	Hyoid bone
15	Internal jugular vein
16	Laryngeal prominence
17	Lesser occipital nerve
18	Levator scapulae
19	Mandible
20	Omohyoid, inferior belly
21	Omohyoid, superior belly
22	Parotid gland
23	Phrenic nerve
24	Platysma
25	Retromandibular vein
26	Scalenus anterior
27	Scalenus medius
28	Sternocleidomastoid, clavicular head
29	Sternocleidomastoid, sternal head
30	Sternohyoid
31	Sternothyroid
32	Submandibular gland
33	Superior thyroid artery
34	Superior thyroid vein
35	Supraclavicular nerve
36	Suprascapular artery
37	Suprascapular vein
38	Thyrohyoid
39	Thyroid gland, lateral lobe
40	Trapezius

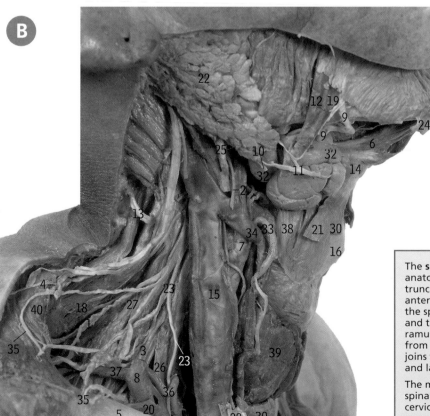

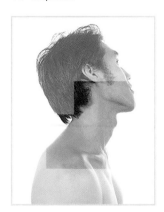

The **spinal part** of the accessory nerve is in official anatomical nomenclature the ramus externus of the truncus nervi accessorii. The cells of origin are in the anterior horn of the upper five or six cervical segments of the spinal cord, and the fibres supply sternocleidomastoid and trapezius. The **cranial part** of the accessory nerve, the ramus internus of the truncus nervi accessorii, is derived from the nucleus ambiguus in the medulla oblongata and joins the vagus nerve to supply muscles of the soft palate and larynx.

The motor nerve supply of trapezius (40) is usually the spinal accessory nerve (1), with the branches from the cervical plexus to the muscle (4) being afferent only, but in some cases the cervical branches do appear to be motor.

Left side of the neck *from the left and front*

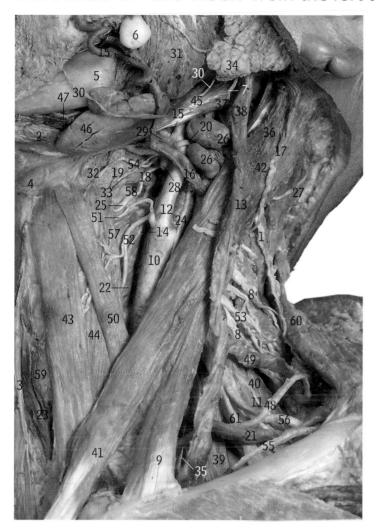

Platysma and the deep cervical fascia have been removed.

In 20 per cent of faces, as in this specimen, the marginal mandibular branch of the facial nerve (30) arches downwards off the face for part of its course and overlies the submandibular gland (46).

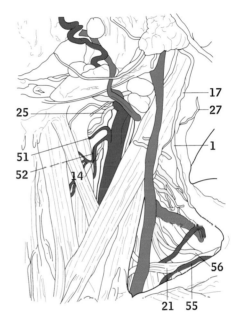

1 Accessory nerve	**17** Great auricular nerve	**31** Masseter	**46** Submandibular gland
2 Anterior belly of digastric	**18** Greater horn of hyoid bone (underlying 25)	**32** Mylohyoid	**47** Submental artery and vein
3 Anterior jugular vein		**33** Nerve to thyrohyoid	**48** Superficial cervical artery
4 Body of hyoid bone	**19** Hyoglossus	**34** Parotid gland	**49** Superficial cervical vein
5 Body of mandible	**20** Hypoglossal nerve	**35** Phrenic nerve (on scalenus anterior)	**50** Superior belly of omohyoid
6 Buccal fat pad	**21** Inferior belly of omohyoid		**51** Superior laryngeal artery
7 Cervical branch of facial nerve	**22** Inferior constrictor of pharynx	**36** Posterior auricular vein	**52** Superior thyroid artery
	23 Inferior thyroid vein	**37** Posterior belly of digastric	**53** Supraclavicular nerve (cut upper edge)
8 Cervical nerves to trapezius	**24** Internal carotid artery and superior root of ansa cervicalis	**38** Posterior branch of retromandibular vein	**54** Suprahyoid artery
9 Clavicular head of sternocleidomastoid		**39** Scalenus anterior	**55** Suprascapular artery
10 Common carotid artery	**25** Internal laryngeal nerve	**40** Scalenus medius	**56** Suprascapular nerve
11 Dorsal scapular nerve	**26** Jugulodigastric lymph nodes	**41** Sternal head of sternocleidomastoid	**57** Thyrohyoid
12 External carotid artery	**27** Lesser occipital nerve		**58** Thyrohyoid membrane
13 External jugular vein	**28** Lingual artery	**42** Sternocleidomastoid	**59** Thyroid gland
14 External laryngeal nerve	**29** Lingual vein	**43** Sternohyoid	**60** Trapezius
15 Facial artery	**30** Marginal mandibular branch of facial nerve	**44** Sternothyroid	**61** Upper trunk of brachial plexus
16 Facial vein		**45** Stylohyoid	

 Carotid artery bruits, cervical lymph node enlargement, see p. 89.

Right lower face and upper neck

Ⓐ *parotid and upper cervical regions* Ⓑ *submandibular region*

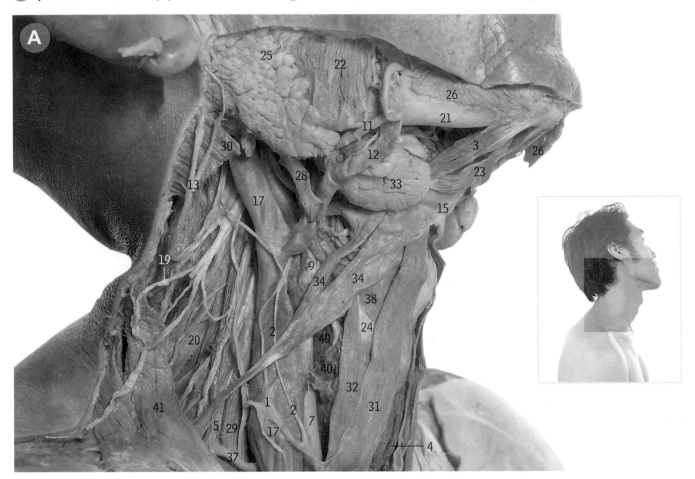

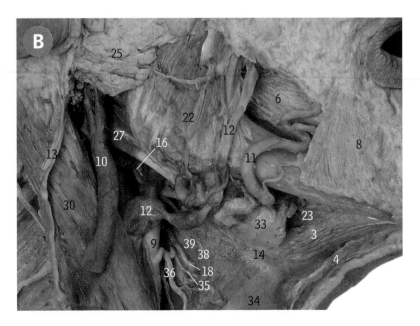

1 Ansa cervicalis, inferior root	**23** Mylohyoid
2 Ansa cervicalis, superior root	**24** Oblique line of the thyroid cartilage
3 Anterior belly of digastric	**25** Parotid gland and facial nerve branches at anterior border
4 Anterior jugular vein	**26** Platysma
5 Brachial plexus (roots)	**27** Posterior belly of digastric
6 Buccinator	**28** Retromandibular vein
7 Common carotid artery	**29** Scalenus anterior
8 Depressor anguli oris	**30** Sternocleidomastoid
9 External carotid artery	**31** Sternohyoid
10 External jugular vein	**32** Sternothyroid
11 Facial artery	**33** Submandibular gland
12 Facial vein	**34** Superior belly of omohyoid (bifid)
13 Great auricular nerve	**35** Superior laryngeal artery
14 Greater horn of hyoid bone	**36** Superior thyroid artery
15 Hyoid bone	**37** Suprascapular artery
16 Hypoglossal nerve	**38** Thyrohyoid
17 Internal jugular vein	**39** Thyrohyoid membrane
18 Internal laryngeal nerve	**40** Thyroid gland
19 Lesser occipital nerve	**41** Trapezius
20 Levator scapulae	
21 Mandible	
22 Masseter	

 Mumps, parotidectomy (removal of parotid gland), parotid tumours, see pp 90, 91.

Right side of the neck *deep dissection*

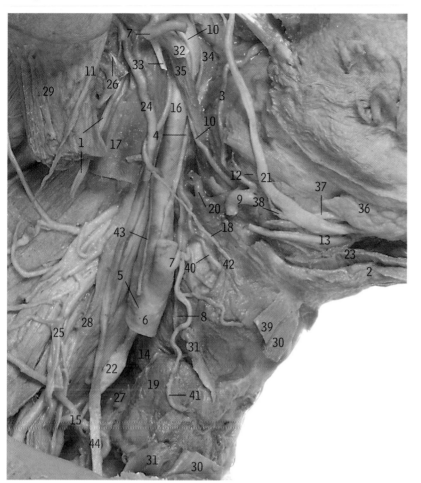

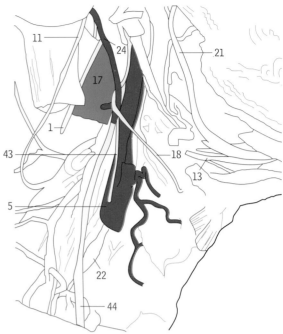

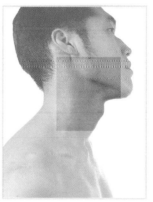

1	Accessory nerve	**23**	Mylohyoid
2	Anterior belly of digastric	**24**	Occipital artery
3	Ascending palatine artery	**25**	Phrenic nerve
4	Ascending pharyngeal artery	**26**	Posterior belly of digastric
5	Carotid sinus	**27**	Recurrent laryngeal nerve
6	Common carotid artery	**28**	Scalenus anterior
7	External carotid artery	**29**	Sternocleidomastoid
8	External laryngeal nerve	**30**	Sternohyoid
9	Facial artery	**31**	Sternothyroid
10	Glossopharyngeal nerve	**32**	Styloglossus
11	Great auricular nerve	**33**	Stylohyoid (cut end displaced
12	Hyoglossus		medially)
13	Hypoglossal nerve	**34**	Stylohyoid ligament
14	Inferior constrictor	**35**	Stylopharyngeus
15	Inferior thyroid artery	**36**	Sublingual gland
16	Internal carotid artery	**37**	Submandibular duct
17	Internal jugular vein	**38**	Submandibular ganglion
18	Internal laryngeal nerve	**39**	Superior belly of omohyoid
19	Lateral lobe of thyroid gland	**40**	Superior laryngeal artery
20	Lingual artery	**41**	Superior thyroid artery
21	Lingual nerve	**42**	Thyrohyoid and nerve
22	Middle cervical sympathetic	**43**	Upper root of ansa cervicalis
	ganglion	**44**	Vagus nerve

The hypoglossal nerve (13) passes downwards, curling around the occipital artery (24) and lying superficial to the external carotid (7) and lingual (20) arteries.

The glossopharyngeal nerve (10) passes downwards and forwards, curling round the lateral side of stylopharyngeus (35).

The removal of parts of the sternohyoid (30), omohyoid (39) and sternothyroid (31) displays the lateral lobe of the thyroid gland (19). Note the inferior thyroid artery (15) behind the lower part of the lobe, with the recurrent laryngeal nerve (27) passing deep to this looping vessel to enter the pharynx beneath the inferior constrictor (14).

Carotid endarterectomy, see p. 89.

Left prevertebral region

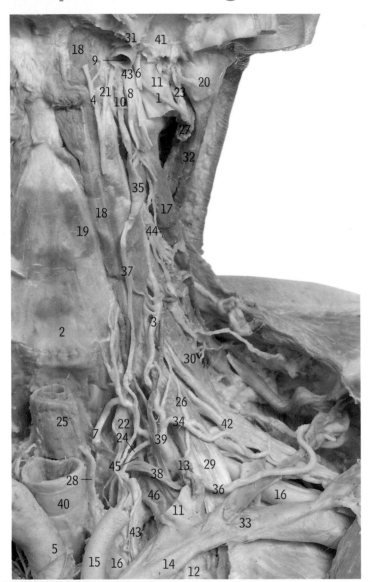

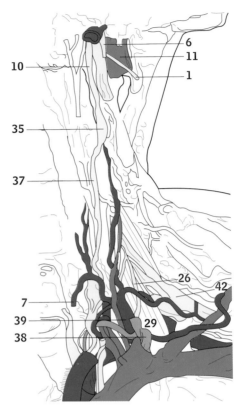

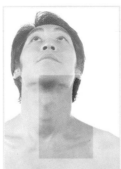

1 Accessory nerve	**17** Levator scapulae	**31** Spine of sphenoid bone
2 Anterior longitudinal ligament	**18** Longus capitis	**32** Sternocleidomastoid
3 Ascending cervical vessels	**19** Longus colli	**33** Subclavian vein
4 Ascending pharyngeal artery	**20** Mastoid process	**34** Superficial cervical artery
5 Brachiocephalic trunk	**21** Meningeal branch of ascending	**35** Superior cervical ganglion
6 Glossopharyngeal nerve	pharyngeal artery	**36** Suprascapular artery
7 Inferior thyroid artery	**22** Middle cervical ganglion	**37** Sympathetic trunk
8 Inferior vagal ganglion	**23** Occipital artery	**38** Thoracic duct
9 Internal carotid artery	**24** Oesophageal branch (large)	**39** Thyrocervical trunk
10 Internal carotid nerve (sympathetic)	of the inferior thyroid artery	**40** Trachea
11 Internal jugular vein	**25** Oesophagus	**41** Tympanic part of temporal bone
12 Internal thoracic artery	**26** Phrenic nerve	**42** Upper trunk of brachial plexus
13 Jugular lymphatic trunk	**27** Posterior belly of digastric	**43** Vagus nerve
14 Left brachiocephalic vein	**28** Recurrent laryngeal nerve	**44** Ventral ramus of third cervical nerve
15 Left common carotid artery	**29** Scalenus anterior	**45** Vertebral artery
16 Left subclavian artery	**30** Scalenus medius	**46** Vertebral vein

Cervical sympathectomy, see p. 89.

Root of the neck

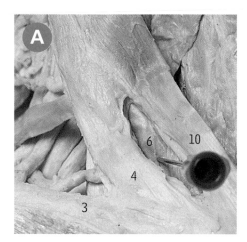

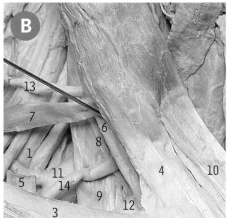

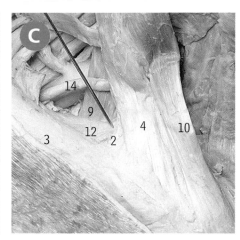

A Dissection of puncture of the right internal jugular vein between the two heads of sternocleidomastoid, with the needle directed backwards and slightly laterally.

B Dissection of puncture of the right internal jugular vein at the posterior border of sternocleidomastoid, with the needle directed towards the jugular notch of the sternum.

C Dissection of puncture of the right brachiocephalic vein, with the needle directed towards the sternal angle.

1 Brachial plexus
2 Brachiocephalic vein
3 Clavicle
4 Clavicular head of sternocleidomastoid
5 External jugular vein
6 Internal jugular vein
7 Omohyoid
8 Phrenic nerve
9 Scalenus anterior
10 Sternal head of sternocleidomastoid
11 Subclavian artery
12 Subclavian vein
13 Superficial cervical artery
14 Suprascapular artery

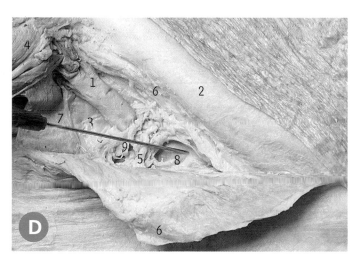

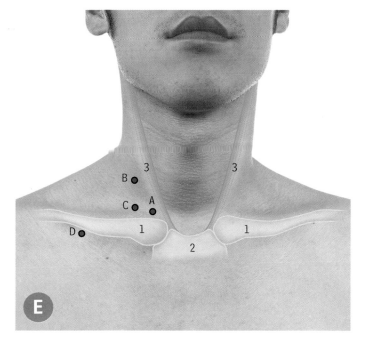

D Dissection of infraclavicular puncture of the subclavian vein, from below the midpoint of the clavicle on a line directed to just above the jugular notch. Part of pectoralis major is detached from the clavicle and the clavipectoral fascia divided to show the subclavian vein deep to it and passing under cover of the clavicle.

1 Cephalic vein
2 Clavicle
3 Clavipectoral fascia
4 Deltoid
5 Lateral pectoral nerve
6 Pectoralis major
7 Pectoralis minor
8 Subclavian vein
9 Thoraco-acromial vessels

E Root of neck surface anatomy. A, B, C and D are the puncture sites as shown above.

1 Clavicle   2 Sternum   3 Sternocleidomastoid

 Internal jugular vein catheterization, subclavian vein catheterization, see pp 90, 91.

Face *surface markings on the front and right side*

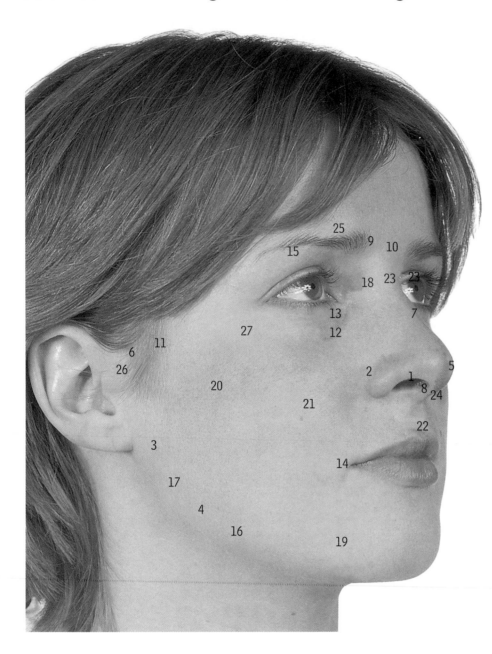

1 Ala of external nose
2 Alar groove of external nose
3 Angle of mandible
4 Anterior border of masseter and facial vessels
5 Apex of external nose
6 Auriculotemporal nerve and superficial temporal vessels
7 Dorsum of external nose
8 External aperture of external nose
9 Frontal notch and supratrochlear nerve and vessels
10 Glabella of external nose
11 Head of mandible
12 Infra-orbital foramen, nerve and vessels
13 Infra-orbital margin
14 Lateral angle of mouth
15 Lateral part of supra-orbital margin
16 Lower border of body of mandible
17 Lower border of ramus of mandible
18 Medial palpebral ligament anterior to lacrimal sac
19 Mental foramen, nerve and vessels
20 Parotid duct emerging from gland
21 Parotid duct turning medially at anterior border of masseter
22 Philtrum
23 Root of external nose
24 Septum of external nose
25 Supra-orbital notch (or foramen), nerve and vessels
26 Tragus
27 Zygomatic arch

The pulsation of the superficial temporal artery (6) is palpable in front of the tragus of the ear (26).

The parotid duct (20 and 21) lies under the middle third of a line drawn from the tragus of the ear (26) to the midpoint of the philtrum (22).

The pulsation of the facial artery (4) is palpable where the vessel crosses the lower border of the mandible at the anterior margin of the masseter muscle, about 2.5 cm (1 in) in front of the angle of the mandible (3).

Ophthalmic herpes zoster, the philtrum, see pp 90, 91.

Face *superficial dissection from the front and the right*

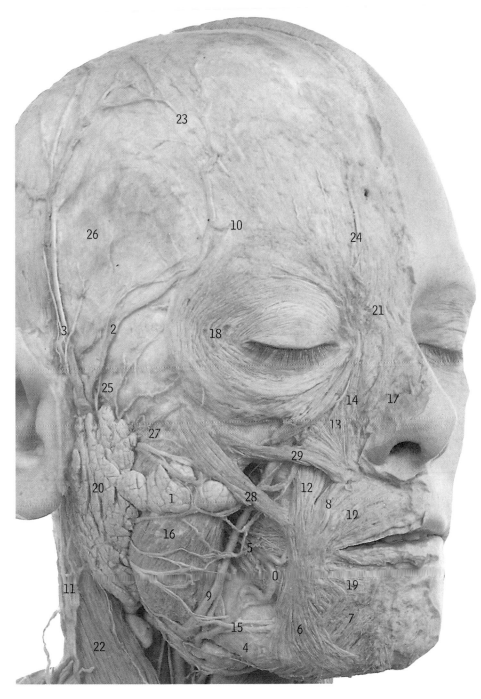

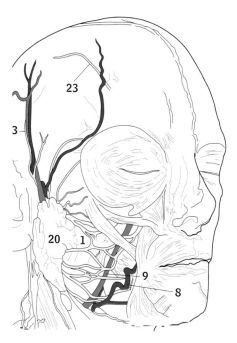

1 Accessory parotid gland overlying parotid duct	**7** Depressor labii inferioris	**15** Marginal mandibular branch of facial nerve	**24** Supratrochlear nerve
2 Anterior branch of superficial temporal artery	**8** Facial artery		**25** Temporal branch of facial nerve
	9 Facial vein	**16** Masseter	
3 Auriculotemporal nerve and superficial temporal vessels	**10** Frontalis part of occipitofrontalis	**17** Nasalis	**26** Temporalis underlying temporal fascia
		18 Orbicularis oculi	
4 Body of mandible	**11** Great auricular nerve	**19** Orbicularis oris	**27** Zygomatic branch of facial nerve
5 Buccinator and buccal branches of facial nerve	**12** Levator anguli oris	**20** Parotid gland	
	13 Levator labii superioris	**21** Procerus	**28** Zygomaticus major
6 Depressor anguli oris	**14** Levator labii superioris alaeque nasi	**22** Sternocleidomastoid	**29** Zygomaticus minor
		23 Supra-orbital nerve	

 Bell's palsy, intracranial spread of infections, surgical flaps of the scalp, see pp 89, 90, 91.

Right temporal fossa *superficial view*

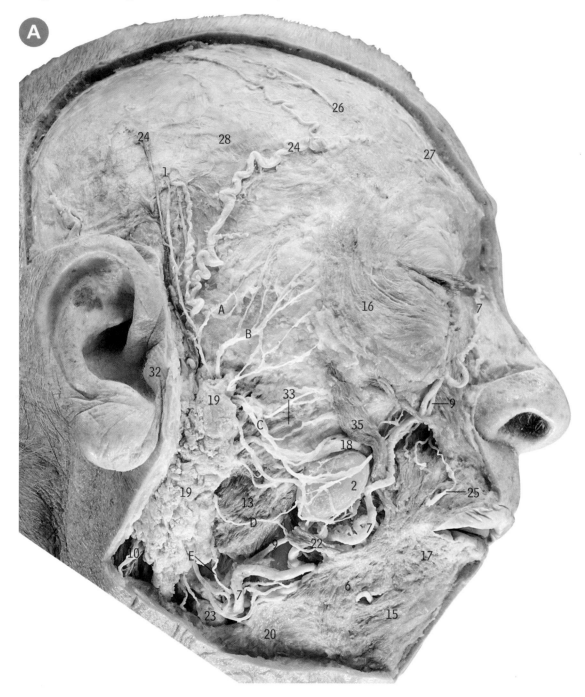

After removal of skin and some fat (A, B, C, D, E = superficial, temporal zygomatic, buccal, mandibular and cervical branches of facial nerve, respectively).

1 Auriculotemporal nerve	**9** Facial vein	**19** Parotid gland	**28** Temporal fascia
2 Buccal fat pad	**10** Great auricular nerve	**20** Platysma	**29** Temporal line, inferior
3 Buccal nerve (V$_3$)	**11** Infraorbital nerve	**21** Retromandibular vein	**30** Temporal line, superior
4 Buccinator	**12** Mandible, body	**22** Risorius, overlying facial	**31** Temporalis
5 Capsule of	**13** Masseter	artery and vein	**32** Tragus
temporomandibular joint	**14** Mental nerve	**23** Submandibular gland	**33** Transverse facial artery
6 Depressor anguli oris	**15** Mentalis	**24** Superficial temporal vessels	**34** Zygomatic arch
7 Facial artery	**16** Orbicularis oculi	**25** Superior labial artery	**35** Zygomaticus major
8 Facial nerve	**17** Orbicularis oris	**26** Supraorbital nerve	
(A, B, C, D, E branches)	**18** Parotid duct	**27** Supratrochlear nerve	

Temporal fossa *deeper view*

B

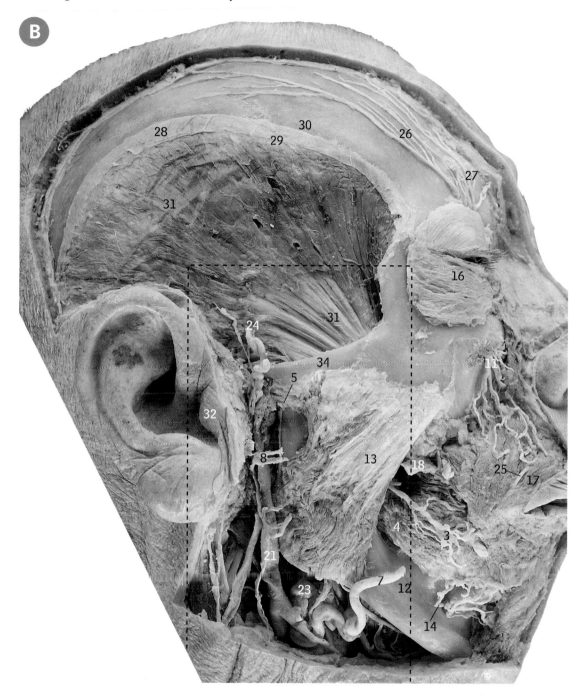

After removal of temporal fascia, parotid gland and most branches of the facial nerve.
Dotted line indicates field of deeper dissections shown on next page.

Infratemporal fossa *progressively deeper dissections*

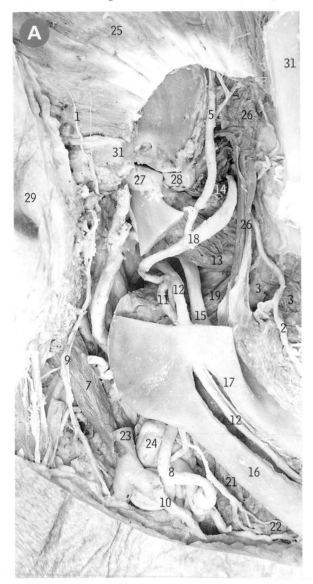

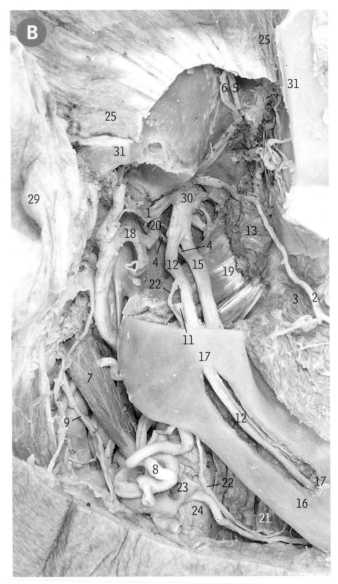

A Removal of the masseter, part of the zygomatic arch, most of the superficial, inferior parts of temporalis, the superior half of the mandibular ramus (except the neck and condyle) and the pterygoid venous plexus reveals the superficial contents of the infratemporal fossa.

B Removal of the deep head of temporalis, the lateral pterygoid and the neck and condyle of the mandible exposes the deepest structures.

1 Auriculotemporal nerve	**13** Lateral pterygoid, inferior head	**24** Submandibular gland
2 Buccal nerve (V₃)		**25** Temporalis
3 Buccinator	**14** Lateral pterygoid, superior head	**26** Temporalis, deep head (sphenomandibularis)
4 Chorda tympani	**15** Lingual nerve	**27** Temporomandibular joint, capsule
5 Deep temporal artery	**16** Mandible, body	
6 Deep temporal nerve	**17** Mandibular canal (opened)	**28** Temporomandibular joint, disc
7 Digastric, posterior belly	**18** Maxillary artery	
8 Facial artery	**19** Medial pterygoid	**29** Tragus
9 Facial nerve, cervical branch	**20** Middle meningeal artery	**30** Trigeminal nerve, mandibular division (V₃)
10 Facial vein	**21** Mylohyoid	
11 Inferior alveolar artery	**22** Nerve to mylohyoid	**31** Zygomatic arch
12 Inferior alveolar nerve	**23** Retromandibular vein	

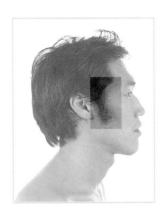

Deep head of temporalis *coronal section*

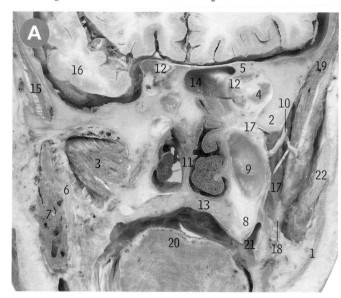

1 Buccinator
2 Greater wing of sphenoid
3 Lateral pterygoid
4 Lateral rectus
5 Lesser wing of sphenoid
6 Mandible
7 Masseter
8 Maxilla
9 Maxillary air (paranasal) sinus
10 Maxillary artery, muscular branches
11 Nasal septum
12 Optic nerve
13 Palate
14 Sphenoidal sinus
15 Temporal bone
16 Temporal lobe, brain
17 Temporalis, deep head
     (sphenomandibularis – Zenker 1955)
18 Temporalis, insertion
19 Temporalis, superficial head
20 Tongue
21 Vestibule of oral cavity
22 Zygoma

Deep head of temporalis *coronal MR image*

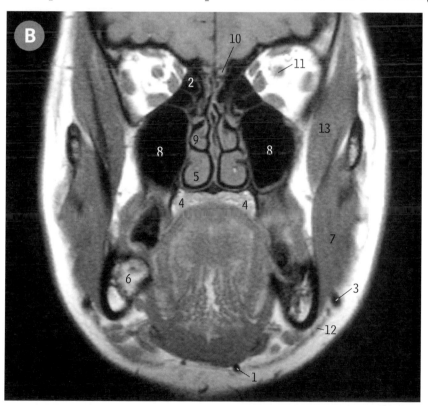

1 Anterior jugular vein
2 Ethmoid air cells
3 External jugular vein
4 Hard palate
5 Inferior concha
6 Mandible
7 Masseter
8 Maxillary sinus
9 Middle concha
10 Olfactory nerve
11 Optic nerve
12 Platysma
13 Temporalis

Inferior alveolar nerve block, see p. 90.

Right trigeminal, facial and petrosal nerves *with associated ganglia*

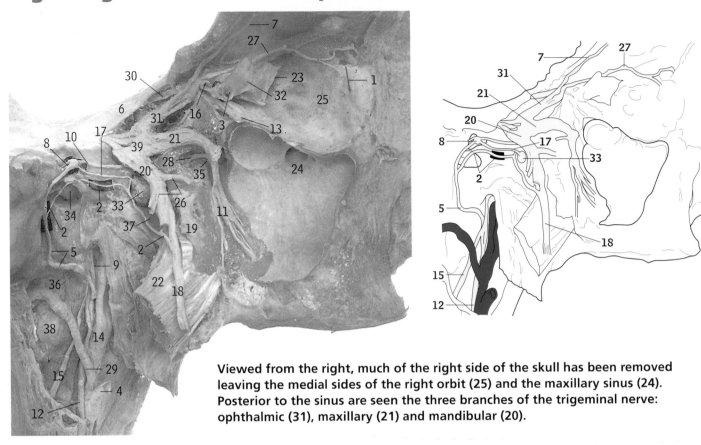

Viewed from the right, much of the right side of the skull has been removed leaving the medial sides of the right orbit (25) and the maxillary sinus (24). Posterior to the sinus are seen the three branches of the trigeminal nerve: ophthalmic (31), maxillary (21) and mandibular (20).

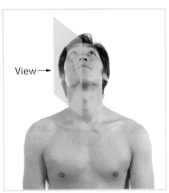

View→

1 Bristle in lacrimal canaliculus	**14** Internal carotid artery	**26** Muscular branches of
2 Chorda tympani	**15** Internal jugular vein and	mandibular nerve
3 Ciliary ganglion	accessory nerve	**27** Nasociliary nerve
4 External carotid artery	**16** Lacrimal nerve	**28** Nerve of pterygoid canal
5 Facial nerve	**17** Lesser petrosal nerve	**29** Occipital artery
6 Free margin of tentorium	**18** Lingual nerve	**30** Oculomotor nerve
cerebelli	**19** Lower head of lateral	**31** Ophthalmic nerve
7 Frontal nerve	pterygoid and lateral	**32** Optic nerve
8 Genicular ganglion of	pterygoid plate	**33** Otic ganglion
facial nerve	**20** Mandibular nerve	**34** Position of tympanic
9 Glossopharyngeal nerve	**21** Maxillary nerve	membrane
10 Greater petrosal nerve	**22** Medial pterygoid	**35** Pterygopalatine ganglion
11 Greater and lesser	**23** Medial rectus	**36** Rectus capitis lateralis
palatine nerves	**24** Medial wall of maxillary	**37** Tensor veli palatini
12 Hypoglossal nerve	sinus and ostium	**38** Transverse process of atlas
13 Inferior rectus	**25** Medial wall of orbit	**39** Trigeminal ganglion

The greater petrosal nerve (10) is a branch of the geniculate ganglion of the facial nerve (8) and can be remembered as the nerve of tear secretion (though it also supplies nasal glands). It carries preganglionic fibres from the superior salivary nucleus in the pons, and runs in the groove on the floor of the middle cranial fossa (page 21, 25) to enter the foramen lacerum and become the nerve of the pterygoid canal (28) which joins the pterygopalatine ganglion (35). Postganglionic fibres leave the ganglion to join the maxillary nerve and enter the orbit by the zygomatic branch which communicates with the lacrimal nerve, supplying the gland (page 65, B11).

The lesser petrosal nerve (17), although having a communication with the facial nerve, is a branch of the glossopharyngeal nerve, being derived from the tympanic branch which supplies the mucous membrane of the middle ear by the tympanic plexus (page 70, C19). Its fibres are derived from the inferior salivary nucleus in the pons, and after leaving the middle ear and running in its groove on the floor

of the middle cranial fossa (17, and page 21, 26), the nerve reaches the otic ganglion (33) via the foramen ovale. From the ganglion secretomotor fibres join the mandibular nerve (20) to be distributed to the parotid gland by filaments from the auriculotemporal nerve.

The chorda tympani (2) arises from the facial nerve before the latter leaves the stylomastoid foramen (5, upper leader line). It crosses the upper part of the tympanic membrane (34) underneath its mucosal covering and runs through the temporal bone, emerging from the petrotympanic fissure (page 19, 35) to join the lingual nerve (18). It carries preganglionic fibres to the submandibular ganglion (page 69, C35) for the submandibular and sublingual salivary glands, and also taste fibres for the anterior two-thirds of the tongue.

The otic ganglion (33), which normally adheres to the deep surface of the mandibular nerve (20), has been teased off from the nerve and a black marker has been placed behind it.

Pharynx *posterior surface, from behind*

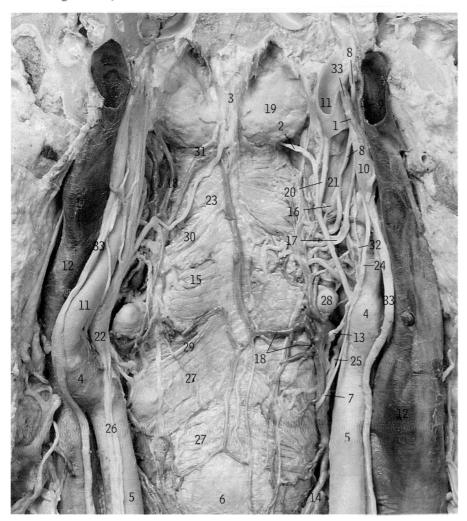

The vertebral column has been removed to reveal the carotid sheath and constrictor muscles of the pharynx.

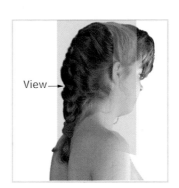

View→

1	Accessory nerve	**17**	Pharyngeal branch of vagus nerve
2	Ascending pharyngeal artery	**18**	Pharyngeal veins
3	Attachment of pharyngeal raphe to pharyngeal tubercle of base of skull	**19**	Pharyngobasilar fascia
		20	Posterior meningeal artery
4	Carotid sinus	**21**	Stylopharyngeus
5	Common carotid artery	**22**	Superior cervical sympathetic ganglion
6	Cricopharyngeal part of inferior constrictor	**23**	Superior constrictor
		24	Superior laryngeal branch of vagus nerve
7	External laryngeal nerve	**25**	Superior thyroid artery
8	Glossopharyngeal nerve	**26**	Sympathetic trunk
9	Hypoglossal nerve	**27**	Thyropharyngeal part of inferior constrictor
10	Inferior ganglion of vagus nerve		
11	Internal carotid artery	**28**	Tip of greater horn of hyoid bone
12	Internal jugular vein	**29**	Upper border of inferior constrictor
13	Internal laryngeal nerve	**30**	Upper border of middle constrictor
14	Lateral lobe of thyroid gland	**31**	Upper border of superior constrictor
15	Middle constrictor	**32**	Vagal branch to carotid body
16	Pharyngeal branch of glossopharyngeal nerve	**33**	Vagus nerve

Gag reflex, see p. 90.

Posterior pharyngeal wall *from behind*

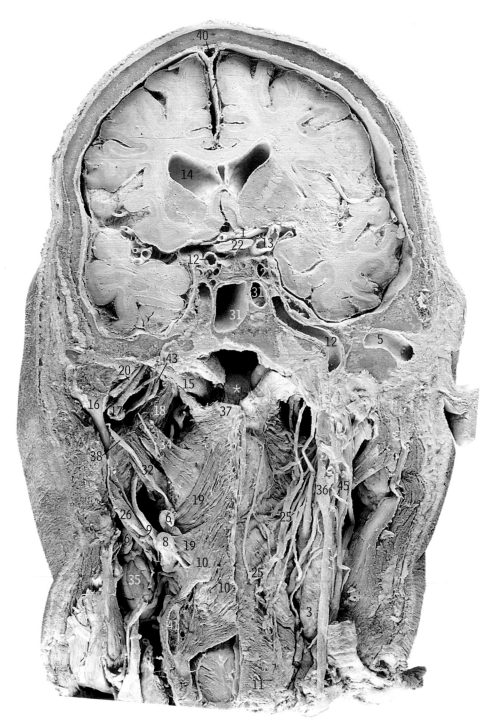

Slightly oblique coronal section of the head and neck in the plane of the posterior pharyngeal wall, with the right side slightly posterior to the left.

Sections of the posterior pharyngeal wall have been removed (asterisks – superiorly the pharyngobasilar fascia and inferiorly the lower border of the inferior constrictor) to reveal parts of the nasopharynx and the laryngopharynx, respectively.

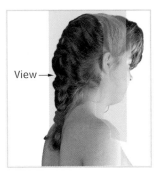

View →

'Opened' pharynx *from behind*

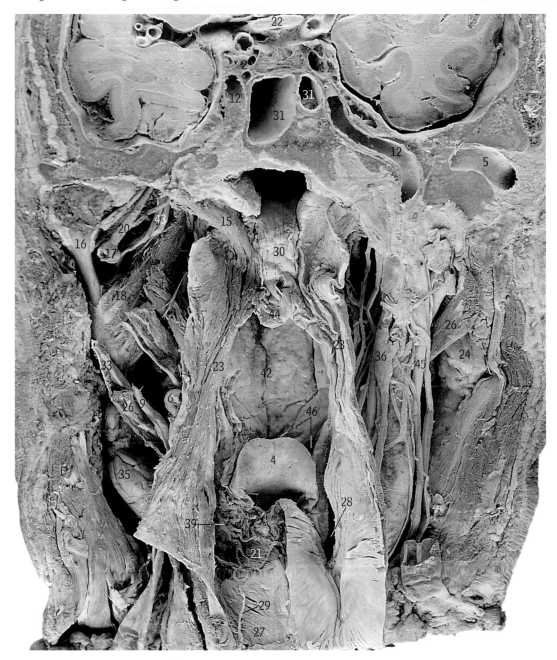

Close-up of interior of the pharynx, after incising and reflecting posterior pharyngeal wall and removing the mucosa from the left pharyngeal walls.

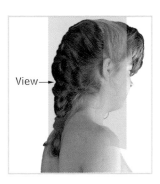

View→

1 Anterior cerebral artery	**13** Internal carotid giving off middle cerebral	**25** Pharyngeal plexus of veins	**37** Superior constrictor
2 Cavernous sinus	**14** Lateral ventricle	**26** Posterior belly of digastric	**38** Superior pharyngeal branch of vagus
3 Common carotid	**15** Levator veli palatini	**27** Posterior crico-arytenoid	**39** Superior laryngeal nerve, internal branch
4 Epiglottis	**16** Mandible, neck	**28** Piriform fossa (recess)	**40** Superior sagittal sinus
5 External auditory canal	**17** Maxillary artery	**29** Recurrent laryngeal nerve	**41** Thyroid cartilage lamina, cut
6 Facial artery	**18** Medial pterygoid	**30** Soft palate, nasal surface	**42** Tongue, dorsum, posterior third
7 Falx cerebri	**19** Middle constrictor	**31** Sphenoidal sinus	**43** Trigeminal nerve, mandibular division
8 Hyoid-tip of greater horn	**20** Middle meningeal artery	**32** Styloglossus muscle	**44** Uvula
9 Hypoglossal nerve	**21** Oblique arytenoid	**33** Stylohyoid muscle	**45** Vagus
10 Inferior constrictor	**22** Optic chiasm	**34** Stylopharyngeus, with glossopharyngeal nerve	**46** Vallecula
11 Inferior constrictor-cricopharyngeus part	**23** Palatopharyngeus	**35** Submandibular gland	
12 Internal carotid	**24** Parotid gland	**36** Superior cervical ganglion	

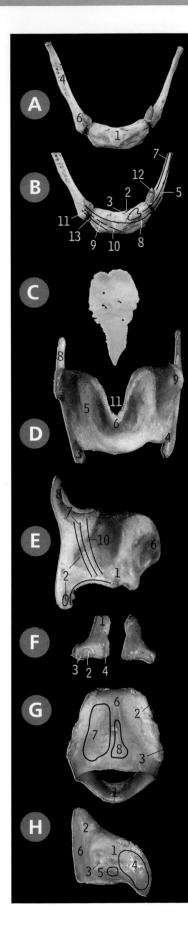

Hyoid bone

(A) from above and in front

(B) with muscle attachments

1 Body	8 Mylohyoid
2 Genioglossus	9 Omohyoid
3 Geniohyoid	10 Sternohyoid
4 Greater horn	11 Stylohyoid
5 Hyoglossus	12 Stylohyoid
6 Lesser horn	ligament
7 Middle	13 Thyrohyoid
constrictor	

Epiglottis

(C) cartilage, from the front

Thyroid

(D) cartilage, from the front

(E) from the right, with attachments

1 Cricothyroid
2 Inferior constrictor
3 Inferior horn
4 Inferior tubercle
5 Lamina
6 Laryngeal prominence (Adam's apple)
7 Sternothyroid
8 Superior horn
9 Superior tubercle
10 Thyrohyoid
11 Thyroid notch

Arytenoid cartilages

(F) from behind

1 Apex
2 Articular surface for cricoid cartilage
3 Muscular process
4 Vocal process

Cricoid cartilage

and muscle attachments

(G) from behind and below

(H) from the right

1 Arch
2 Articular surface for arytenoid cartilage
3 Articular surface for inferior horn of thyroid cartilage
4 Cricothyroid
5 Inferior constrictor
6 Lamina
7 Posterior crico-arytenoid
8 Tendon of oesophagus

Laryngeal *surface anatomy*

(I) lateral view   (J) anterior view

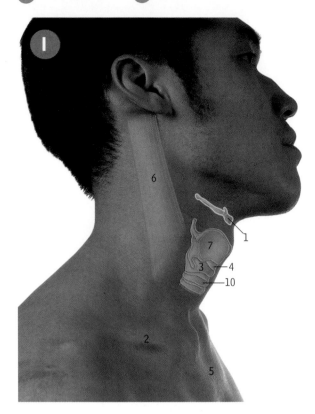

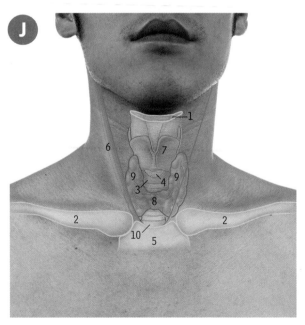

1 Body of hyoid bone	7 Thyroid cartilage, laryngeal prominence
2 Clavicle	
3 Cricoid cartilage	8 Thyroid gland, lateral lobe
4 Cricothyroid ligament/membrane	
	9 Thyroid gland, isthmus
5 Manubrium	10 Tracheal ring
6 Sternomastoid muscle	

Tongue and the inlet of the larynx *from above*

The V-shaped sulcus terminalis (10), behind the row of vallate papillae (11), is not well marked in this tongue.

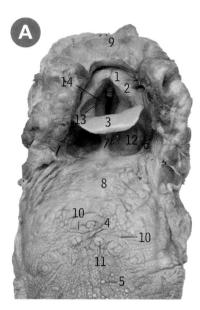

A

1 Corniculate cartilage in aryepiglottic fold
2 Cuneiform cartilage in aryepiglottic fold
3 Epiglottis
4 Foramen caecum
5 Fungiform papilla
6 Lateral glosso-epiglottic fold
7 Median glosso-epiglottic fold
8 Pharyngeal part of dorsum of tongue
9 Posterior wall of pharynx
10 Sulcus terminalis
11 Vallate papilla
12 Vallecula
13 Vestibular fold
14 Vocal fold

Larynx *from behind*

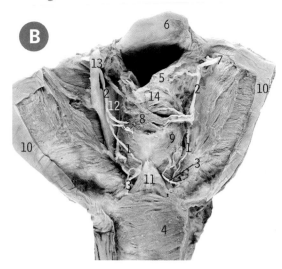

B

1 Anastomosis between internal and recurrent laryngeal nerves
2 Branch of internal laryngeal nerve
3 Branches of recurrent laryngeal nerve
4 Circular fibres of oesophagus
5 Corniculate cartilage in aryepiglottic fold
6 Epiglottis
7 Internal branch of superior laryngeal nerve, piercing mucosa and thyrohyoid membrane
8 Oblique arytenoid muscle
9 Posterior crico-arytenoid muscle
10 Posterior pharyngeal wall
11 Tendon of oesophagus
12 Thyroid cartilage, lamina, posterior surface
13 Thyroid cartilage, superior horn
14 Transverse arytenoid muscle

Intrinsic muscles of the larynx

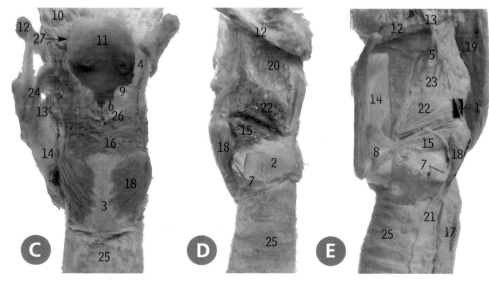

C *from behind* **D** *from the right* **E** *from the left*

In D the right lamina of the thyroid cartilage has been removed, and in E part of the thyroid lamina has been turned forwards.

1 Anastomosis of internal and recurrent laryngeal nerves
2 Arch of cricoid cartilage
3 Area on lamina of cricoid cartilage for tendon of oesophagus
4 Aryepiglottic fold
5 Aryepiglottic muscle
6 Corniculate cartilage
7 Cricothyroid joint
8 Cricothyroid muscle (reflected from cricoid attachment)
9 Cuneiform cartilage
10 Dorsum of tongue
11 Epiglottis
12 Greater horn of hyoid bone
13 Internal laryngeal nerve
14 Lamina of thyroid cartilage
15 Lateral crico-arytenoid muscle
16 Oblique arytenoid muscle
17 Oesophagus
18 Posterior crico-arytenoid muscle
19 Posterior wall of pharynx
20 Quadrangular membrane
21 Recurrent laryngeal nerve
22 Thyro-arytenoid muscle
23 Thyro-epiglottic muscle
24 Thyrohyoid membrane
25 Trachea
26 Transverse arytenoid muscle
27 Vallecula

Recurrent laryngeal nerve damage, see p. 91.

Larynx *in sagittal section, from the right*

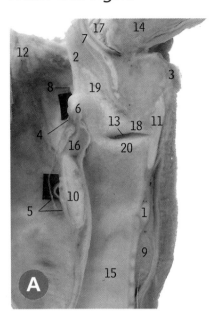

A

The vocal fold (vocal cord, 20) lies below the vestibular fold (false vocal cord, 18)

1 Arch of cricoid cartilage
2 Aryepiglottic fold and inlet of larynx
3 Body of hyoid bone
4 Branches of internal laryngeal nerve anastomosing with recurrent laryngeal nerve
5 Branches of recurrent laryngeal nerve
6 Corniculate cartilage and apex of arytenoid cartilage
7 Epiglottis
8 Internal laryngeal nerve entering piriform recess

9 Isthmus of thyroid gland
10 Lamina of cricoid cartilage
11 Lamina of thyroid cartilage
12 Pharyngeal wall
13 Sinus of larynx
14 Tongue
15 Trachea
16 Transverse arytenoid muscle
17 Vallecula
18 Vestibular fold
19 Vestibule of larynx
20 Vocal fold

The space between the vestibular and vocal folds is the sinus of the larynx (A13), and this is continuous with the saccule, a small pouch that extends upwards for a few millimetres between the vestibular fold and the inner surface of the thyroarytenoid muscle.

The fissure between the two vestibular folds (A18) is the rima of the vestibule. The fissure between the vocal folds is the rima of the glottis.

The vestibular folds are sometimes called the false vocal cords.

The intrinsic muscles of the larynx are supplied by the recurrent laryngeal nerve, except the cricothyroid (page 41, 6) which is supplied by the external laryngeal nerve (page 43, 14).

Larynx *internal view, hemisection*

B

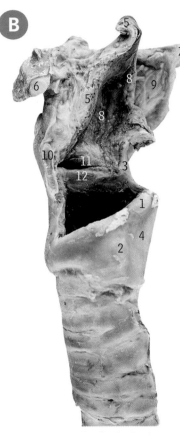

1 Articular facet on cricoid for left arytenoid cartilage
2 Articulation site of thyroid and cricoid cartilages
3 Arytenoid cartilage, right, medial surface
4 Cricoid cartilage, lamina
5 Epiglottis, hemisected
6 Hyoid arch, cross-section
7 Hyoid, greater horn
8 Quadrangular membrane
9 Thyrohyoid membrane
10 Thyroid cartilage, lamina, cross-section
11 Vestibular fold (false vocal cord)
12 Vocal fold (true vocal cord)

Medial view of the membranes and ligaments of the right side of the superior larynx, after removal of the left half above the cricoid cartilage.

The mucous membrane of the larynx above the level of the vocal folds is supplied by the internal laryngeal nerve, and below the vocal folds by the recurrent laryngeal nerve (A4 and 5 above).

The recurrent laryngeal nerve (E21 on page 59) enters the larynx by passing beneath the lower border of the inferior constrictor of the pharynx, and here it lies immediately behind the cricothyroid joint (E7 on page 59).

The anterior part of the vocal fold (A20 and B12 above) is formed by the upper margin of the cricovocal membrane, and the posterior part by the vocal process of the arytenoid cartilage (page 58, F4).

The vestibular fold (false vocal cord, A18 above) is formed by the lower margin of the quadrangular membrane (B8), whose upper margin forms the aryepiglottic fold (A2 above).

The central (anterior) part of the cricothyroid membrane is usually known as the conus elasticus but sometimes this term is used for the cricovocal membrane.

Cranial fossae Ⓐ *with dura mater intact* Ⓑ *with some dura removed*

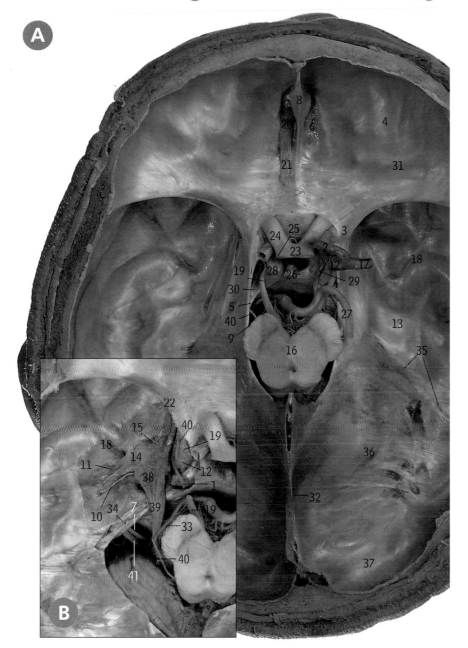

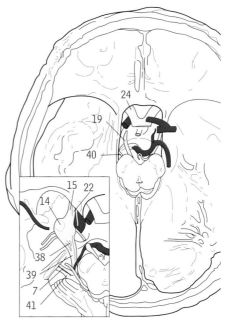

1 Abducent nerve	**16** Midbrain (superior colliculus level)	**31** Sphenoparietal sinus (at posterior border of lesser wing of sphenoid bone)
2 Anterior cerebral artery	**17** Middle cerebral artery	
3 Anterior clinoid process	**18** Middle meningeal vessels	**32** Straight sinus (at junction of falx cerebri and tentorium cerebelli)
4 Anterior cranial fossa	**19** Oculomotor nerve	
5 Attached margin of tentorium cerebelli	**20** Olfactory bulb	**33** Superior cerebellar artery
6 Cribriform plate of ethmoid bone	**21** Olfactory tract	**34** Superior petrosal sinus
7 Facial nerve	**22** Ophthalmic nerve	**35** Superior petrosal sinus (at attached margin of tentorium cerebelli)
8 Falx cerebri attached to crista galli	**23** Optic chiasma	
9 Free margin of tentorium cerebelli	**24** Optic nerve	**36** Tentorium cerebelli
10 Hiatus for greater petrosal nerve	**25** Optic tract	**37** Transverse sinus (at attached margin of tentorium cerebelli)
11 Hiatus for lesser petrosal nerve	**26** Pituitary stalk	
12 Internal carotid artery	**27** Posterior cerebral artery	**38** Trigeminal ganglion
13 Lateral part of middle cranial fossa	**28** Posterior clinoid process	**39** Trigeminal nerve
14 Mandibular nerve	**29** Posterior communicating artery	**40** Trochlear nerve
15 Maxillary nerve	**30** Roof of cavernous sinus	**41** Vestibulocochlear nerve

Cavernous sinus thrombosis, see p. 89.

Sagittal section of the head

A *right half, from the left*

B *MR (magnetic resonance) image*

The falx cerebri (10) separates the two cerebral hemispheres. The tentorium cerebelli (39) separates the posterior parts of the cerebral hemispheres from the cerebellum (5).

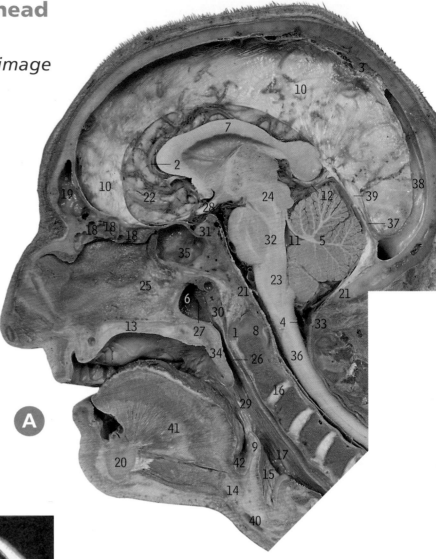

A

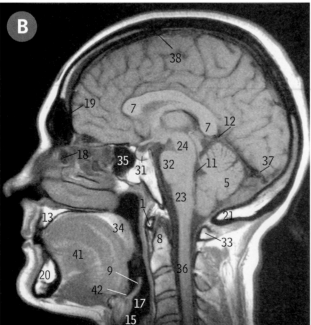

B

1 Anterior arch of atlas	**22** Medial surface of right
2 Anterior cerebral artery	cerebral hemisphere
3 Arachnoid granulations	**23** Medulla oblongata
4 Cerebellomedullary cistern	**24** Midbrain
(cisterna magna)	**25** Nasal septum (bony part)
5 Cerebellum	**26** Nasopharynx
6 Choana (posterior nasal	**27** Opening of auditory tube
aperture)	**28** Optic chiasma
7 Corpus callosum	**29** Oral part of pharynx
8 Dens of axis	(oropharynx)
9 Epiglottis	**30** Pharyngeal (nasopharyngeal)
10 Falx cerebri	tonsil
11 Fourth ventricle	**31** Pituitary gland
12 Great cerebral vein	**32** Pons
13 Hard palate	**33** Posterior arch of atlas
14 Hyoid bone	**34** Soft palate
15 Inlet of larynx	**35** Sphenoidal sinus
16 Intervertebral disc between axis	**36** Spinal cord
and third cervical vertebra	**37** Straight sinus
17 Laryngeal part of pharynx	**38** Superior sagittal sinus
18 Left ethmoidal air cells	**39** Tentorium cerebelli
19 Left frontal sinus	**40** Thyroid cartilage
20 Mandible	**41** Tongue
21 Margin of foramen magnum	**42** Vallecula

Adenoid (pharyngeal tonsil) enlargement, see p. 89.

Ⓐ Cerebral dura mater and cranial nerves

1 Abducent nerve
2 Arachnoid granulations
3 Attached margin of tentorium cerebelli
4 Choana (posterior nasal aperture)
5 Clivus
6 Dens of axis
7 Falx cerebri
8 Free margin of tentorium cerebelli
9 Glossopharyngeal, vagus and accessory nerves
10 Inferior sagittal sinus
11 Internal carotid artery
12 Margin of foramen magnum
13 Medulla oblongata
14 Motor root of facial nerve
15 Nasal septum
16 Oculomotor nerve
17 Olfactory tract
18 Optic nerve
19 Pituitary gland
20 Posterior arch of atlas
21 Rootlets of hypoglossal nerve
22 Sensory root (nervus intermedius) of facial nerve
23 Sphenoidal sinus
24 Sphenoparietal sinus
25 Spinal cord
26 Spinal part of accessory nerve
27 Straight sinus
28 Superior sagittal sinus
29 Tentorium cerebelli
30 Transverse sinus
31 Trigeminal nerve
32 Trochlear nerve
33 Vertebral artery
34 Vestibulocochlear nerve

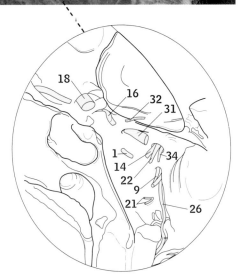

In this oblique view from the left and behind, the brain has been removed and a window has been cut in the posterior part of the falx cerebri (7) to show the upper surface of the tentorium cerebelli (29).

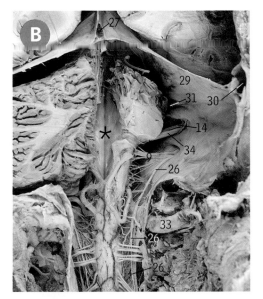

Ⓑ Right posterior cranial fossa

viewed from behind

After removal of posterior skull, dura, upper cervical vertebral laminae, all of right cerebellar hemisphere and much of left to expose the floor of the 4th ventricle (asterisk).

Subdural haemorrhages, see p. 91.

Right eye
surface features

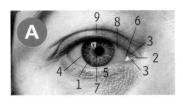

With the eyelids in the normal open position, the lower margin of the upper lid (9) overlaps approximately the upper half of the iris (1); the margin of the lower lid (5) is level with the lower margin of the iris (1).

1 Iris behind cornea
2 Lacrimal caruncle
3 Lacrimal papilla
4 Limbus (corneoscleral junction)
5 Lower lid
6 Plica semilunaris
7 Pupil behind cornea
8 Sclera
9 Upper lid

The cornea is the transparent anterior part of the outer coat of the eyeball and is continuous with the sclera (8) at the limbus (4).

The pupil (7) is the central aperture of the iris (1), the circular pigmented diaphragm that lies in front of the lens.

Each lacrimal papilla (3) contains the lacrimal punctum, the minute opening of the lacrimal canaliculus (B8) which runs medially to open into the lacrimal sac, lying deep to the medial palpebral ligament (B10) and continuing downwards as the nasolacrimal duct (B12) within the nasolacrimal canal.

Nasolacrimal duct

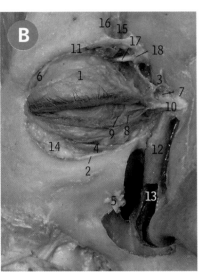

1 Aponeurosis of levator palpebrae superioris
2 Cut edge of orbital septum and periosteum
3 Dorsal nasal artery
4 Inferior oblique
5 Infra-orbital nerve
6 Lacrimal gland
7 Lacrimal sac (upper extremity)
8 Lower lacrimal canaliculus
9 Lower lacrimal papilla and punctum
10 Medial palpebral ligament
11 Muscle fibres of levator palpebrae superioris
12 Nasolacrimal duct
13 Opening of nasolacrimal duct (anterior wall removed) in inferior meatus of nose
14 Orbital fat pad
15 Supra-orbital artery
16 Supra-orbital nerve
17 Tendon of superior oblique
18 Trochlea

Macrodacryocystogram

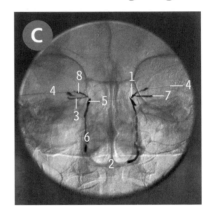

1 Common canaliculus
2 Hard palate
3 Inferior canaliculus
4 Lacrimal catheters
5 Lacrimal sac
6 Nasolacrimal duct
7 Site of lacrimal punctum
8 Superior canaliculus

In B, the facial muscles and part of the skull have been dissected away to display the nasolacrimal duct (12) opening into the meatus of the nose (13).

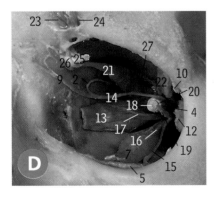

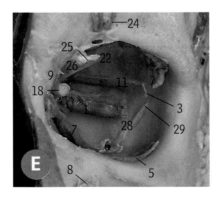

Left orbit

D from the front and left

E from the front and right

The views in D and E show muscles and nerves in relation to the orbital walls after removal of the eye. In D note the extension of the subarachnoid space (20) and the dural sheath (4) round the optic nerve (18).

1 Abducent nerve
2 Anterior ethmoidal nerve
3 Communication between 11 and 28
4 Dural sheath of optic nerve
5 Inferior oblique
6 Inferior orbital fissure
7 Inferior rectus
8 Infra-orbital nerve
9 Infratrochlear nerve
10 Lacrimal gland
11 Lacrimal nerve
12 Lateral rectus
13 Medial rectus
14 Nasociliary nerve
15 Nerve to inferior oblique
16 Nerve to inferior rectus
17 Nerve to medial rectus
18 Optic nerve surrounding central artery of retina
19 Short ciliary nerves
20 Subarachnoid space
21 Superior oblique
22 Superior rectus
23 Supra-orbital artery
24 Supra-orbital nerve
25 Tendon of superior oblique
26 Trochlea
27 Trochlear nerve
28 Zygomatic nerve
29 Zygomatico-orbital foramen

Central retinal artery, corneal reflex, ophthalmoscopy, pupillary reflex, see pp 89, 90, 91.

Orbits *from above*

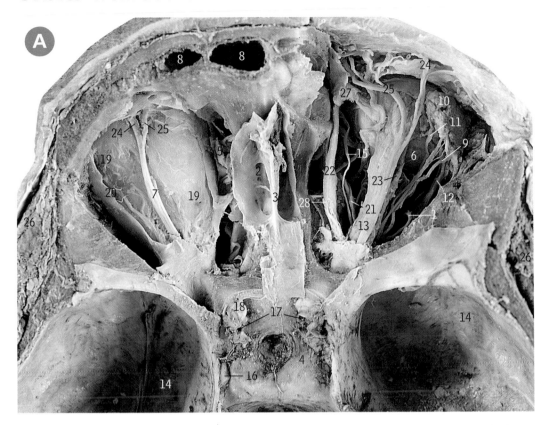

1	Abducent nerve – VI
2	Cribriform plate of ethmoid
3	Crista galli
4	Diaphragma sellae
5	Ethmoid sinus
6	Eyeball
7	Frontal nerve
8	Frontal sinus
9	Lacrimal artery
10	Lacrimal gland
11	Lacrimal nerve
12	Lateral rectus
13	Levator palpebrae superioris
14	Middle cranial fossa
15	Nasociliary nerve
16	Oculomotor nerve – III
17	Ophthalmic artery
18	Optic nerve – II
19	Orbital fat
20	Periorbita
21	Posterior ethmoidal nerve and vessels
22	Superior oblique
23	Superior rectus
24	Supraorbital nerve
25	Supratrochlear nerve
26	Temporalis
27	Trochlea
28	Trochlear nerve – IV

Below the floor of the anterior cranial fossa lie the orbits. On the left the orbital plate of the frontal bone has been removed to show the most superficial structures. On the right, the orbit has been more deeply dissected by removing periorbital fat.

Orbits *from above*

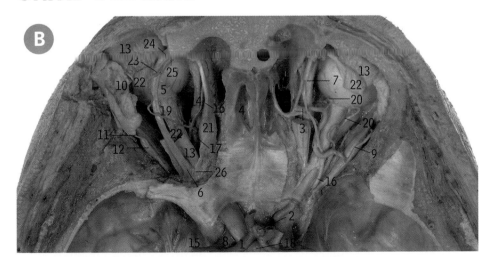

1	Anterior cerebral artery
2	Anterior communicating artery
3	Anterior ethmoidal artery and nerve
4	Cribriform plate of ethmoid bone
5	Eyeball
6	Frontal nerve
7	Infratrochlear nerve and ophthalmic artery
8	Internal carotid artery
9	Lacrimal artery
10	Lacrimal gland
11	Lacrimal nerve
12	Lateral rectus
13	Levator palpebrae superioris
14	Medial rectus
15	Middle cerebral artery
16	Nasociliary nerve
17	Ophthalmic artery
18	Optic chiasma
19	Optic nerve (with overlying short ciliary nerves in left orbit)
20	Posterior ciliary artery
21	Superior oblique
22	Superior rectus
23	Supra-orbital artery
24	Supra-orbital nerve
25	Supratrochlear nerve
26	Trochlear nerve

Both orbits have been exposed from above, and most of levator palpebrae superioris (13) and the superior rectus (22) have been removed. On the right, as is usual, the ophthalmic artery (17) and nasociliary nerve (16) cross above the optic nerve (19) from lateral to medial; on the left the artery has crossed below the nerve, which is uncommon. The supra-orbital artery (23) is unusually small on the left and is absent on the right.

Right orbit C *from above* D *from the right*

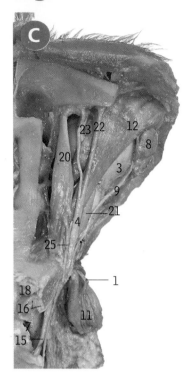

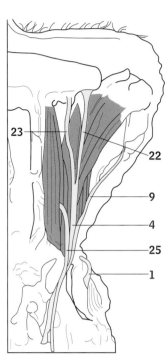

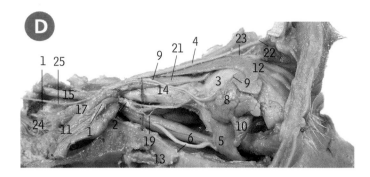

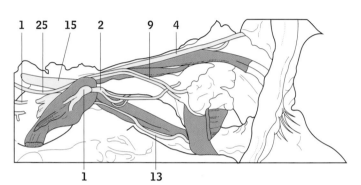

1	Abducent nerve	**8**	Lacrimal gland
2	Ciliary ganglion	**9**	Lacrimal nerve
3	Eyeball	**10**	Lateral rectus
4	Frontal nerve	**11**	Lateral rectus (reflected backwards)
5	Inferior oblique	**12**	Levator palpebrae superioris
6	Inferior rectus	**13**	Nerve to inferior oblique
7	Internal carotid artery		

14	Nerve to medial rectus	**20**	Superior oblique
15	Oculomotor nerve	**21**	Superior rectus
16	Ophthalmic artery	**22**	Supra-orbital nerve
17	Ophthalmic nerve	**23**	Supratrochlear nerve
18	Optic nerve	**24**	Trigeminal ganglion
19	Short ciliary nerves (superficial to marker)	**25**	Trochlear nerve

Right extra-ocular muscles E *from the right*

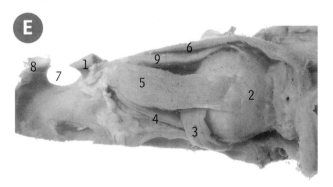

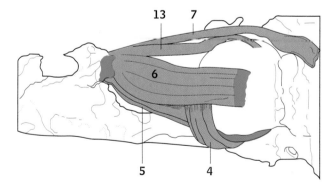

1	Anterior clinoid process	**6**	Levator palpebrae superioris
2	Eyeball	**7**	Pituitary fossa (sella turcica)
3	Inferior oblique	**8**	Posterior clinoid process
4	Inferior rectus	**9**	Superior rectus
5	Lateral rectus		

The upper and lateral walls of the orbit have been removed, together with all fat, vessels and nerves, leaving only the muscles.

Abducent nerve paralysis, oculomotor nerve paralysis, trochlear nerve paralysis, see pp 89, 90, 92.

Nose *in sagittal section, from the left*

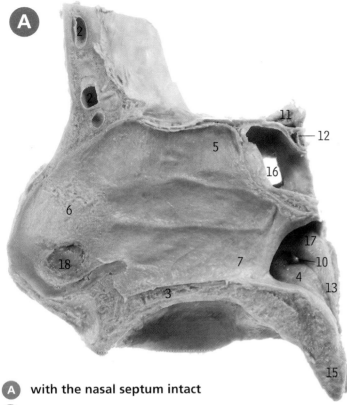

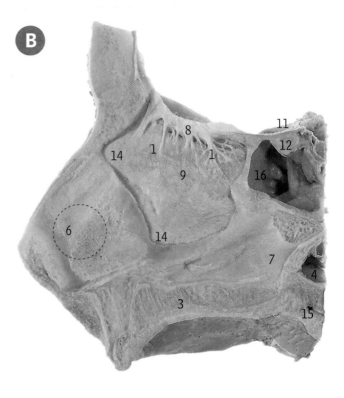

Dotted line indicates Little's area.

A with the nasal septum intact

B with the nasal septum removed

1 Dural covering, olfactory fibres	**5** Nasal septum: perpendicular plate of ethmoid	**9** Olfactory epithelium	**14** Septal bone, cut edge
2 Frontal sinus		**10** Opening of auditory tube	**15** Soft palate
3 Hard palate	**6** Nasal septum: septal cartilage	**11** Optic nerve	**16** Sphenoidal sinus
4 Nasal part of pharynx (nasopharynx)	**7** Nasal septum: vomer	**12** Pituitary gland	**17** Tubal elevation
	8 Olfactory bulb	**13** Salpingopharyngeal fold	**18** Vestibule

Palatine tonsils

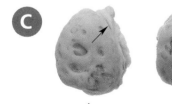

2 cm

The pits on the medial surfaces of these operation specimens from a child aged 14 years are the openings of the tonsillar crypts. The arrows indicate the intratonsillar clefts (the remains of the embryonic second pharyngeal pouch).

The palatine tonsils (commonly called 'the tonsils') are masses of lymphoid tissue that are frequently enlarged in childhood but become much reduced in size in later life. Together with the lymphoid tissue in the posterior part of the tongue (lingual tonsil) and in the posterior wall of the nasopharynx (pharyngeal tonsil) and the tubal tonsil they form a protective 'ring' of lymphoid tissue (Waldeyer's ring) at the upper end of the respiratory and alimentary tracts.

Cerebrospinal fluid rhinorrhea, epistaxis, tonsillitis, see pp 89, 91.

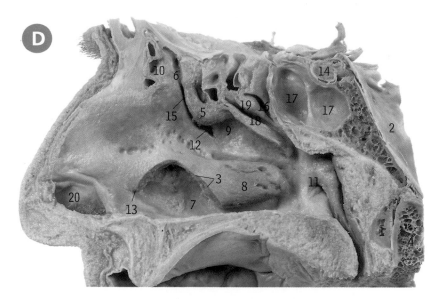

D Lateral wall of the right nasal cavity

1   Anterior arch of atlas
2   Clivus
3   Cut edge of nasal concha
4   Dens of axis
5   Ethmoidal bulla
6   Ethmoidal infundibulum
7   Inferior meatus
8   Inferior nasal concha
9   Middle meatus
10 Opening of anterior ethmoidal air cells
11 Opening of auditory tube
12 Opening of maxillary sinus
13 Opening of nasolacrimal duct
14 Pituitary gland
15 Semilunar hiatus
16 Sphenoethmoidal recess
17 Sphenoidal sinus
18 Superior meatus
19 Superior nasal concha
20 Vestibule

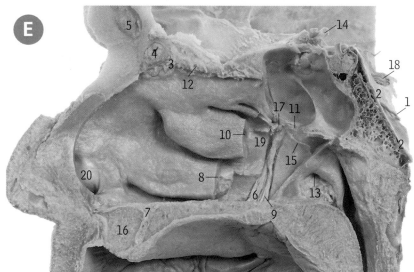

E Right nasal cavity and pterygopalatine ganglion
from the left

1   Abducent nerve
2   Clivus
3   Cribriform plate of ethmoid
4   Ethmoidal air cell (anterior)
5   Frontal sinus
6   Greater palatine nerve
7   Incisive foramen
8   Inferior nasal concha, cut edge of mucoperiosteum
9   Lesser palatine nerves
10 Middle nasal concha, cut
11 Nerve of pterygoid canal
12 Olfactory nerve fibres
13 Opening of auditory tube
14 Optic nerve
15 Pharyngeal branch to ganglion
16 Premaxilla
17 Pterygopalatine ganglion
18 Trigeminal nerve
19 Vertical plate of ethmoid
20 Vestibule

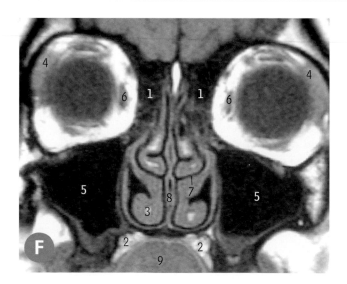

F Conchae
coronal MR image

1   Ethmoid air cells
2   Hard palate
3   Inferior concha
4   Lacrimal gland
5   Maxillary sinus
6   Medial rectus muscle
7   Middle meatus
8   Nasal septum
9   Tongue

Middle ear pressure equalization, nasogastric intubation, see p. 90.

Right trigeminal nerve branches *from the midline*

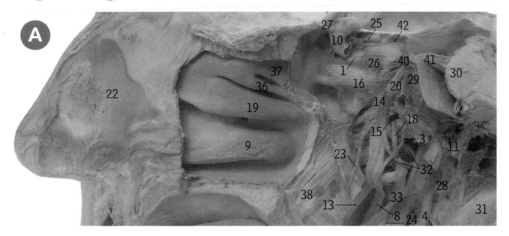

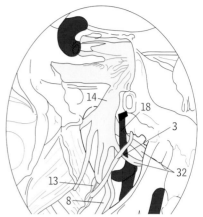

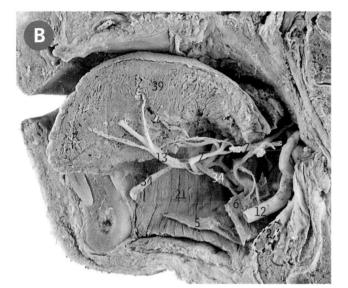

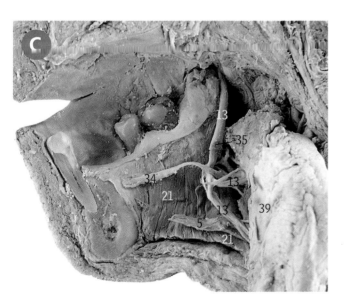

A sagittal section just left of midline

B **C** sagittal sections just right of the midline after removal of geniohyoid muscle, sublingual gland and oral mucosa. Tongue reflected medially in C.

1 Abducent nerve
2 Body of hyoid bone
3 Chorda tympani
4 External carotid artery
5 Geniohyoid
6 Hyoglossus
7 Hypoglossal nerve
8 Inferior alveolar nerve
9 Inferior nasal concha
10 Internal carotid artery
11 Jugular bulb
12 Lingual artery
13 Lingual nerve
14 Mandibular branch of trigeminal nerve
15 Marker in auditory tube
16 Maxillary branch of trigeminal nerve
17 Medial pterygoid
18 Middle meningeal artery
19 Middle nasal concha
20 Motor root of trigeminal nerve
21 Mylohyoid
22 Nasal septum (cartilaginous part)
23 Nerve to medial pterygoid
24 Nerve to mylohyoid
25 Oculomotor nerve
26 Ophthalmic branch of trigeminal nerve
27 Optic nerve
28 Parotid gland
29 Petrous part of temporal bone
30 Pons
31 Posterior belly of digastric
32 Roots of auriculotemporal nerve
33 Sphenomandibular ligament and maxillary artery
34 Submandibular duct
35 Submandibular ganglion
36 Superior nasal concha
37 Supreme nasal concha
38 Tensor veli palatini
39 Tongue
40 Trigeminal ganglion
41 Trigeminal nerve
42 Trochlear nerve

Hypoglossal nerve paralysis, see p. 90.

Right external ear

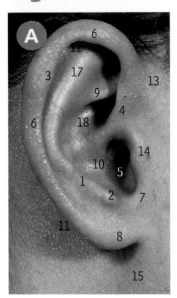

1 Antihelix
2 Antitragus
3 Auricular tubercle
4 Crus of helix
5 External acoustic meatus
6 Helix
7 Intertragic notch
8 Lobule
9 Lower crus of antihelix
10 Lower part of concha
11 Mastoid process
12 Scaphoid fossa
13 Superficial temporal vessels
    and auriculotemporal nerve
14 Tragus
15 Transverse process of atlas
16 Triangular fossa
17 Upper crus of antihelix
18 Upper part of concha

Right tympanic membrane
as seen using auriscope

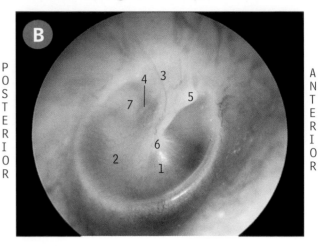

1 Cone of light (light reflex)   5 Malleus, lateral process
2 Pars flaccida   6 Umbo
3 Pars tensa   7 Incus, long limb
4 Chorda tympani

Image supplied courtesy of Prof. T. Wright,
Institute of Laryngology and Otology, London.

Right temporal bone and ear

The bone has been
bisected and opened out
like a book, with some
removal of the upper
part of the petrous part.
The section has opened
up the tympanic (middle
ear) cavity. On the left
side of the figure the
lateral wall of the middle
ear, which includes the
tympanic membrane (26),
is seen from the medial
side, while on the right
the main features of the
medial wall are in view.

1 Aditus to mastoid antrum
2 Anterior semicircular canal
3 Bony part of auditory tube
4 Canal for facial nerve (yellow)
5 Carotid canal (red)
6 Epitympanic recess
7 Groove for greater petrosal
   nerve (yellow)
8 Groove for middle
   meningeal vessels
9 Incus
10 Jugular bulb (blue)
11 Lateral semicircular canal
12 Lesser petrosal nerve
13 Malleus
14 Mastoid air cells
15 Mastoid antrum
16 Mastoid process
17 Part of carotid canal (red)
18 Part of jugular bulb (blue)
19 Promontory with overlying
   tympanic plexus
20 Stapes in oval window and
    stapedius muscle
21 Styloid process
22 Stylomastoid foramen
23 Tegmen tympani
24 Tensor tympani muscle
    in its canal
25 Tympanic branch of
    glossopharyngeal nerve
    entering its canaliculus
26 Tympanic membrane

Hyperacusis, otalgia (referred pain), see p. 90.

Ear *right temporal bone*

A middle ear and the facial nerve and branches

B enlarged view of A

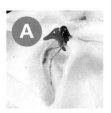
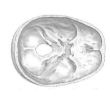

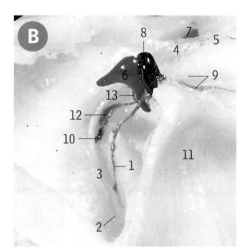

This dissection is seen from the right and above, looking forwards and medially. Bone has been removed to show the upper parts of the malleus (8) and incus (6), which normally project up into the epitympanic recess. The upper part of the facial canal (2) has been opened to show the facial nerve (3) giving off the chorda tympani (1) and the nerve to stapedius (10). The geniculate ganglion of the facial nerve (4) is seen giving off the greater petrosal nerve (5).

1 Chorda tympani
2 Facial canal leading to stylomastoid foramen
3 Facial nerve
4 Geniculate ganglion of facial nerve
5 Greater petrosal nerve
6 Incus
7 Internal acoustic meatus
8 Malleus
9 Margin of auditory tube
10 Nerve to stapedius
11 Paraffin wax (for support) overlying tympanic membrane
12 Stapedius
13 Stapes

> The stapedius (12) tendon emerges from a small conical projection on the posterior wall of the tympanic cavity, the pyramid (here dissected away).

Ear

C right temporal bone; middle ear and inner ear, enlarged

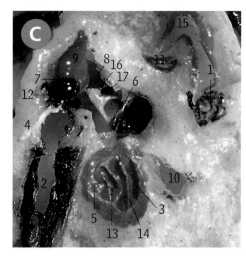

This dissection is viewed from above, looking slightly backwards and laterally. Within the cavity of the middle ear are the three auditory ossicles – malleus (12), incus (9) and stapes (17). The tympanic membrane and external acoustic meatus are not seen but lie below the label 7. The cochlea has been opened up to show its internal bony structure (3, 5, 13 and 14).

1 Anterior semicircular canal
2 Auditory tube
3 Bony canal of cochlea
4 Chorda tympani
5 Cupola of cochlea
6 Footplate of stapes in oval window of vestibule
7 Incudomallealar joint
8 Incudostapedial joint
9 Incus
10 Internal acoustic meatus
11 Lateral semicircular canal
12 Malleus
13 Modiolus of cochlea
14 Osseous spiral lamina of cochlea
15 Posterior semicircular canal
16 Stapedius muscle
17 Stapes

> The spiral organ (the end organ of hearing) lies on the basilar membrane, which stretches between the free edge of the osseous spiral lamina (14) and the side of the bony cochlear canal.
>
> The modiolus (13) is the central axis of the cochlea, and the cupola (5) is its apex.

Right ear

D from above, diagram of parts

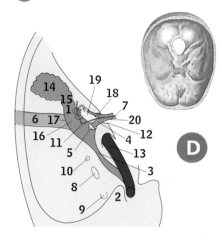

The schematic diagram of part of the right side of the base of the skull (D) indicates the position of the parts of the ear within the temporal bone. (The auditory ossicles have been omitted from the middle ear cavity, 16.) The external acoustic meatus (6) is at a right angle to the side of the skull, and the internal acoustic meatus (12) is level with it on the inner side of the temporal bone. The line (from front to back) of the auditory tube (3), middle ear cavity (16), mastoid antrum (1 and 15) and mastoid air cells (14) lies at about 60° to the line of the external meatus. The cochlear part of the inner ear (5) is in front of the vestibular part (19). The facial nerve (7) runs immediately above the vestibulocochlear nerve (20) and takes a right-angled turn backwards at the geniculate ganglion (11) to pass below the lateral semicircular canal in the medial wall of the middle ear and then turns downwards in the medial wall of the aditus to the antrum (1) to reach the stylomastoid foramen.

1 Aditus to mastoid antrum
2 Anterior clinoid process
3 Auditory tube
4 Cochlear nerve
5 Cochlear part of inner ear
6 External acoustic meatus
7 Facial nerve
8 Foramen ovale
9 Foramen rotundum
10 Foramen spinosum
11 Geniculate ganglion of facial nerve
12 Internal acoustic meatus
13 Internal carotid artery emerging from foramen lacerum
14 Mastoid air cells
15 Mastoid antrum
16 Middle ear
17 Tympanic membrane
18 Vestibular nerve
19 Vestibular part of inner ear
20 Vestibulocochlear nerve

Cranial vault and falx
from below

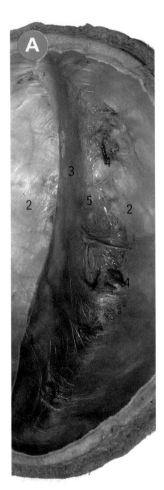

Brain *from above*

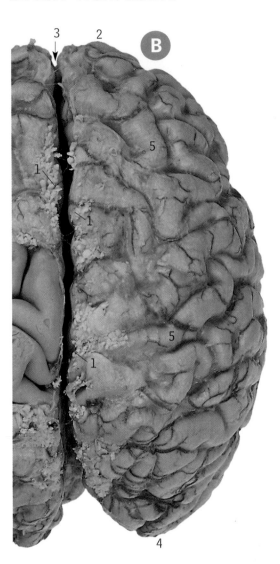

Brain *right cerebral hemisphere, from above*

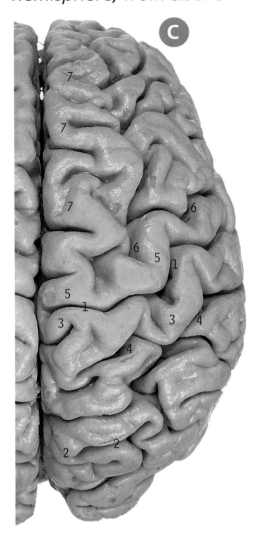

Looking up into the cranial vault from below, the falx cerebri (3) is seen to be continuous with the dura over the vault (2), and has been cut off at the back (1) from the tentorium cerebelli.

1 Cut edge of falx cerebri
2 Dura mater over cranial vault
3 Falx cerebri
4 Superior cerebral veins
5 Superior sagittal sinus

The right cerebral hemisphere is seen with the overlying arachnoid mater and arachnoid granulations (1) adjacent to the longitudinal fissure (3). Over the small part of the left hemisphere shown, a window has been cut in the arachnoid revealing the subarachnoid space.

1 Arachnoid granulations
2 Frontal pole
3 Longitudinal fissure
4 Occipital pole
5 Superolateral surface

Removal of the arachnoid and the underlying vessels displays the gyri and sulci. Only a small number are named here; the most important are the central sulcus (1) and the precentral and postcentral gyri (5 and 3).

1 Central sulcus
2 Parieto-occipital sulcus
3 Postcentral gyrus
4 Postcentral sulcus
5 Precentral gyrus
6 Precentral sulcus
7 Superior frontal gyrus

 Subarachnoid haemorrhage, see p. 91.

Brain Ⓐ *from the right* Ⓑ *right cerebral hemisphere, from the right*

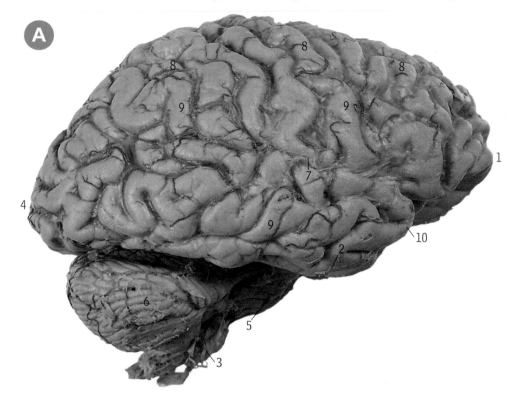

As in B (page 72), the arachnoid mater has been left intact and vessels are seen beneath it; the larger ones are veins (as at 7).

1 Frontal pole
2 Inferior cerebral veins
3 Medulla oblongata and vertebral artery
4 Occipital pole
5 Pons and basilar artery
6 Right cerebellar hemisphere
7 Superficial middle cerebral vein overlying lateral sulcus
8 Superior cerebral veins
9 Superolateral surface of right cerebral hemispheres
10 Temporal pole

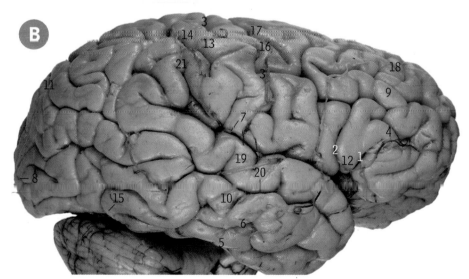

The arachnoid mater has been removed, leaving some of the larger branches of the middle cerebral artery (unlabelled) after they have emerged from the lateral sulcus (7). Only the main gyri and sulci are named here: the most important are the precentral and postcentral gyri (16 and 13) and the central and lateral sulci (3 and 7).

1 Anterior ramus of lateral sulcus
2 Ascending ramus of lateral sulcus
3 Central sulcus
4 Inferior frontal gyrus
5 Inferior temporal gyrus
6 Inferior temporal sulcus
7 Lateral sulcus (posterior ramus)
8 Lunate sulcus
9 Middle frontal gyrus
10 Middle temporal gyrus
11 Parieto-occipital sulcus
12 Pars triangularis
13 Postcentral gyrus
14 Postcentral sulcus
15 Pre-occipital notch
16 Precentral gyrus
17 Precentral sulcus
18 Superior frontal gyrus
19 Superior temporal gyrus
20 Superior temporal sulcus
21 Supramarginal gyrus

The central sulcus (C1 (page 72) and B3 (above)) marks the boundary between the frontal and parietal lobes.

An arbitrary line from the pre-occipital notch (B15) to the parieto-occipital sulcus (B11) marks the boundary between the parietal and occipital lobes, and the part of the hemisphere in front of this line and below the lateral sulcus (strictly, the posterior ramus of the lateral sulcus, B7) forms the temporal lobe.

The precentral and postcentral gyri (B16 and 13) contain the classically described 'motor' and 'sensory' areas of the cortex.

The motor speech areas (usually in the left cerebral hemisphere) are in the region of the ascending and anterior rami of the lateral sulcus and the pars triangularis (B2, 1 and 12).

The auditory areas of the cortex probably comprise parts of the superior temporal gyrus (B19), especially the upper surface of it within the lateral sulcus (B7).

Ⓐ **Brain** *from below*

This is the view of the under-surface of the brain as typically seen when first removed from the skull, without any dissection. Arachnoid mater, torn in places and with blood vessels beneath it, remains on the outer surface.

1 Abducent nerve
2 Anterior perforated substance
3 Arachnoid mater overlying mamillary bodies
4 Basilar artery
5 Cerebellar hemisphere
6 Crus of cerebral peduncle (midbrain)
7 Facial nerve
8 Frontal pole
9 Gyrus rectus
10 Inferior surface of frontal lobe
11 Inferior surface of temporal lobe
12 Internal carotid artery
13 Longitudinal fissure
14 Medulla oblongata
15 Oculomotor nerve
16 Olfactory bulb
17 Olfactory tract
18 Optic chiasma
19 Optic nerve
20 Pituitary stalk (infundibulum)
21 Pons
22 Posterior communicating artery
23 Spinal part of accessory nerve
24 Temporal pole
25 Trigeminal nerve
26 Uncus
27 Vertebral artery
28 Vestibulocochlear nerve

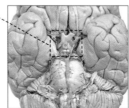

Ⓑ **Optic tract and geniculate bodies**

from below

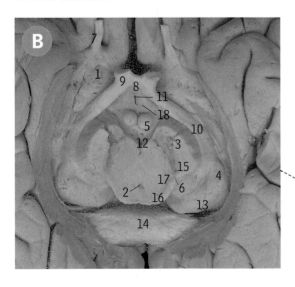

The brainstem has been mostly removed, leaving only the upper part of the midbrain. The most medial parts of each cerebral hemisphere have also been dissected away. To find the geniculate bodies (4 and 6), which are on the under-surface of the posterior part (pulvinar, 13) of the thalamus, identify the optic chiasma (8) and then follow the optic tract (10) backwards round the side of the midbrain (3).

1 Anterior perforated substance
2 Aqueduct of midbrain
3 Crus of midbrain
4 Lateral geniculate body
5 Mamillary body
6 Medial geniculate body
7 Olfactory tract
8 Optic chiasma
9 Optic nerve
10 Optic tract
11 Pituitary stalk (infundibulum)
12 Posterior perforated substance
13 Pulvinar of thalamus
14 Splenium of corpus callosum
15 Substantia nigra of midbrain
16 Tectum of midbrain
17 Tegmentum of midbrain
18 Tuber cinereum

A Brain *from below*

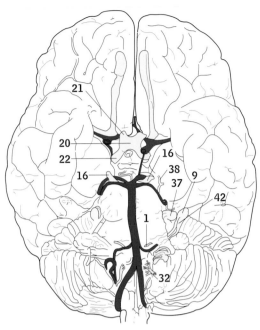

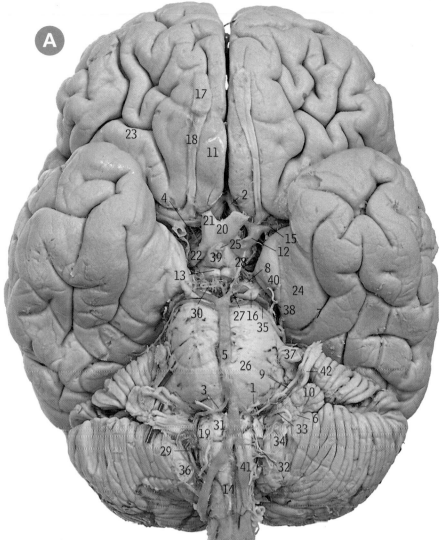

1 Abducent nerve
2 Anterior cerebral artery
3 Anterior inferior cerebellar artery
4 Anterior perforated substance
5 Basilar artery
6 Choroid plexus from lateral recess of fourth ventricle
7 Collateral sulcus
8 Crus of cerebral peduncle
9 Facial nerve
10 Flocculus of cerebellum
11 Gyrus rectus
12 Internal carotid artery
13 Mamillary body
14 Medulla oblongata
15 Middle cerebral artery
16 Oculomotor nerve
17 Olfactory bulb
18 Olfactory tract
19 Olive of medulla oblongata
20 Optic chiasma
21 Optic nerve
22 Optic tract
23 Orbital sulcus
24 Parahippocampal gyrus
25 Pituitary stalk (infundibulum)
26 Pons
27 Posterior cerebral artery
28 Posterior communicating artery
29 Posterior inferior cerebellar artery
30 Posterior perforated substance
31 Pyramid of medulla oblongata
32 Rootlets of hypoglossal nerve (superficial to marker)
33 Roots of glossopharyngeal, vagus and accessory nerves
34 Spinal part of accessory nerve
35 Superior cerebellar artery
36 Tonsil of cerebellum
37 Trigeminal nerve
38 Trochlear nerve
39 Tuber cinereum and median eminence
40 Uncus
41 Vertebral artery
42 Vestibulocochlear nerve

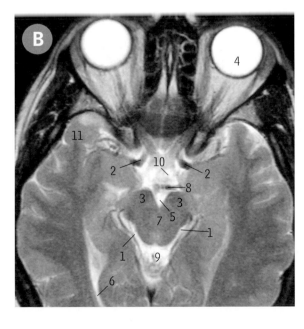

B Brain
axial MR image showing cisterns

1 Ambient cistern
2 Carotid artery
3 Cerebral peduncle
4 Globe
5 Interpeduncular cistern
6 Lateral ventricle, posterior horn
7 Midbrain
8 Posterior cerebral artery
9 Quadrigeminal cistern
10 Suprachiasmatic cistern
11 Temporal lobe

Right half of the brain *in a midline sagittal section, from the left*

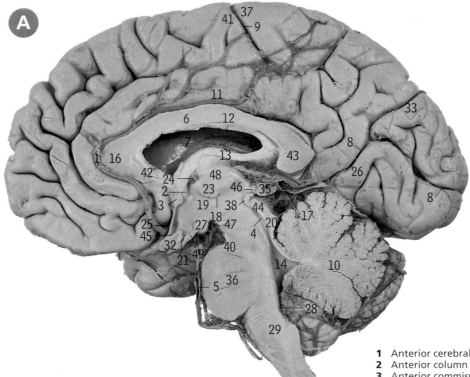

A

In this typical half-section of the brain, the medial surface of the right cerebral hemisphere is seen, together with the sectioned brainstem (midbrain, 4, 20, 44, 47; pons, 36; and medulla oblongata, 29). The septum pellucidum, which is a midline structure and whose cut edge (12) is seen below the body of the corpus callosum (6), has been removed to show the interior of the body of the lateral ventricle (7). The third ventricle has the thalamus (48) and hypothalamus (19) in its lateral wall, while in its floor from front to back are the optic chiasma (32), the base of the pituitary stalk (21), the median eminence (49), the mamillary bodies (27), and the posterior perforated substance (40).

Carotid arteriogram

digitally subtracted arterial phase of carotid arteriogram, lateral projection

B

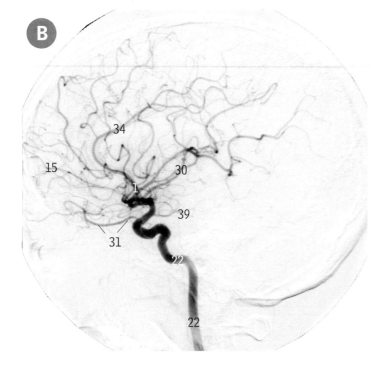

1 Anterior cerebral artery	**26** Lingual gyrus
2 Anterior column of fornix	**27** Mamillary body
3 Anterior commissure	**28** Median aperture of
4 Aqueduct of midbrain	fourth ventricle
5 Basilar artery	**29** Medulla oblongata
6 Body of corpus callosum	**30** Middle cerebral artery
7 Body of lateral ventricle	**31** Ophthalmic artery
8 Calcarine sulcus	**32** Optic chiasma
9 Central sulcus	**33** Parieto-occipital sulcus
10 Cerebellum	**34** Pericallosal artery
11 Cingulate gyrus	**35** Pineal body
12 Cut edge of septum	**36** Pons
pellucidum	**37** Postcentral gyrus
13 Fornix	**38** Posterior commissure
14 Fourth ventricle	**39** Posterior communicating
15 Frontopolar artery	artery
16 Genu of corpus callosum	**40** Posterior perforated
17 Great cerebral vein	substance
18 Hypothalamic sulcus	**41** Precentral gyrus
19 Hypothalamus	**42** Rostrum of corpus callosum
20 Inferior colliculus of	**43** Splenium of corpus callosum
midbrain	**44** Superior colliculus of
21 Infundibular recess	midbrain
(base of pituitary stalk)	**45** Supra-optic recess
22 Internal carotid artery	**46** Suprapineal recess
23 Interthalamic connexion	**47** Tegmentum of midbrain
24 Interventricular foramen	**48** Thalamus
and choroid plexus	**49** Tuber cinereum and
25 Lamina terminalis	median eminence

The third ventricle is the cavity which has in its lateral wall the thalamus (A48) and hypothalamus (A19).

The fourth ventricle (A14) is largely between the pons (A36) and cerebellum (A10), although its lower end is behind the upper part of the medulla oblongata (A29) (see page 79, E).

The aqueduct of the midbrain (A4) connects the third and fourth ventricles; cerebrospinal fluid normally flows through it from the third to the fourth ventricle.

The interventricular foramen (A24) connects the third to the lateral ventricle, and is bounded in front by the anterior column of the fornix (A2) and behind by the thalamus (A48).

Brain *medial surface of the right cerebral hemisphere*

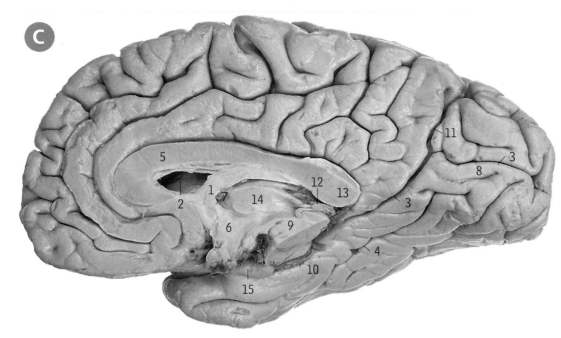

The brainstem has been removed through the midbrain (9) so that the lower part of the hemisphere can be seen; in A, on page 76, the brainstem hides this part.

1 Anterior column of fornix
2 Anterior horn of lateral ventricle
3 Calcarine sulcus
4 Collateral sulcus
5 Corpus callosum
6 Hypothalamus in lateral wall of third ventricle
7 Interventricular foramen
8 Lingual gyrus
9 Midbrain
10 Parahippocampal gyrus
11 Parieto-occipital sulcus
12 Pineal body
13 Splenium of corpus callosum
14 Thalamus in lateral wall of third ventricle
15 Uncus

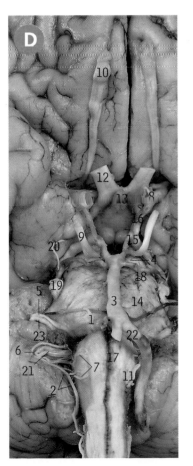

Cranial nerves

In this ventral view of the central part of the brain, the right vertebral artery (on the left of the picture) has been removed almost at the junction with its fellow (22). The filaments of the first nerve (olfactory) are not seen entering the olfactory bulb (10) as they are torn off when removing the brain. The roots forming the glossopharyngeal, vagus and accessory nerves (6, 21 and 2) cannot be clearly identified from one another, but the spinal part of the accessory nerve (2) is seen running up beside the medulla to join the cranial part.

1 Abducent nerve
2 Accessory nerve, spinal root
3 Basilar artery
4 Crus of cerebral peduncle
5 Facial nerve
6 Glossopharyngeal nerve
7 Hypoglossal nerve
8 Internal carotid artery
9 Oculomotor nerve
10 Olfactory bulb
11 Olive of medulla oblongata
12 Optic nerve
13 Pituitary stalk
14 Pons
15 Posterior cerebral artery
16 Posterior communicating artery
17 Pyramid of medulla oblongata
18 Superior cerebellar artery
19 Trigeminal nerve
20 Trochlear nerve
21 Vagus nerve
22 Vertebral artery
23 Vestibulocochlear nerve

The oculomotor nerve (D9) emerges on the medial side of the crus of the cerebral peduncle (D4), and the trochlear nerve (D20) winds round the lateral side of the peduncle. Both nerves pass between the posterior cerebral and superior cerebellar arteries (D15 and 18).

The trochlear nerve (D20) is the only cranial nerve to emerge from the dorsal surface of the brainstem.

The trigeminal nerve (D19) emerges from the lateral side of the pons (D14).

The abducent nerve (D1) emerges between the pons and the pyramid (D14 and 17).

The facial and vestibulocochlear nerves (D5 and 23) emerge from the lateral pontomedullary angle.

The glossopharyngeal and vagus nerves (D6, 21, 2) and the cranial root of the accessory nerve emerge from the medulla oblongata lateral to the olive (D11).

The hypoglossal nerve (D7) emerges as two series of rootlets from the medulla oblongata between the pyramid (D17) and the olive (D11).

The spinal part of the accessory nerve emerges from the lateral surface of the upper five or six cervical segments of the spinal cord, dorsal to the denticulate ligament (page 79, F27).

Arteries of the base of the brain Ⓐ *injected arteries*
Ⓑ *arterial circle (Willis) and basilar artery* Ⓒ *MR angiogram of arterial circle (Willis)*

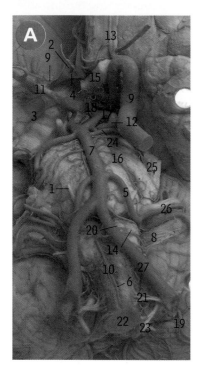

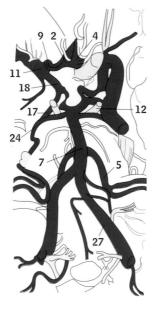

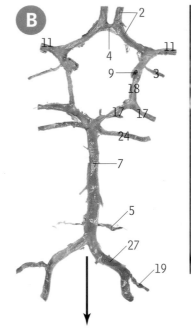

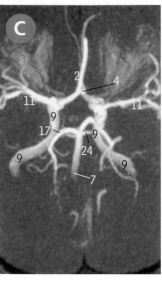

Part of the right cerebral hemisphere (on the left of the picture) has been removed to show the right middle cerebral artery (11).

The anastomising vessels have been removed from the base of the brain and spread out in their relative positions

1 Abducent nerve	**8** Filaments of glossopharyngeal, vagus and accessory nerves	**15** Optic nerve	**23** Spinal part of accessory nerve
2 Anterior cerebral		**16** Pons	
3 Anterior choroidal	**9** Internal carotid	**17** Posterior cerebral	**24** Superior cerebellar
4 Anterior communicating	**10** Medulla oblongata	**18** Posterior communicating	**25** Trigeminal nerve
5 Anterior inferior cerebellar	**11** Middle cerebral	**19** Posterior inferior cerebellar	**26** Unusually large branch of 5 overlying facial and vestibulocochlear nerves
6 Anterior spinal	**12** Oculomotor nerve	**20** Pyramid	
7 Basilar with pontine branches	**13** Olfactory tract	**21** Rootlets of first cervical nerve	
	14 Olive	**22** Spinal cord	**27** Vertebral

Brainstem and cerebellum in sagittal section *from the left*

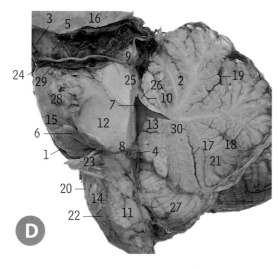

The left half of the cerebellum has been removed by sagittal section in the midline and by transecting the left cerebellar peduncles (8, 12 and 25).

1 Abducent nerve	**17** Postpyramidal fissure
2 Anterior lobe	**18** Prepyramidal fissure
3 Basal cerebral vein	**19** Primary fissure
4 Choroid plexus in lateral recess	**20** Pyramid of medulla oblongata
5 Crus of cerebral peduncle	**21** Pyramid of vermis
6 Facial and vestibulocochlear nerves	**22** Rootlets of hypoglossal nerve
7 Fourth ventricle	**23** Roots of glossopharyngeal, vagus and accessory nerves
8 Inferior cerebellar peduncle	**24** Superior cerebellar artery
9 Inferior colliculus	**25** Superior cerebellar peduncle
10 Lingula	**26** Superior medullary velum
11 Medulla oblongata	**27** Tonsil
12 Middle cerebellar peduncle	**28** Trigeminal nerve
13 Nodule of vermis	**29** Trochlear nerve
14 Olive	**30** Uvula of vermis
15 Pons	
16 Posterior cerebral artery	

E Brainstem and floor of the fourth ventricle

In this view of the dorsal surface of the brainstem, it has been cut off from the rest of the brain at the top of the midbrain, just above the superior colliculi (15). The cerebellum has been removed by transecting the superior (14), middle (12) and inferior (6) cerebellar peduncles.

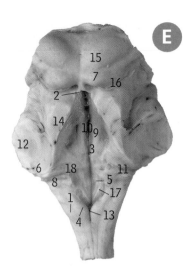

1 Cuneate tubercle
2 Cut edge of superior medullary velum
3 Facial colliculus
4 Gracile tubercle
5 Hypoglossal triangle
6 Inferior cerebellar peduncle
7 Inferior colliculus
8 Lateral recess
9 Medial eminence
10 Median sulcus
11 Medullary striae
12 Middle cerebellar peduncle
13 Obex
14 Superior cerebellar peduncle
15 Superior colliculus
16 Trochlear nerve
17 Vagal triangle
18 Vestibular area

F Brainstem and upper part of the spinal cord *from behind*

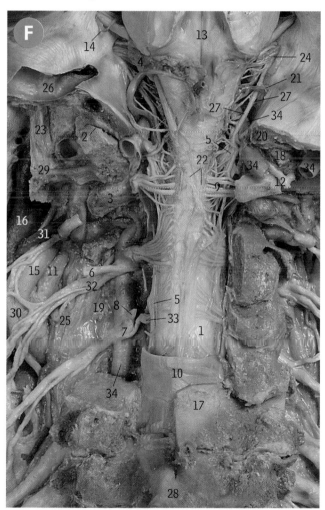

The posterior parts of the skull and upper vertebrae have been removed to show the continuity of the brainstem with the spinal cord, from which dorsal nerve rootlets are seen to emerge (as at 9). The spinal part of the accessory nerve (27) runs up through the foramen magnum (20) to join the cranial part in the jugular foramen (24). Ventral nerve rootlets (as at 33), ventral to the denticulate ligament (5), unite to form a ventral nerve root which joins with a dorsal nerve root (8, whose formative rootlets dorsal to the ligament have been cut off from the cord in order to make the ventral roots visible) to form a spinal nerve immediately beyond the dorsal root ganglion (7). The nerve immediately divides into ventral and dorsal rami (as at 32 and 6).

1 Arachnoid mater
2 Atlanto-occipital joint
3 Capsule of lateral atlanto-axial joint
4 Choroid plexus emerging from lateral recess of fourth ventricle
5 Denticulate ligament
6 Dorsal ramus of third cervical nerve
7 Dorsal root ganglion of fourth cervical nerve
8 Dorsal root of fourth cervical nerve
9 Dorsal rootlets of second cervical nerve
10 Dura mater
11 External carotid artery
12 First cervical nerve and posterior arch of atlas
13 Floor of the fourth vehicle
14 Internal acoustic meatus with facial and vestibulocochlear nerves and labyrinthine artery
15 Internal carotid artery
16 Internal jugular vein
17 Lamina of sixth cervical vertebra
18 Lateral mass of atlas
19 Longus capitus
20 Margin of foramen magnum
21 Posterior inferior cerebellar artery
22 Posterior spinal arteries
23 Rectus capitis lateralis
24 Roots of glossopharyngeal, vagus and cranial part of accessory nerves and jugular foramen
25 Scalenus anterior
26 Sigmoid sinus
27 Spinal part of accessory nerve
28 Spinous process of seventh cervical vertebra
29 Transverse process of atlas
30 Vagus nerve
31 Vein from vertebral venous plexuses
32 Ventral ramus of third cervical nerve
33 Ventral rootlets of fourth cervical nerve
34 Vertebral artery

The lower part of the diamond-shaped floor of the fourth ventricle containing the hypoglossal and vagal triangles (E5 and 17) is part of the medulla oblongata; the rest of the floor is part of the pons.

The gracile and cuneate tubercles (E4 and 1) are caused by the underlying gracile and cuneate nuclei, where the fibres of the gracile and cuneate tracts (posterior white columns) end by synapsing with the cells of the nuclei. The fibres from these cells form the medial lemniscus which runs through the brainstem to the thalamus.

The facial colliculus (E3), at the lower end of the medial eminence (E9) in the floor of the fourth ventricle, is caused by fibres of the facial nerve overlying the abducent nerve nucleus; it is not produced by the facial nerve nucleus, which lies at a deeper level in the pons.

After emerging from the foramen in the transverse process of the atlas the vertebral artery (F34) winds backwards round the lateral mass of the atlas (F18) on its posterior arch before turning upwards to enter the skull.

Cerebral hemispheres Ⓐ *sectioned horizontally* Ⓑ *axial MR image*

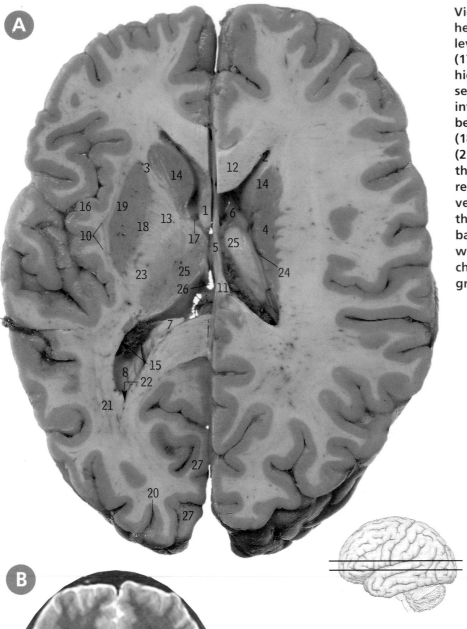

Ⓐ

Viewed from above, the left cerebral hemisphere has been sectioned on a level with the interventricular foramen (17), and that on the right about 1.5 cm higher. The most important feature seen in the left hemisphere is the internal capsule (3, 13 and 23), situated between the caudate (14) and lentiform (18 and 19) nuclei and the thalamus (25). On the right side a large part of the corpus callosum (11) has been removed, so opening up the lateral ventricle (6) from above and showing the caudate nucleus (14 and 4) arching backwards over the thalamus (25), with the thalamostriate vein (24) and choroid plexus (9) in the shallow groove between them.

1 Anterior column of fornix
2 Anterior horn of lateral ventricle
3 Anterior limb of internal capsule
4 Body of caudate nucleus
5 Body of fornix
6 Body of lateral ventricle
7 Bulb
8 Calcar avis
9 Choroid plexus
10 Claustrum
11 Corpus callosum
12 Forceps minor (corpus callosum)
13 Genu of internal capsule
14 Head of caudate nucleus
15 Inferior horn of lateral ventricle
16 Insula
17 Interventricular foramen
18 Lentiform nucleus: globus pallidus
19 Lentiform nucleus: putamen
20 Lunate sulcus
21 Optic radiation
22 Posterior horn of lateral ventricle
23 Posterior limb of internal capsule
24 Thalamostriate vein
25 Thalamus
26 Third ventricle
27 Visual area of cortex

Ⓑ

The anterior limb of the internal capsule (3) is bounded medially by the head of the caudate nucleus (14) and laterally by the lentiform nucleus (putamen and globus pallidus, 18 and 19).

The genu of the internal capsule (13) lies at the most medial edge of the globus pallidus (18).

The posterior limb of the internal capsule (23) is bounded medially by the thalamus (25) and laterally by the lentiform nucleus (18 and 19).

Corticonuclear fibres (motor fibres from the cerebral cortex to the motor nuclei of cranial nerves) pass through the genu of the internal capsule (13).

Corticospinal fibres (motor fibres from the cerebral cortex to anterior horn cells of the spinal cord) pass through the anterior two-thirds of the posterior limb of the internal capsule (23).

The genu and the posterior limb of the internal capsule, supplied by the striate branches of the anterior and middle cerebral arteries, are of the greatest clinical importance as they are the common sites for cerebral haemorrhage or thrombosis ('stroke').

Brain Ⓐ coronal section, from the front Ⓑ coronal MR image

Ⓐ

This coronal section is not quite vertical but passes slightly backwards, through the third ventricle (25) and bodies of the lateral ventricles (3) from a level about 0.5 cm behind the interventricular foramina, and down through the pons (17) and the pyramid of the medulla (19). It has been cut in this way to show the path of the important corticospinal (motor) fibres passing down through the internal capsule (11) and pons (17) to form the pyramid of the medulla (19). Compare with features in the MR image.

Ⓑ

1	Body of caudate nucleus	6	Choroid plexus of third ventricle	13	Lentiform nucleus: globus pallidus	19	Pyramid of medulla oblongata
2	Body of fornix	7	Choroidal fissure	14	Lentiform nucleus: putamen	20	Septum pellucidum
3	Body of lateral ventricle	8	Corpus callosum	15	Olive of medulla oblongata	21	Substantia nigra
4	Choroid plexus of inferior horn of lateral ventricle	9	Hippocampus	16	Optic tract	22	Tail of caudate nucleus
5	Choroid plexus of lateral ventricle	10	Insula	17	Pons	23	Thalamostriate vein
		11	Internal capsule	18	Posterior cerebral artery	24	Thalamus
		12	Interpeduncular cistern			25	Third ventricle

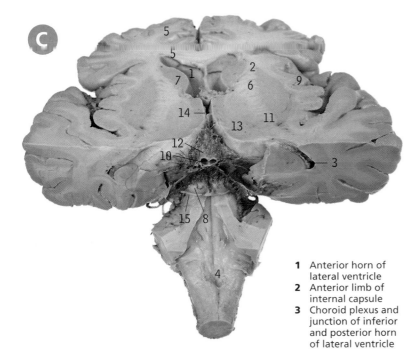

Ⓒ Sectioned cerebral hemispheres and the brainstem

from above and behind

The cerebral hemispheres have been sectioned horizontally just above the level of the interventricular foramina, and the posterior parts of the hemispheres have been removed, together with the whole of the cerebellum, to show the tela choroidea (12) of the posterior part of the roof of the third ventricle and the underlying internal cerebral veins (10).

1	Anterior horn of lateral ventricle	4	Floor of fourth vehicle	10	Internal cerebral vein
2	Anterior limb of internal capsule	5	Forceps minor	11	Posterior limb of internal capsule
3	Choroid plexus and junction of inferior and posterior horn of lateral ventricle	6	Genu of internal capsule	12	Tela choroidea of roof of third ventricle
		7	Head of caudate nucleus	13	Thalamus
		8	Inferior colliculus	14	Third ventricle
		9	Insula	15	Trochlear nerve

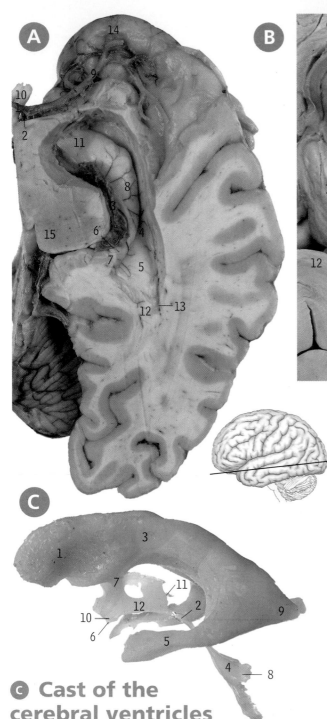

A

B

Ⓐ Inferior horn of right lateral ventricle

Brain substance above the front part of the lateral sulcus has been removed, displaying the middle cerebral artery (9) running laterally over the upper surface of the front of the temporal lobe (14). Part of the temporal lobe has been opened up from above to show the hippocampus (11 and 8) in the floor of the inferior horn.

1	Anterior cerebral artery	9	Middle cerebral artery
2	Anterior choroidal artery	10	Optic nerve
3	Choroid plexus	11	Pes hippocampi
4	Collateral eminence	12	Posterior horn
5	Collateral trigone	13	Tapetum
6	Fimbria	14	Temporal pole of temporal lobe
7	Fornix	15	Thalamus
8	Hippocampus		

Ⓑ Right cerebral hemisphere dissection *from above*

Much of the cerebral substance has been dissected away to show the caudate nucleus (3), thalamus (13) and lentiform nucleus (9). The intervening gap (8) is occupied by the internal capsule. The optic radiation (10) has also been dissected out; it runs backwards lateral to the posterior horn of the lateral ventricle. Compare this three-dimensional view of these structures with the brain sections on page 81.

1	Bulb	6	Forceps minor	11	Posterior horn of lateral ventricle
2	Calcar avis	7	Fornix	12	Splenium of corpus callosum
3	Caudate nucleus	8	Internal capsule	13	Thalamus
4	Collateral trigone	9	Lentiform nucleus		
5	Forceps major	10	Optic radiation		

C

Ⓒ Cast of the cerebral ventricles

from the left

In this side view the left lateral ventricle largely overlaps the right one.

1	Anterior horn of lateral ventricle	8	Lateral recess
2	Aqueduct of midbrain	9	Posterior horn of lateral ventricle
3	Body of lateral ventricle	10	Supra-optic recess of third ventricle
4	Fourth ventricle	11	Suprapineal recess of third ventricle
5	Inferior horn of lateral ventricle	12	Third ventricle (with gap for interthalamic connexion)
6	Infundibular recess of third ventricle		
7	Interventricular foramen		

The third ventricle (C12) communicates at its upper front end with each lateral ventricle through the interventricular foramen (C7).

The main part of the lateral ventricle is the body (C3). The part in front of the interventricular foramen (C7) is the anterior horn (C1) which extends into the frontal lobe of the brain. At its posterior end the body divides into the posterior horn (C9) which extends backwards into the occipital lobe, and the inferior horn (C5) which passes downwards and forwards into the temporal lobe.

The lower posterior part of the third ventricle (C12) communicates with the fourth ventricle (C4) through the aqueduct of the midbrain (C2).

The floor of the inferior horn consists of the hippocampus (A11 and 8) medially and the collateral eminence (A4) laterally. At its junction with the posterior horn (A12 and B11) the eminence broadens into the collateral trigone (A5, B4).

The collateral eminence (A4) is produced by the inward projection of the collateral sulcus (page 77, C4).

In the medial wall of the posterior horn, the bulb (B1) is produced by fibres of the corpus callosum, and the calcar avis (B2) by the inward projection of the calcarine sulcus (page 77, C3).

Cranial nerve *I – olfactory*

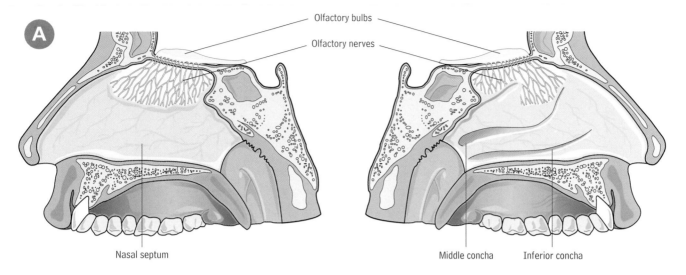

A

Olfactory bulbs
Olfactory nerves
Nasal septum
Middle concha   Inferior concha

See pages 63, 74 and 75.

Cranial nerve *II – optic*

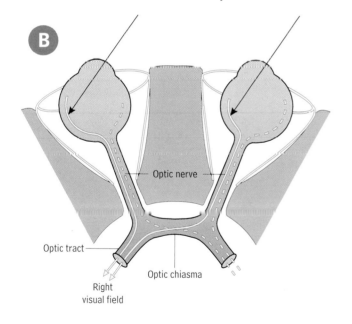

B

Optic nerve
Optic tract
Optic chiasma
Right visual field

See pages 7, 65, 75 and 77.

Fundus of eye
ophthalmoscopic photograph of a retina

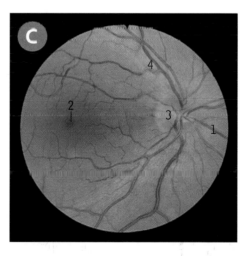

C

1 Inferior nasal branches of central vein and artery
2 Macula with central fovea
3 Optic disc
4 Superior temporal branches of central vein and artery

Photo reproduced courtesy of Miss Gilli Vafidis FRCOphth, Central Middlesex Hospital, London

Anosmia, see p. 89.

Cranial nerves *III– oculomotor, IV – trochlear, VI – abducens*

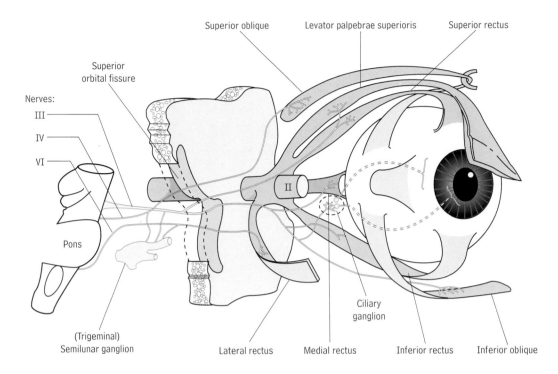

Superior oblique

Levator palpebrae superioris

Superior rectus

Superior orbital fissure

Nerves:

III

IV

VI

Pons

II

(Trigeminal) Semilunar ganglion

Lateral rectus

Medial rectus

Ciliary ganglion

Inferior rectus

Inferior oblique

See pages 63–65 for III.
See pages 63A for IV.
See pages 63–66 for VI.

Abducent nerve paralysis, accommodation reflex, oculomotor nerve paralysis, trochlear nerve paralysis, see pp 89, 90, 92.

Cranial nerve

Ⓐ V – trigeminal (overview)

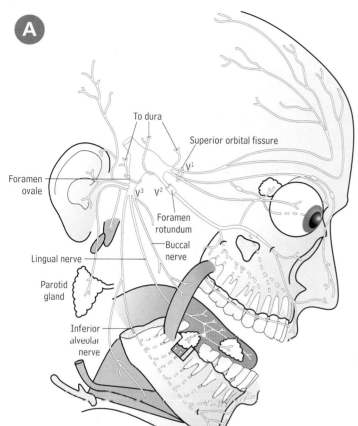

Ⓑ V¹ ophthalmic division of trigeminal

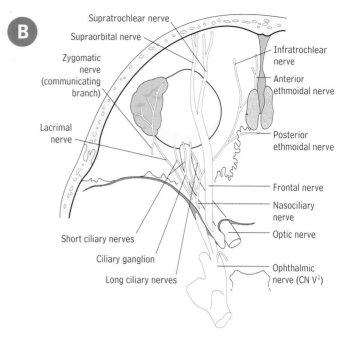

Supratrochlear nerve
Supraorbital nerve
Zygomatic nerve (communicating branch)
Infratrochlear nerve
Anterior ethmoidal nerve
Lacrimal nerve
Posterior ethmoidal nerve
Frontal nerve
Nasociliary nerve
Optic nerve
Short ciliary nerves
Ciliary ganglion
Long ciliary nerves
Ophthalmic nerve (CN V¹)

See page 61B for V.
See pages 61B and 66D for V¹.

To dura
Superior orbital fissure
V¹
Foramen ovale
V³ V²
Foramen rotundum
Buccal nerve
Lingual nerve
Parotid gland
Inferior alveolar nerve

Ⓒ V² maxillary division of trigeminal

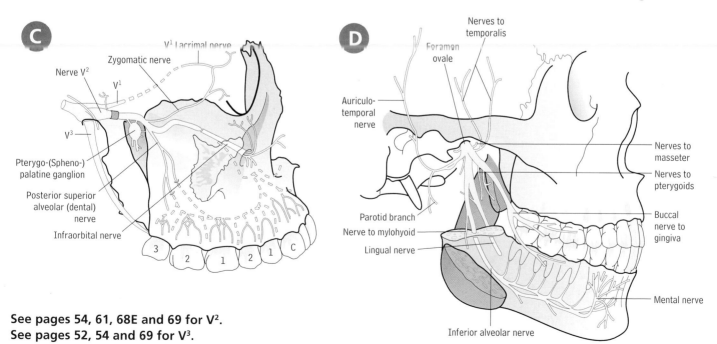

V¹ Lacrimal nerve
Zygomatic nerve
Nerve V²
V¹
V³
Pterygo-(Spheno-) palatine ganglion
Posterior superior alveolar (dental) nerve
Infraorbital nerve
3 2 1 2 1 C

See pages 54, 61, 68E and 69 for V².
See pages 52, 54 and 69 for V³.

Ⓓ V³ mandibular division of trigeminal

Nerves to temporalis
Foramen ovale
Auriculo-temporal nerve
Nerves to masseter
Nerves to pterygoids
Buccal nerve to gingiva
Parotid branch
Nerve to mylohyoid
Lingual nerve
Mental nerve
Inferior alveolar nerve

Cranial nerve *VII – facial*

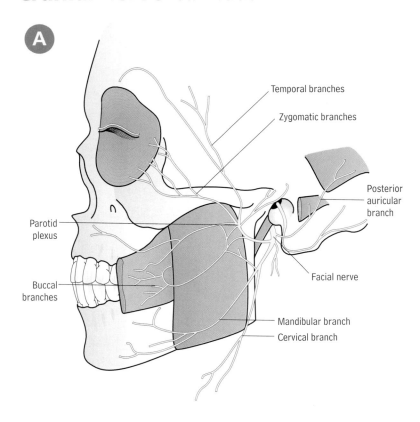

See pages 49, 50, 63, 70 and 71.

Cranial nerve *VIII – vestibulocochlear*

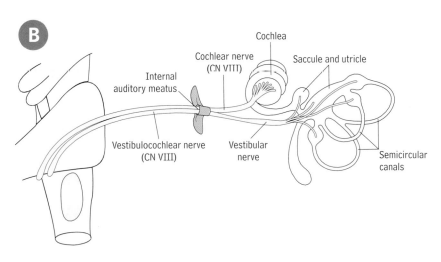

See pages 63, 70, 71 and 75.

 Bell's palsy, hyperacusis, otalgia, see pp 89, 90.

Cranial nerve Ⓐ IX – glossopharyngeal Ⓑ X – vagus

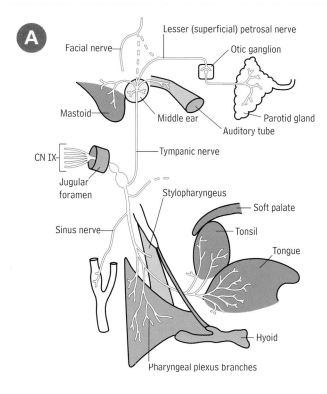

See pages 63, 75, 77 and 79.

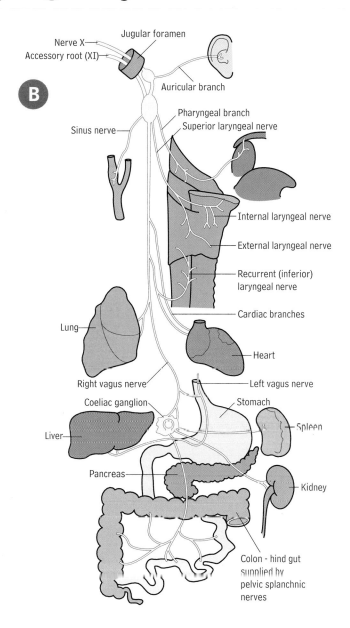

See pages 45, 46, 55 and 77–79.

Parotid tumours, recurrent laryngeal nerve damage, vagus nerve injuries, see p. 91, 92.

Cranial nerve Ⓐ *XI – accessory* Ⓑ *XII – hypoglossal*

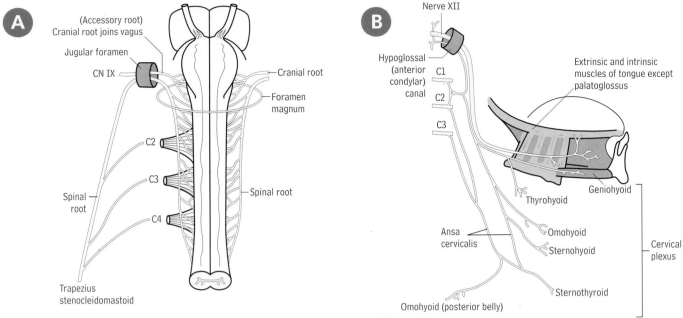

A

- (Accessory root) Cranial root joins vagus
- Jugular foramen
- CN IX
- Cranial root
- Foramen magnum
- C2
- C3
- C4
- Spinal root
- Spinal root
- Trapezius stenocleidomastoid

See page 79.

B

- Nerve XII
- Hypoglossal (anterior condylar) canal
- C1
- C2
- C3
- Extrinsic and intrinsic muscles of tongue except palatoglossus
- Geniohyoid
- Thyrohyoid
- Ansa cervicalis
- Omohyoid
- Sternohyoid
- Sternothyroid
- Cervical plexus
- Omohyoid (posterior belly)

See pages 40, 53 and 63.

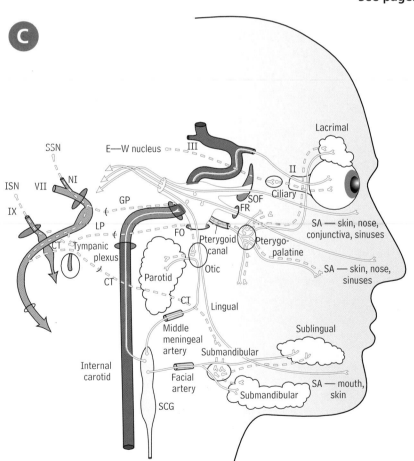

C

Lacrimal, SSN, E–W nucleus, III, ISN, VII, NI, II, Ciliary, GP, SOF, FR, LP, FO, Pterygoid canal, Pterygo-palatine, SA — skin, nose, conjunctiva, sinuses, Tympanic plexus, Otic, CT, Parotid, SA — skin, nose, sinuses, CT, Lingual, Middle meningeal artery, Sublingual, Internal carotid, Submandibular, Facial artery, Submandibular, SA — mouth, skin, SCG

Ⓒ Cranial autonomics

CT — chorda tympani
E–W — Edinger–Westphal
FO — foramen ovale
FR — foramen rotundum
GP — greater petrosal
ISN — inferior salivatory nucleus
LP — lesser petrosal
NI — nervus intermedius
SA — somatic afferent
SCG — superior cervical ganglion
SOF — superior orbital fissure
SSN — superior salivatory nucleus

 Accessory nerve paralysis, gag reflex, hypoglossal nerve paralysis, see pp 89, 90.

Head, neck and brain
Clinical notes

Abducent nerve paralysis. The abducent nerve innervates only the lateral rectus muscle of the eye, and damage results in an inability to move the eye laterally in the horizontal plane. This symptom may be an indication of increased intracranial pressure, owing to the long intracranial course of the sixth nerve. (pages 66 and 84)

Accessory nerve paralysis. Lesions of the cranial branch of this nerve are rare but associated with vagus nerve problems and may be related to bulbar palsy. This is because all accessory nerve motor fibres are transferred to the vagus as it exits the skull. The spinal portion is more commonly damaged in the mid-portion of the posterior triangle of the neck from stab wounds, or from spread of malignancy along the accessory lymph node chain. This injury can cause paralysis of the sternocleidomastoid and trapezius muscles, with weakness in shoulder raising and a permanent droop on that side and also difficulty in turning the head towards the opposite side. (pages 41 and 88)

Accommodation reflex is contraction of the pupil when trying to focus on a near object and is controlled by the parasympathetic nerve fibres carried in the third cranial nerve from the Edinger–Westphal nucleus of the midbrain (synapse in ciliary ganglion) which act on the sphincter pupillae muscle to cause reduction in pupil diameter and on the ciliary muscle to cause relaxation of the suspensory ligament, allowing the lens to adopt a more spherical shape for near focusing. (page 84)

Adenoid (pharyngeal tonsil) enlargement. The adenoids, properly known as the nasopharyngeal tonsils, lie on the posterior nasopharyngeal wall near the openings of the auditory tubes. If repeatedly swollen they may cause prolonged otitis media and need to be removed to allow drainage of the middle ear by the auditory tube. (page 82)

Anosmia is loss of smell commonly following forehead trauma, fracture of the cribriform plate of the ethmoid bone and resultant damage to the olfactory nerves. (pages 21 and 83)

Bell's palsy is a facial nerve palsy of unknown aetiology first described by Sir Charles Bell. The site of this lower motor neurone lesion may be diagnosed precisely by careful evaluation as to whether the stapedius, petrosal nerves and chorda tympani are involved. (pages 49 and 86)

'Blow-out' fractures of orbit are usually produced by direct trauma to the eye. The eye itself is rarely ruptured but the thin orbital floor is often fractured and the eye and its surrounding fat are pushed into the roof of the maxillary sinus. This may be a cause of double vision (diplopia). (page 26)

Burr holes through the skull have been performed for many years (trephination), originally 'to let out the evil spirits', and are now used by neurosurgeons to release intracranial pressure. (page 17)

Carotid artery bruits. Extra and abnormal sounds heard through the stethoscope just lateral to the larynx are often the result of turbulent arterial blood flow due to stenosis of the carotid artery. Early detection of narrowing of this essential artery is often accomplished by colour Doppler ultrasound. (page 43)

Carotid endarterectomy is the removal of atherosclerotic plaque from the narrowed lumen of common and internal carotid arteries. (page 45)

Cavernous sinus thrombosis. Owing to the great number of structures passing through or in the lateral wall of the cavernous sinus, a blockage or infection in this region has serious consequences which may include damage to the third, fourth, fifth and sixth cranial nerves. Infections around the face and forehead may travel into the cavernous sinus, via the ophthlamic viens. (page 61)

Central retinal artery occlusion is caused by a small thrombus or embolus within this branch of the ophthalmic artery. Blindness ensues unless there is immediate treatment. (page 64)

Cerebrospinal fluid rhinorrhea. CSF dripping from the nose is most probably due to a traumatic tear of the olfactory nerve fibres as they pass through the cribriform plate of the ethmoid bone. A fracture of the ethmoid is most common in traffic accidents. To test whether the 'runny nose' is a cold or CSF, a simple dipstick will reveal a high glucose content in CSF. A late complication may be anosmia. (page 67)

Cervical lymph node enlargement. Any infection in the head and neck can cause lymph node enlargement, the most common site being the jugulodigastric nodes located just below the angle of the jaw. (page 43)

Cervical sympathectomy is performed through either the neck or the axilla to sever the sympathetic nerves to the upper limb. A common reason is to prevent gangrene of the fingertips in Raynaud's disease. (page 46)

Corneal reflex is closure of the eyelid after stimulation of the thin anterior transparent membrane of the eye and is controlled by two cranial nerves: the sensory component is via the ophthalmic division of the trigeminal nerve and the motor component (closing of the eye) by the facial. (page 64)

Epistaxis. Nose bleeds are most commonly found on the anteromedial septum (Little's area), a site of rich anastomoses (Kiesselbach) from external and internal carotid branches (facial, palatine and ophthalmic). (page 67)

Extradural haemorrhage in the skull is usually due to trauma at the pterion on the same or opposite side of the cranium, which causes tearing of the middle meningeal artery or of one of its divisions. (pages 14 and 27)

Gag reflex. Stimulation of the posterior third of the tongue or posterior oropharynx sends afferent stimuli via the glossopharyngeal (ninth cranial) nerve. The efferent pathway involves the vagus (tenth cranial) and accessory (eleventh cranial) nerves, causing elevation of the soft palate and contraction of the pharyngeal muscles. Putting a spatula against the back of the mouth will normally elicit this reflex and thus test three different cranial nerves. (pages 55 and 88)

Goitre is a non-specific enlargement of the thyroid gland, making it easily palpable and often visible. There are numerous causes but world-wide the most common is a dietary deficiency of iodine. A very large goitre may cause compression of lower cervical and superior mediastinal structures including the trachea, making breathing difficult. (page 41)

Hydrocephalus. This condition of cranial enlargement is due to increased CSF pressure which produces dilatation of the cerebral ventricles. Typically, there is enlargement of the skull, prominence of the forehead and deterioration in mental capacity due to brain atrophy. (page 25)

Hyperacusis is a very acute sense of hearing (lowered threshold), most commonly caused by damage to the stapedius muscle (seventh cranial nerve) or the tensor tympani muscle (fifth cranial nerve). Occasionally this is a symptom associated with Bell's palsy. (pages 70 and 86)

Hypoglossal nerve paralysis. Because all intrinsic and most extrinsic muscles of the tongue are supplied by the twelfth cranial nerve, its paralysis causes atrophy of the ipsilateral half of the tongue. On protrusion the tip of the tongue deviates towards the paralysed, injured side, owing to the unapposed action of the genioglossus muscle of the other side. (pages 69 and 88)

Inferior alveolar nerve block is a common dental procedure that anaesthetizes this nerve as it enters the mandibular foramen on the medial side of the ramus of the mandible. Using an intra-oral approach the anaesthetic is deposited near the lingula, producing anaesthesia of the ipsilateral mandibular dentition, lip and cheek. (page 53)

Internal jugular vein catheterization is often performed by anaesthetists on unconscious patients, and has two common routes: the first is directly through the sternocleidomastoid muscle halfway down the neck; the second is through the gap between the two heads of the sternocleidomastoid muscle, deep to which lies the termination of the internal jugular vein. The needle is passed at 45° to the skin in the direction of the ipsilateral nipple. It provides emergency intravenous access for example during cardiac arrest. (page 47)

Intracranial spread of infections: face. Ophthalmic veins connect the cavernous sinus to facial veins. These valveless connections mean that superficial facial infections can easily become serious intracranial ones. (page 49)

Intracranial spread of infections: scalp. Emissary veins traverse the skull, connecting scalp veins and intracranial sinuses. Foramina for the largest of these veins can be found in the occipital bone and near the mastoid process. (page 19)

Mastoiditis, infection of the mastoid air cells, is rarely seen now since the common use of antibiotics. However, once the mastoid air cells are infected it is difficult to eradicate the condition and there is always the risk of spread internally towards the sigmoid sinus. (page 26)

Middle ear pressure equalization. The auditory tube is normally closed and opens to atmospheric pressure momentarily during swallowing, allowing equilibration of pressures between the middle ear and the atmosphere. Changes in external pressures (in an aeroplane or when diving) require pressure equilibration to avoid the severe pain of a stretched tympanic membrane. (page 68)

Mumps is an acute infection of the parotid and submandibular salivary glands. It is extremely painful and both opening the mouth and chewing may be restricted. (page 44)

Nasogastric intubation involves passing a small plastic tube via the nose and nasopharynx into the stomach and may be used to obtain gastric secretions for analysis or to remove an accumulation of gastric secretions when the bowel is obstructed. (page 68)

Oculomotor nerve paralysis. If complete, this condition affects most eye muscles and especially the levator palpebrae superioris and the sphincter pupillae. Consequently, the upper eyelid droops (ptosis), there is a fully dilated non-reactive pupil, and the eyeball tends to be looking downwards and outwards owing to the unopposed action of the lateral rectus and superior oblique muscles. (pages 66 and 84)

Ophthalmic herpes zoster, also known as shingles, is a cutaneous viral eruption that maps out the distribution of the ophthalmic division of the trigeminal nerve (scalp, forehead, upper eyelid, nose and possibly as far down as the philtrum). Involvement of the corneal membrane is an indication for immediate antiviral treatment. (page 48)

Ophthalmoscopy is examination of the eye using an ophthalmoscope to visualize internal structures. The major structures seen include the pale optic disc, the macula, the radiating retinal vessels and the fovea centralis – the pale depression in the centre of the macula for acute vision. Pathological findings include abnormalities of the optic disc such as papilloedema, or rupture of vessels caused by small aneurysms; in diabetes, exudates may be seen on the retina. High blood pressure may also be diagnosed by observing the state of the retinal vessels. (pages 64 and 83)

Otalgia (referred pain). Pain from the ear itself is a common complaint but referred otalgia can be a diagnostic nightmare. Any structure that has the same nerve supply as the pinna or middle ear may have its pain referred to the ear. These include numerous branches of C2, C3 of the cervical plexus, and the fifth, seventh, ninth and tenth cranial nerves. Conditions that can cause this complaint include myocardial infarction, oesophagitis, tonsillitis, arthritis of the cervical spine, malocclusion, dental caries, sinusitis and carcinoma of the larynx or pharynx. A painful ear with a normal ear examination is therefore an anatomical challenge. (page 70)

Parotid tumours may involve the retromandibular vein or the superficial temporal artery which lie within its substance, but the most common effect is involvement of the facial nerve as its numerous branches pass from deep to superficial through this gland. A facial paralysis associated with a swelling in the parotid gland is a condition to be taken seriously. The pain of a tumour here may often be referred to the temporomandibular joint via the auriculotemporal nerve which carries the parotid's secretomotor fibres. (pages 44 and 87)

Parotidectomy (surgical removal of the parotid gland) requires tedious dissection to minimize damage to branches of the facial nerve. The use of a facial nerve stimulator (a special pair of forceps conducting a low voltage) helps the surgeon avoid these branches. The deep portion of the gland abuts the pharyngeal wall. (page 44)

Philtrum, this is the small flat area bounded by two vertical ridges below the nose where the two maxillary processes meet the frontonasal process in the developing face. It is along the ridges of the philtrum that the common congenital abnormality of harelip occurs. (page 48)

Pituitary tumour. Presenting with endocrine derangements, a tumour in the pituitary fossa (sella turcica) may affect the optic chiasma, causing bitemporal hemianopia. Surgical access to the sella via the sphenoidal sinus does not leave a visible facial scar. An advanced tumour may be seen on a lateral skull X-ray as enlargement and erosion of the fossa. (page 27)

Pupillary reflex is constriction of the pupil on exposure of the retina to bright light. The sensory pathway is via the second cranial nerve; the motor pathway is from the parasympathetic fibres of the third cranial nerve that originate in the Edinger-Westphal nucleus. Other stimuli may also alter the size of the pupil; for example, emotional stimulation, fear and excitement cause dilatation of the pupil via the sympathetic fibres. (page 64)

Recurrent laryngeal nerve damage. A complication of thyroid surgery, this condition causes paralysis of the vocal cords. When the paralysis is bilateral the voice is almost absent as the two vocal folds cannot be adducted. A unilateral recurrent laryngeal nerve injury may not be detected in normal speech. (pages 59 and 87)

Scalp wounds. Cuts in the scalp tend to bleed profusely owing to its numerous anastomoses of branches of the internal and external carotid arteries. The fibrous arrangement of the connective tissue in the scalp tends to keep arteries open when cut. However, the rich blood supply also means that scalp wounds heal rapidly. (page 25)

Sialolithiasis. Formation of salivary calculi or stones depends on the composition of the fluid being secreted by each salivary gland. Most commonly found in the submandibular gland and rarely in the parotid, these small calcium stones may completely block the duct system and cause a painful swelling of the gland. Surgical removal is usually via the floor of the mouth. (page 41)

Subarachnoid haemorrhage. Because the subarachnoid space contains the CSF, this condition may be diagnosed at lumbar puncture. It can be due to rupture of a congenital ('berry') aneurysm, often in the region of the arterial 'Circle of Willis'. (page 72)

Subclavian vein catheterization takes advantage of the vascular relations on the superior aspect of the first rib to place a central venous line, normally by an infraclavicular route. The tip of the needle should be pointed as anteriorly as possible towards the jugular notch to avoid injury to posterior structures (apex of the lung, subclavian artery and the brachial plexus). A supraclavicular approach puts the needle into the origin of the brachiocephalic vein. (page 47)

Subdural haemorrhages, being of venous origin, develop slowly following trauma but can have consequences as serious as those of extradural (arterial) haemorrhages. (page 63)

Surgical flaps of the scalp. Plastic surgeons have devised numerous flaps based upon different vascular pedicles within the scalp. All depend on the rich blood supply of the scalp, which contains numerous anastomoses between internal and external carotid branches. Approximately 10–12 named arteries supply the scalp periphery, so that any one single artery will often be enough to give nourishment for recovery from scalp injuries and flap construction. (page 49)

Temporomandibular joint (TMJ) reduction. Following dislocation of the TMJ, the mandibular condyle rests anterior to the articular tubercle of the temporal bone and the resultant spasm in the masticatory muscles is painful. Reduction of the condyle into the mandibular fossa requires inferior and posterior movements, accomplished by firmly grasping the mandibular body, and can be aided by local anaesthesia or muscle relaxants. (page 16)

Tonsillitis. This common condition results from infection of the palatine tonsils (which lie between the palatoglossal and palatopharyngeal folds). The inflamed cherry-like tonsil may be packed with pus, particularly in the crypts of this lymphoid mass, or even develop into an abscess (quinsy). Pain from this condition is often referred to the ear via the glossopharyngeal nerve which lies in the tonsillar bed (the ninth cranial nerve also supplies sensation to the middle ear). Swallowing is also made difficult. Haemorrhage after surgical removal may be severe from the tonsillar branch of the facial artery or from the external palatine vein. (page 67)

Torticollis is an abnormal sustained contraction of the neck musculature causing the head to be pulled to one side. It is commonly seen after a difficult forceps delivery, when the infant may develop a cervical swelling – usually a haematoma of the sternocleidomastoid. (page 39)

Tracheostomy is an opening (stoma) into the trachea often used for patients who cannot breathe on their own. Anatomically, it involves splitting the strap muscles i.e. sternohyoid, passing through the deep cervical fascia and removing or clamping the isthmus of the thyroid gland. A low tracheostomy below the isthmus may endanger an unusually high left brachiocephalic vein (especially in children) or the rare thyroidea ima artery. A safer emergency procedure is to pass a needle or tube through the cricothyroid membrane, just above the cricoid cartilage. (page 40)

Trochlear nerve paralysis. This rare condition affects only the superior oblique muscle of the eye and commonly presents as a squint or with the patient complaining of diplopia on looking downwards or at the end of the nose. (page 66 and 84)

Vagus nerve injuries are most commonly seen associated with surgery in the region of the carotid sheath. The resultant injury may cause a speech problem (recurrent laryngeal branch) or gastrointestinal disturbances. (page 87)

Vertebral column and spinal cord

3

Back and vertebral column
A *surface anatomy* **B** *axial skeleton* **C** *vertebral column*

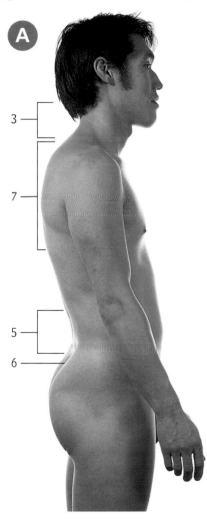

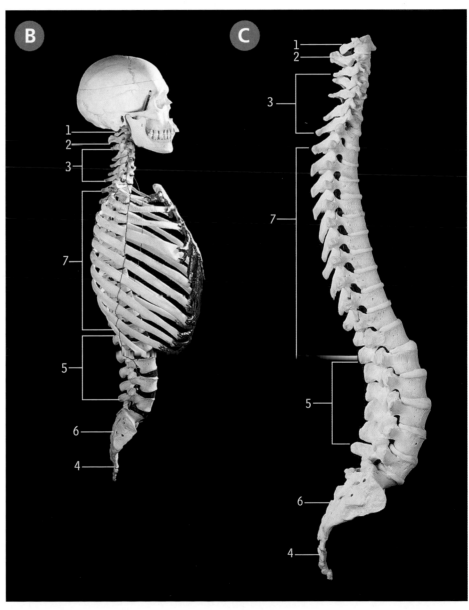

1 Atlas vertebra
2 Axis vertebra
3 Cervical vertebrae, lordosis
4 Coccyx
5 Lumbar vertebrae, lordosis
6 Sacrum
7 Thoracic vertebrae, kyphosis

Back and shoulder

A *surface anatomy* **B** *muscles*

1 Coccyx	**7** Medial border scapula (dotted)
2 Deltoid	**8** Rhomboid major
3 External oblique	**9** Rhomboid minor
4 Gluteus maximus	**10** Sacrum
5 Iliac crest	**11** Trapezius
6 Latissimus dorsi	**12** Thoracolumbar fascia

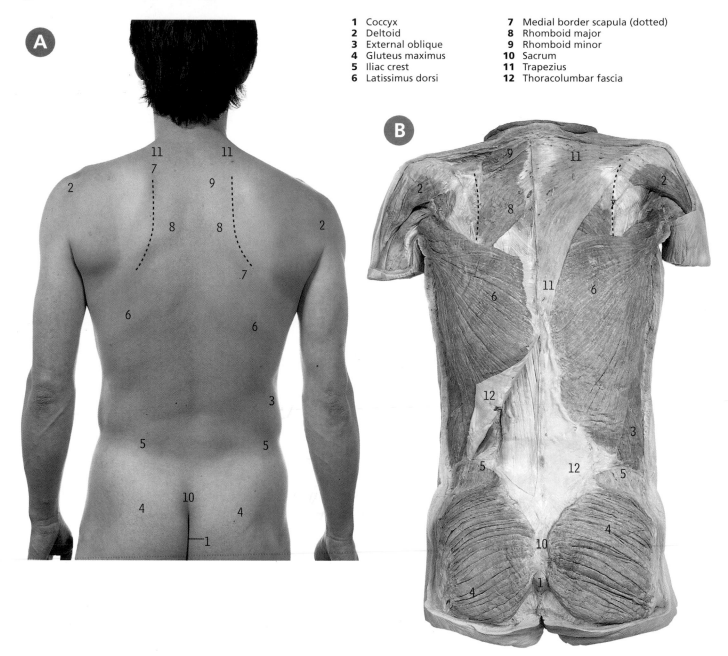

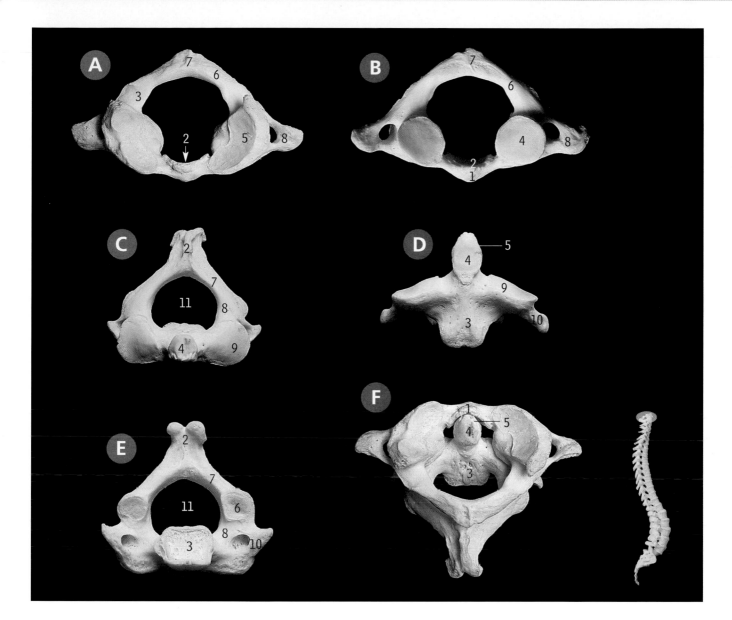

First cervical vertebra *atlas*

A from above

B from below

1 Anterior arch and tubercle	**5** Lateral mass with superior
2 Facet for dens of axis	articular facet
3 Groove for vertebral artery	**6** Posterior arch
4 Lateral mass with inferior	**7** Posterior tubercle
articular facet	**8** Transverse process and foramen

The superior articular facets (5) are concave and kidney-shaped.

The inferior articular facets (4) are circular and almost flat.

The anterior arch (1) is straighter and shorter than the posterior arch (6) and contains on its posterior surface the facet for the dens of the axis (2).

The atlas is the only vertebra that has no body.

Second cervical vertebra *axis*

C from above

D from the front

E from below

F articulated with the atlas, from above

1 Anterior arch of atlas	**7** Lamina
2 Bifid spinous process	**8** Pedicle
3 Body	**9** Superior articular surface
4 Dens	**10** Transverse process and
5 Impression for alar ligament	foramen
6 Inferior articular facet	**11** Vertebral foramen

The axis is unique in having the dens (4) which projects upwards from the body, representing the body of the atlas.

Fifth cervical vertebra

a typical cervical vertebra

A from above

B from the front

C from the left

1 Anterior tubercle of transverse process
2 Bifid spinous process
3 Body
4 Foramen of transverse process
5 Inferior articular process
6 Intertubercular lamella of transverse process
7 Lamina
8 Pedicle
9 Posterior tubercle of transverse process
10 Posterolateral lip (uncus)
11 Superior articular process
12 Vertebral foramen

Seventh cervical vertebra

vertebra prominens

D from above

1 Anterior tubercle of transverse process
2 Body
3 Foramen of transverse process
4 Intertubercular lamella of transverse process
5 Lamina
6 Pedicle
7 Posterior tubercle of transverse process
8 Posterolateral lip (uncus)
9 Spinous process with tubercle
10 Superior articular process
11 Vertebral foramen

All cervical vertebrae (first to seventh) have a foramen in each transverse process (as A4).

Typical cervical vertebrae (third to sixth) have superior articular processes that face backwards and upwards (A11, C11), posterolateral lips on the upper surface of the body (A10), a triangular vertebral foramen (A12) and a bifid spinous process (A2).

The anterior tubercle of the transverse process of the sixth cervical vertebra is large and known as the carotid tubercle.

The seventh cervical vertebra (vertebra prominens) has a spinous process that ends in a single tubercle (D9).

The rib element of a cervical vertebra is represented by the anterior root of the transverse process, the anterior tubercle, the intertubercular lamella (with its groove for the ventral ramus of a spinal nerve) and the anterior part of the posterior tubercle (as at D1, 4 and 7).

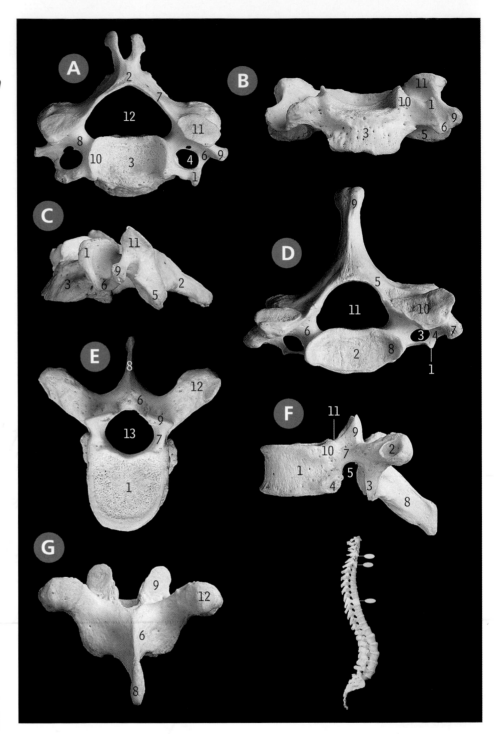

Seventh thoracic vertebra

typical

E from above

F from the left

G from behind

1 Body
2 Costal facet of transverse process
3 Inferior articular process
4 Inferior costal facet
5 Inferior vertebral notch
6 Lamina
7 Pedicle
8 Spinous process
9 Superior articular process
10 Superior costal facet
11 Superior vertebral notch
12 Transverse process
13 Vertebral foramen

Typical thoracic vertebrae (second to ninth) are characterized by costal facets on the bodies (F10, 4), costal facets on the transverse processes (F2), a round vertebral foramen (E13), a spinous process that points downwards as well as backwards (F8, G8) and superior articular processes that are vertical, flat and face backwards and laterally (E9, F9, G9).

First thoracic vertebra

A from above

B from the front and the left

1 Body
2 Inferior articular process
3 Inferior costal facet
4 Lamina
5 Pedicle
6 Posterolateral lip (uncus)
7 Spinous process
8 Superior articular process
9 Superior costal facet
10 Transverse process with costal facet
11 Vertebral foramen

Tenth and eleventh thoracic vertebra

C tenth thoracic vertebra, from the left

D eleventh thoracic vertebra, from the left

1 Body
2 Costal facet
3 Inferior articular process
4 Inferior vertebral notch
5 Pedicle
6 Spinous process
7 Superior articular process
8 Transverse process

Twelfth thoracic vertebra

E from the left

F from above

G from behind

1 Body
2 Costal facet
3 Inferior articular process
4 Inferior tubercle
5 Lateral tubercle
6 Pedicle
7 Spinous process
8 Superior articular process
9 Superior tubercle

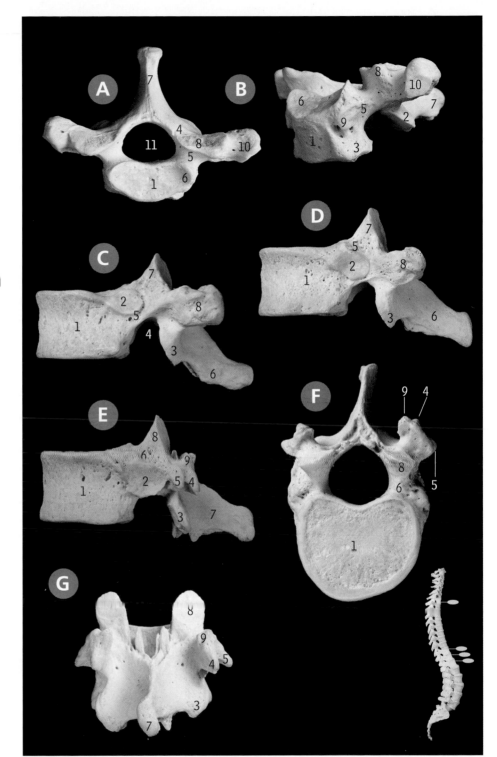

The atypical thoracic vertebrae are the first, tenth, eleventh and twelfth.

The first thoracic vertebra has a posterolateral lip (A6, B6) on each side of the upper surface of the body and a triangular vertebral foramen (features like typical cervical vertebrae), and complete (round) superior costal facets (B9) on the sides of the body.

The tenth, eleventh and twelfth thoracic vertebrae are characterized by a single complete costal facet on each side of the body that in successive vertebrae comes to lie increasingly far from the upper surface of the body and encroaches increasingly onto the pedicle (C2, D2 and E2). There is also no articular facet on the transverse process.

Spondylolisthesis, see p. 115.

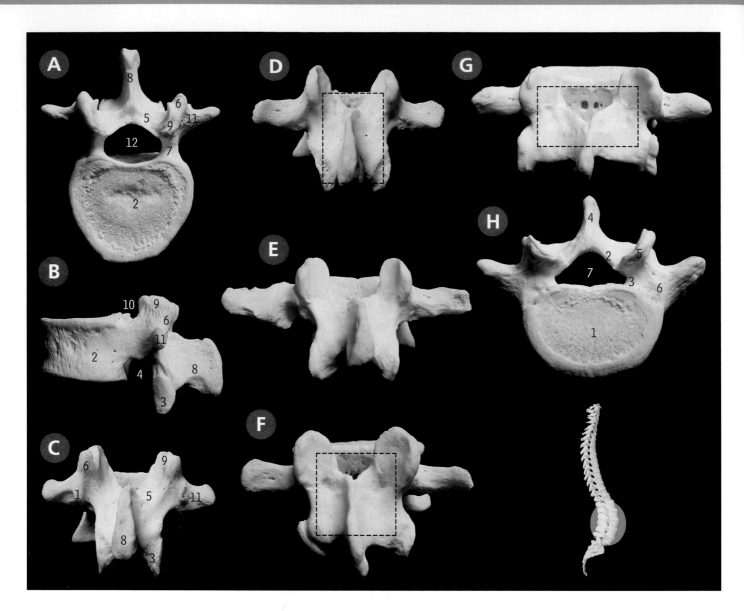

First lumbar vertebra

A from above

B from the left

C from behind

1 Accessory process
2 Body
3 Inferior articular process
4 Inferior vertebral notch
5 Lamina
6 Mamillary process
7 Pedicle
8 Spinous process
9 Superior articular process
10 Superior vertebral notch
11 Transverse process
12 Vertebral foramen

Lumbar vertebrae are characterized by the large size of the bodies, the absence of costal facets on the bodies and the transverse processes, a triangular vertebral foramen (A12), a spinous process that points backwards and is quadrangular or hatchet-shaped (B8) and superior articular processes that are vertical, curved, face backwards and medially (A9) and possess a mamillary process at their posterior rim (A6).

The rib element of a lumbar vertebra is represented by the transverse process (A11).

The level at which facet joint orientation changes between the thoracic and lumbar regions is variable.

Posterior view:

D second lumbar vertebra

E third lumbar vertebra

F fourth lumbar vertebra

G fifth lumbar vertebra

View from above:

H fifth lumbar vertebra

1 Body
2 Lamina
3 Pedicle
4 Spinous process
5 Superior articular process
6 Transverse process fusing with pedicle and body
7 Vertebral foramen

Viewed from behind, the four articular processes of the first and second lumbar vertebrae make a pattern (indicated by the interrupted line) of a vertical rectangle; those of the third or fourth vertebra make a square, and those of the fifth lumbar vertebra make a horizontal rectangle.

The fifth lumbar vertebra is unique in that the transverse process (H6) unites directly with the side of the body (H1) as well as with the pedicle (H3).

Laminectomy, see p. 115.

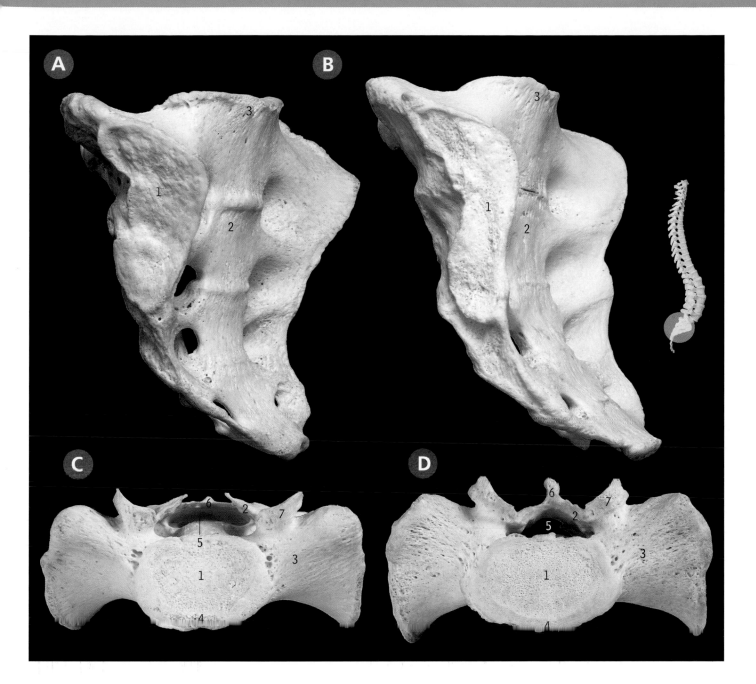

Sacrum *from the front and the right*

A in the female **B** in the male

1 Auricular surface 2 Pelvic surface 3 Promantory

In the female the pelvic surface is relatively straight over the first three sacral vertebrae and becomes more curved below. In the male the pelvic surface is more uniformly curved.

The capsule of the sacro-iliac joint is attached to the margin of the auricular (articular) surface (A1, B1).

Base of the sacrum *upper surface*

C in the female **D** in the male

1 Body of first sacral vertebra
2 Lamina
3 Lateral part (ala)
4 Promontory
5 Sacral canal
6 Spinous tubercle of median sacral crest
7 Superior articular process

In the male the body of the first sacral vertebra (judged by its transverse diameter) forms a greater part of the base of the sacrum than in the female (compare D1 with C1).

In C there is some degree of spina bifida (non-fusion of the laminae, 2, in the vertebral arch of the first sacral vertebra). Compare with the complete arch in D.

Sacrum and coccyx

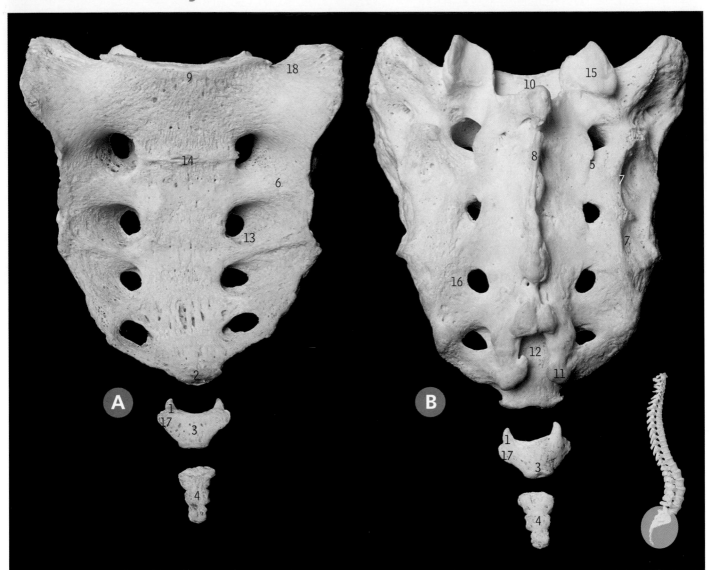

A pelvic surface

1 Coccygeal cornu
2 Facet for coccyx
3 First coccygeal vertebra
4 Fused second to fourth vertebrae
5 Intermediate sacral crest
6 Lateral part
7 Lateral sacral crest
8 Median sacral crest
9 Promontory
10 Sacral canal

B dorsal surface

11 Sacral cornu
12 Sacral hiatus
13 Second pelvic sacral foramen
14 Site of fusion of first and second sacral vertebrae
15 Superior articular process
16 Third dorsal sacral foramen
17 Transverse process
18 Upper surface of lateral part (ala)

The sacrum is formed by the fusion of the five sacral vertebrae. The median sacral crest (B8) represents the fused spinous processes, the intermediate crest (B5) the fused articular processes, and the lateral crest (B7) the fused transverse processes.

The sacral hiatus (B12) is the lower opening of the sacral canal (B10).

The coccyx is usually formed by the fusion of four rudimentary vertebrae but the number varies from three to five. In this specimen the first piece of the coccyx (3) is not fused with the remainder (4).

Coccydynia, see p. 115.

Sacrum *with sacralization of the fifth lumbar vertebra*

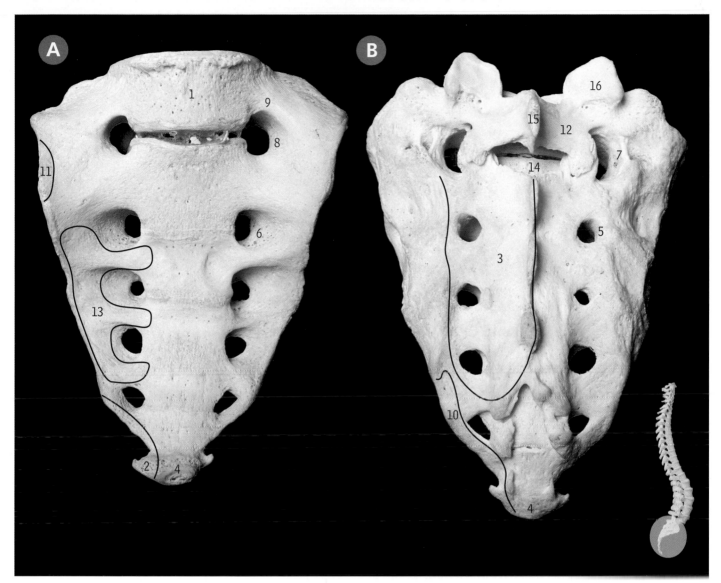

A pelvic surface

B dorsal surface, and sacral muscle attachments

1 Body of fifth lumbar vertebra
2 Coccygeus
3 Erector spinae
4 First coccygeal vertebra fused to apex of sacrum
5 First dorsal sacral foramen
6 First pelvic sacral foramen
7 Foramen for dorsal ramus of fifth lumbar nerve
8 Foramen for ventral ramus of fifth lumbar nerve

9 Fusion of transverse process and lateral part of sacrum
10 Gluteus maximus
11 Iliacus
12 Lamina
13 Piriformis
14 Sacral canal
15 Spinous process of fifth lumbar vertebra
16 Superior articular process of fifth lumbar vertebra

In sacralization of the fifth lumbar vertebra, that vertebra (A1) is (usually incompletely) fused with the sacrum. In the more rare condition of lumbarization of the first sacral vertebra (not illustrated) the first piece of the sacrum is incompletely fused with the remainder.

In this specimen, as well as fusion of the fifth lumbar vertebra with the top of the sacrum, the body of the first coccygeal vertebra (4) is fused with the apex of the sacrum.

Caudal anaesthesia, see p. 115.

Bony pelvis *from in front and above*

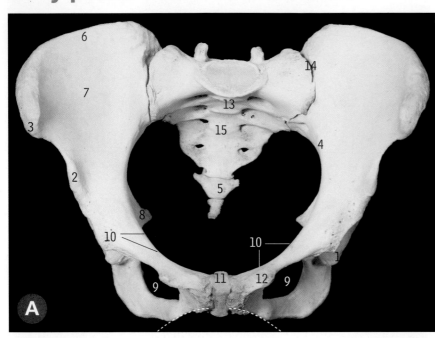

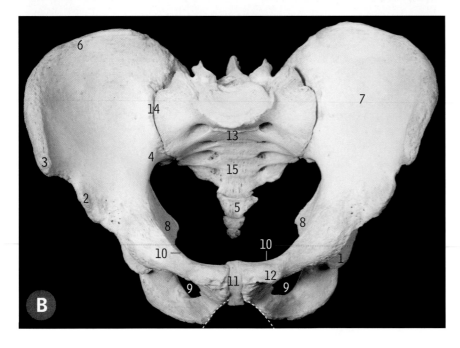

A female

B male

1 Acetabulum
2 Anterior inferior iliac spine
3 Anterior superior iliac spine
4 Arcuate line
5 Coccyx
6 Iliac crest
7 Iliac fossa
8 Ischial spine
9 Obturator foramen
10 Pectineal line
11 Pubic symphysis
12 Pubic tubercle
13 Sacral promontory
14 Sacro-iliac joint
15 Sacrum

The pelvic inlet (brim) is bounded by the sacral promontory, arcuate and pectineal lines, the crest of the pubic bones and anteriorly the pubic symphysis.

The female brim is more circular, the male more heart-shaped.

The female sacrum is wider, shorter and less curved.

The female ischial spines are further apart.

The female subpubic angle (white dotted line on A) is wide (90–120°) and the male subpubic angle (white dotted line on B) only 60–90°.

Vertebrae, ribs and sternum
ossification

Ⓐ typical vertebra in a six-month fetus

Ⓕ axis, primary and secondary centres

Ⓑ at four years

Ⓖ typical rib, secondary centres

Ⓒ Ⓓ during puberty

Ⓔ atlas at four years

Ⓗ sternum at birth, with primary centres

A typical vertebra, which is first cartilaginous, ossifies in early fetal life from three primary centres – one for most of the body (the centrum, A2) and one for each half of the neural arch (A1). The part of the adult body to which the pedicle is attached (B4) is part of the centre for the arch; the site in the developing vertebra where they meet is the neurocentral junction (B5). The two halves of the arch and the neurocentral junctions unite at variable times between birth and six years. Ossification spreads into the transverse processes and spine which grow out from the arch, but secondary centres (B3) appear at their tips during puberty and become fused at about twenty-five years. (Lumbar vertebrae have similar additional secondary centres for the mamillary processes.) There are also ring-like epiphyses on the periphery of the upper and lower surfaces of the vertebral bodies (C6 and D6).

The atlas has a primary centre (E7) for each lateral mass and the adjacent half of the posterior arch, and one for the anterior arch (E8). Fusion is complete by about eight years.

The axis has five primary centres – one for most of the body (F10), one for each lateral mass (F9), and one for each half of the dens and adjacent part of the body (F8). They should all fuse by about three years. There are secondary centres for the tip of the dens (F12, appearing by about two years and fusing at twelve) and the lower surface of the body (F11, appearing during puberty and fusing at about twenty-five years).

The sacrum, representing five fused sacral vertebrae, has many ossification centres, corresponding to the centrum, neural arch halves and costal elements of each vertebra, as well as ring epiphyses for the vertebral bodies and for the auricular surfaces. Most have fused by about twenty years, but some not until middle age or later.

A typical rib has a primary centre for the body with secondary centres for the head (G13) and the articular and non-articular parts of the tubercle (G14 and 15), appearing during puberty and uniting at about twenty years.

The sternum has a variable number of primary centres (H16), one or two in the manubrium and in each of the four pieces of the body. Fusion occurs between puberty and twenty-five years. 'Bullet holes' in the sternum (sternal foramina) may occur when fusion is incomplete.

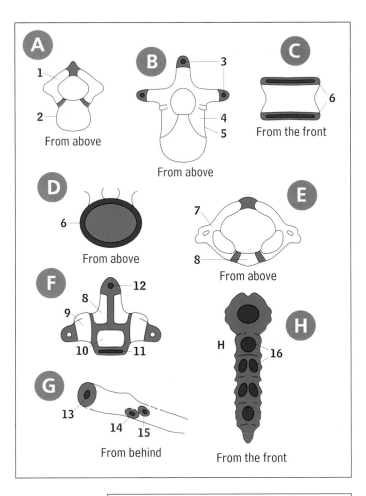

From above

From the front

From above

From above

From above

From behind   From the front

Ⓘ Vertebrae *developmental origins*

Red: costal elements; green: centrum; yellow: neural arch

Parts of the cervical, lumbar and sacral vertebrae represent the ribs that articulate with thoracic vertebrae. These costal elements are indicated here in red.

Cervical: anterior and posterior tubercles and the intertubercular lamella.

Thoracic: the true rib articulates with the vertebra.

Lumbar: the anterior part of the transverse process.

Sacral: the lateral part, including the auricular surface.

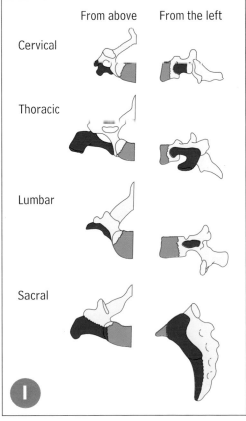

From above   From the left

Cervical

Thoracic

Lumbar

Sacral

Ⓘ

Vertebral column and spinal cord

A *cervical region, from the front*   **B** *cervical region, from behind*

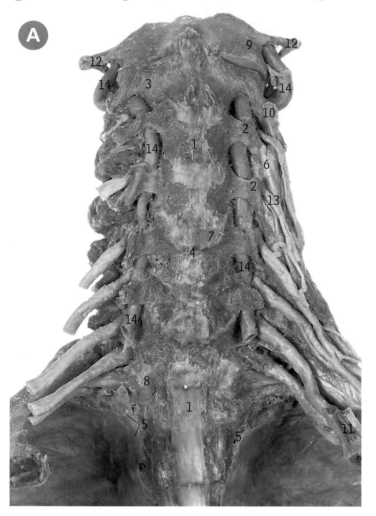

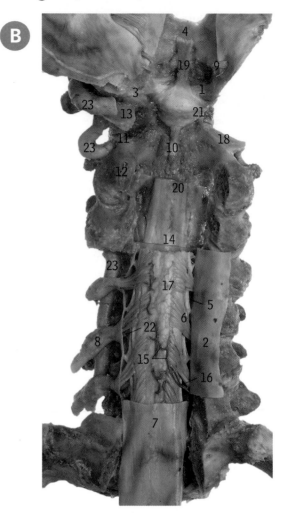

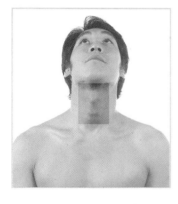

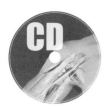

The vertebral artery (14) is seen within foramina of cervical transverse processes.

1   Anterior longitudinal ligament
2   Anterior tubercle of transverse process
3   Axis
4   Body of fifth cervical vertebra
5   Cut edge of the pleura
6   Intertubercular lamella of transverse process
7   Intervertebral disc
8   Joint of head of first rib
9   Lateral mass of atlas
10 Posterior tubercle of transverse process
11 Scalenus anterior muscle
12 Transverse process of atlas
13 Ventral ramus of third cervical nerve
14 Vertebral artery

Much of the skull, the vertebral arches, brainstem and the upper part of the spinal cord have been removed to show the cruciform, transverse and alar ligaments (19, 10, 21 and 1). Lower down, the arachnoid and dura mater (2) have been reflected to show dorsal and ventral nerve roots (as at 6 and 22).

1   Alar ligament
2   Arachnoid and dura mater (reflected)
3   Atlanto-occipital joint
4   Basilar part of occipital bone and position of attachment of tectorial membrane
5   Denticulate ligament
6   Dorsal rootlets of spinal nerve
7   Dura mater
8   Dural sheath over dorsal root ganglion
9   Hypoglossal nerve and canal
10 Inferior longitudinal band of cruciform ligament
11 Lateral atlanto-axial joint

12 Pedicle of axis
13 Posterior arch of atlas
14 Posterior longitudinal ligament
15 Posterior spinal arteries
16 Radicular artery
17 Spinal cord
18 Superior articular surface of axis
19 Superior longitudinal band of cruciform ligament
20 Tectorial membrane
21 Transverse ligament of atlas (transverse part of cruciform ligament)
22 Ventral rootlets of spinal nerve
23 Vertebral artery

Vertebral column and spinal cord

C cervical and upper thoracic regions, from the right

Ventral and dorsal rami of spinal nerves (as at 16 and 4) are seen emerging from intervertebral foramina (as at 7).

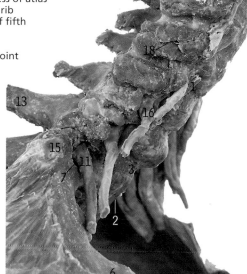

1 Anterior tubercle of transverse process of fifth cervical vertebra	**5** First cervical nerve	**13** Spinous process of seventh cervical vertebra
	6 First rib	**14** Transverse process of atlas
2 Body of first thoracic vertebra	**7** Intervertebral foramen	**15** Tubercle of first rib
	8 Lateral atlanto-axial joint	**16** Ventral ramus of fifth cervical nerve
3 Body of seventh cervical vertebra	**9** Lateral mass of atlas	
	10 Posterior arch of atlas	**17** Vertebral artery
4 Dorsal ramus of first cervical nerve	**11** Seventh cervical nerve	**18** Zygapophyseal joint
	12 Spinous process of second cervical vertebra	

> The first and second spinal nerves pass respectively above and below the posterior arch of the atlas.

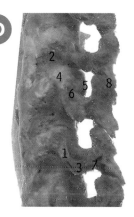

D Cervical region, from the left

Soft tissue has been removed to show the boundaries of intervertebral foramina (as at 5). Compare with the cleared specimens of thoracic vertebrae on page 108, A.

1 Anterior tubercle of transverse process of fifth cervical vertebra
2 Body of third cervical vertebra
3 Intertubercular lamella of transverse process of fifth cervical vertebra
4 Intervertebral disc
5 Intervertebral foramen
6 Pedicle
7 Posterior tubercle of transverse process of fifth cervical vertebra
8 Zygapophyseal joint

> Each intervertebral foramen (as at D5) is bounded in front by a vertebral body and intervertebral disc (D2 and 4), above and below by pedicles (D6), and behind by a zygapophyseal joint (D8).
>
> In the thoracic and lumbar regions there are the same number of pairs of spinal nerves as there are vertebrae (twelve thoracic and five lumbar), and spinal nerves are numbered from the vertebra beneath whose pedicles they emerge. In the cervical region there are seven cervical vertebrae and eight cervical nerves. The first nerve emerges between the occipital bone of the skull and the atlas, and the eighth below the pedicle of the seventh cervical vertebra.

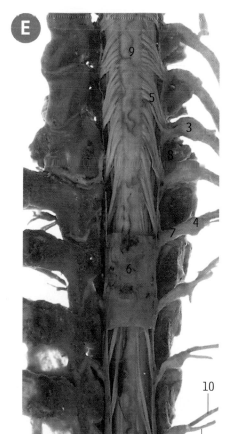

E Lower cervical and upper thoracic regions, from behind

The vertebral arches and most of the dura mater and arachnoid have been removed, to show dorsal nerve rootlets (5) emerging from the spinal cord (9) to unite as a dorsal nerve root and enter the dural sheath (as at 7). Ventral nerve roots do the same from the ventral aspect of the cord but are not seen in this view as they are obscured by the dorsal roots.

1 Angulation of nerve roots entering dural sheath	**6** Dura mater
2 Dorsal ramus of fifth thoracic nerve	**7** Dural sheath of second thoracic nerve
3 Dorsal root ganglion of eighth cervical nerve	**8** Pedicle of first thoracic vertebra
4 Dorsal root ganglion of second thoracic nerve	**9** Spinal cord and posterior spinal vessels
5 Dorsal rootlets of eighth cervical nerve	**10** Ventral ramus of fifth thoracic nerve

Ⓐ Vertebral column and spinal cord
cervical and upper thoracic regions, from the left

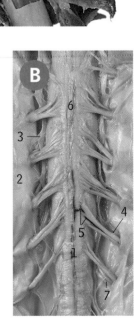

1 Arachnoid mater
2 Body of first thoracic vertebra
3 Denticulate ligament
4 Dorsal ramus of fifth cervical nerve
5 Dorsal root ganglion of eighth cervical nerve
6 Dorsal root ganglion of fifth cervical nerve
7 Dorsal rootlets of fifth cervical nerve
8 Dura mater
9 Foramen magnum
10 Medulla oblongata
11 Occipital bone
12 Posterior arch of atlas
13 Spinal cord
14 Spinal part of accessory nerve
15 Spinous process of axis (abnormally large)
16 Spinous process of seventh cervical vertebra
17 Sympathetic trunk
18 Ventral ramus of fifth cervical nerve
19 Ventral rootlets of fifth cervical nerve

Parts of the vertebral arches and meninges have been removed to show the denticulate ligament (3). Dorsal nerve rootlets lie behind it (as at 7) and ventral nerve rootlets in front of it (as at 19 but largely hidden in this view).

Each spinal nerve is formed by the union of ventral and dorsal nerve roots.

Each nerve root is formed by the union of several rootlets (as at A7).

The union of ventral and dorsal nerve roots to form a spinal nerve occurs immediately distal to the ganglion on the dorsal root (as at A6), within the intervertebral foramen, and the nerve at once divides into a ventral and a dorsal ramus (formerly called ventral and dorsal primary rami) (as at A18 and 4). The spinal nerve proper is thus only a millimetre or two in length, but is often so short that the rami appear to be branches of the ganglion itself.

The lowest cervical and upper thoracic nerve roots become acutely angled in order to enter their dural sheaths.

Ⓑ Spinal cord
cervical region, from the front

For this ventral view of the upper part of the spinal cord (6), the dura and arachnoid mater have been incised longitudinally and turned aside (2) to show the ventral nerve rootlets and roots (as at 7) passing laterally in front of the denticulate ligament (3) to enter meningeal nerve sheaths with dorsal roots (as at 4) and form a spinal nerve. On some roots, branches of radicular vessels (as at 5) are seen anastomosing with anterior spinal vessels (1).

1 Anterior spinal vessels
2 Arachnoid and dura mater
3 Denticulate ligament
4 Dorsal root of sixth cervical nerve
5 Radicular vessels
6 Spinal cord
7 Ventral root of seventh cervical nerve entering dural sheath

The denticulate ligament (B3) is composed of pia mater. The ventral and dorsal nerve roots pass respectively ventral and dorsal to the ligament, which extends laterally from the side of the cord and is attached by its spiky denticulations (as at B3) to the arachnoid and dura mater in the intervals between dural nerve sheaths. The highest denticulation is above the first cervical nerve and the lowest below the twelfth thoracic nerve.

The spinal cord usually ends at the level of the first lumbar vertebra.

The subarachnoid space ends at the level of the second sacral vertebra.

The conus medullaris (C2) is the lower, pointed end of the spinal cord.

The cauda equina (C1) consists of the dorsal and ventral roots of the lumbar, sacral and coccygeal nerves. Note that it is nerve roots which form the cauda, not the spinal nerves themselves; these are not formed until ventral and dorsal roots unite at the level of an intervertebral foramen, immediately distal to the dorsal root ganglion (as at C3).

Lordosis, see p. 115.

Vertebral column and spinal cord

C lumbar and sacral regions, from behind   D lumbar radiculogram

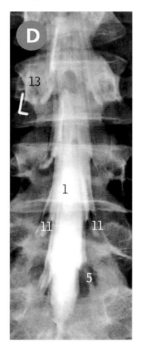

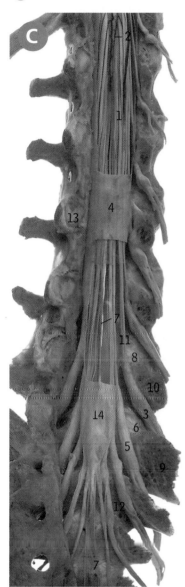

Parts of the vertebral arches and meninges have been removed, to show the cauda equina (1) and nerve roots entering their meningeal sheaths (as at 11), outlined as linear bands by contrast medium in the radiculogram.

1	Cauda equina	**7**	Filum terminale
2	Conus medullaris of spinal cord	**8**	Fourth lumbar intervertebral disc
3	Dorsal root ganglion of fifth lumbar nerve	**9**	Lateral part of sacrum
		10	Pedicle of fifth lumbar vertebra
4	Dura mater	**11**	Roots of fifth lumbar nerve
5	Dural sheath of first sacral nerve roots	**12**	Second sacral vertebra
		13	Superior articular process of third lumbar vertebra
6	Fifth lumbar (lumbosacral) intervertebral disc	**14**	Thecal sac

> If the fifth lumbar intervertebral disc protrudes backwards (the commonest 'slipped disc') it may irritate the roots of the first sacral nerve (C5). This is the general rule for any part of the vertebral column – a protruded disc may irritate the roots of the nerve numbered one below the disc. Note for example that the fifth lumbar nerve roots (C11) within their dural sheath pass laterally immediately below the pedicle of the fifth lumbar vertebra (C10) and so do not come to lie immediately behind the fifth lumbar disc (C6); it is the first sacral roots (C5) which lie in this position. The fifth nerve roots (C11) lie behind the fourth disc (C8).

E Coronal lumbar MR image

F Lower thoracic and upper lumbar regions

The specimen is seen from the left with parts of the vertebral arches and meninges removed, to show (at the front) part of the sympathetic trunk (13) on the vertebral bodies and (at the back) the spinous ligaments (7 and 11).

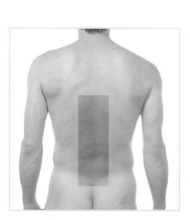

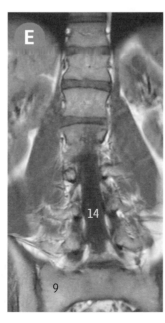

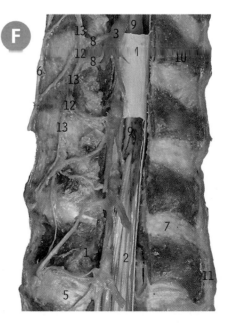

1	Body of first lumbar vertebra
2	Cauda equina
3	Dorsal root ganglion of tenth thoracic nerve
4	Dura mater
5	First lumbar intervertebral disc
6	Greater splanchnic nerve
7	Interspinous ligament
8	Rami communicantes
9	Spinal cord
10	Spinous process of tenth thoracic vertebra
11	Supraspinous ligament
12	Sympathetic ganglion
13	Sympathetic trunk

Epidural anaesthesia, spinal anaesthesia, see p. 115.

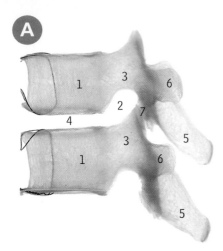

Ⓐ Thoracic vertebrae *cleared specimens*

The pairs of vertebrae are seen from the side and articulated to show the boundaries of an intervertebral foramen (2).

1 Body
2 Intervertebral foramen
3 Pedicle
4 Space for intervertebral disc
5 Spinous process
6 Transverse process
7 Zygapophyseal joint

> The intervertebral foramen (A2) is bounded in front by the lower part of the vertebral body (A1) and the intervertebral disc (A4), above and below by the pedicles (A3), and behind by the zygapophyseal joint (A7).

Ⓑ Back and vertebral column *posterior view*

Vertebral column, lower thoracic region, exposing spinal cord and posterior longitudinal ligament by removal of vertebral arches and meninges.

1 Latissimus dorsi
2 Longissimus
3 Pedicle of thoracic vertebra 9 (cut)
4 Posterior longitudinal ligament
5 Spinal cord
6 Thoracic nerve 10
7 Trapezius
8 Vertebral venous plexus

> The posterior longitudinal ligament (B4) is broad where it is firmly attached to the intervertebral discs, but narrow and less firmly attached to the vertebral bodies, leaving vascular foramina patent and allowing the basivertebral veins which emerge from them to enter the internal vertebral venous plexus.
>
> The anterior longitudinal ligament (D1) is uniformly broad and firmly attached to discs and vertebral bodies.

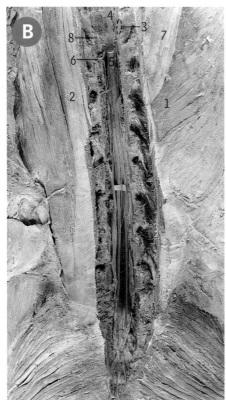

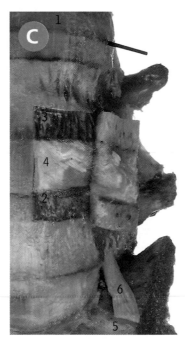

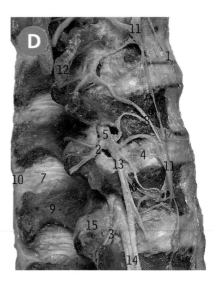

Ⓒ Vertebral column

lower lumbar region, from the front

At the top the anterior longitudinal ligament (1) has a marker behind it, and part of it lower down has been reflected off an intervertebral disc (4) and vertebral bodies (2 and 3).

1 Anterior longitudinal ligament
2 Body of fifth lumbar vertebra
3 Body of fourth lumbar vertebra
4 Fourth lumbar intervertebral disc
5 Lateral part of sacrum
6 Ventral ramus of fifth lumbar nerve

Ⓓ Vertebral column

upper lumbar region, from the right

The side view shows lumbar nerves emerging from intervertebral foramina (as at 5).

1 Anterior longitudinal ligament
2 Dorsal ramus of first lumbar nerve
3 Dorsal ramus of second lumbar nerve
4 First lumbar intervertebral disc
5 First lumbar nerve emerging from intervertebral foramen
6 First lumbar vertebra
7 Interspinous ligament
8 Rami communicantes
9 Spinous process of second lumbar vertebra
10 Supraspinous ligament
11 Sympathetic trunk ganglion
12 Twelfth rib
13 Ventral ramus of first lumbar nerve
14 Ventral ramus of second lumbar nerve
15 Zygapophyseal joint

Compression of spinal nerve, vertebral venous plexus, see p. 115

Ⓐ Vertebral column

*lumbar region,
from the right and behind*

This posterolateral view of the right side of some lumbar vertebrae shows ligamenta flava (as at 4), which pass between the laminae of adjacent vertebrae (as at 2 and 3).

1 Interspinous ligament
2 Lamina of second lumbar vertebra
3 Lamina of third lumbar vertebra
4 Ligamentum flavum
5 Spinous process of second lumbar vertebra
6 Supraspinous ligament
7 Transverse process of third lumbar vertebra
8 Zygapophyseal joint

Spinal cord and cauda equina

Ⓑ *dorsal surface of upper end*

Ⓒ *dorsal surface of lower end with cauda*

The dura and arachnoid mater have been incised longitudinally and turned outwards (B1 and C1) to show the nerve roots entering their dural sheaths (as at B6 and C7). Below the level of the conus medullaris (the lower end of the spinal cord, C3) the nerve roots constitute the cauda equina (C2). Compare B with the ventral surface of the cervical part of the cord (page 106, B).

1 Arachnoid overlying dura mater
2 Cauda equina
3 Conus medullaris
4 Denticulate ligament
5 Dorsal rootlets of fifth cervical nerve
6 Eighth cervical nerve roots entering dural sheath
7 Fifth lumbar nerve roots entering dural sheath
8 Filum terminale
9 Spinal cord

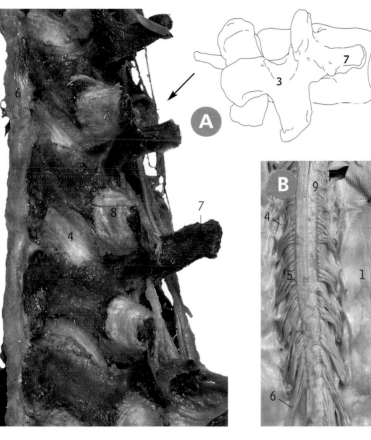

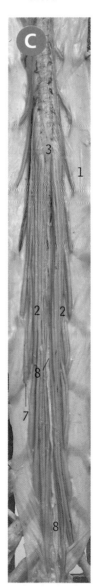

The filum terminale (C8), which consists of connective tissue, not neural elements, extends from the tip of the conus medullaris (C3) through the subarachnoid space to the level of the second sacral vertebra where it fuses with the dura mater and continues downwards to become attached to the first piece of the coccyx.

Ⓓ Intervertebral disc

This disc, on the upper surface of the body of a lumbar vertebra, has been cut horizontally to show the central nucleus pulposus (2) and the concentric fibrocartilaginous laminae of the surrounding annulus fibrosus (1). At the back the annulus has been shaved off to reveal part of the plate of hyaline cartilage (3) on the surface of the vertebra.

1 Annulus fibrosus
2 Nucleus pulposus
3 Plate of hyaline cartilage

The nucleus pulposus of an intervertebral disc represents the remains of the notochord.

The annulus fibrosus of an intervertebral disc is derived from the mesenchyme between adjacent vertebral bodies.

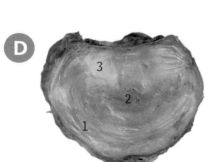

Discectomy, herniated disc, lumbar puncture, see p. 115.

Back *surface anatomy*

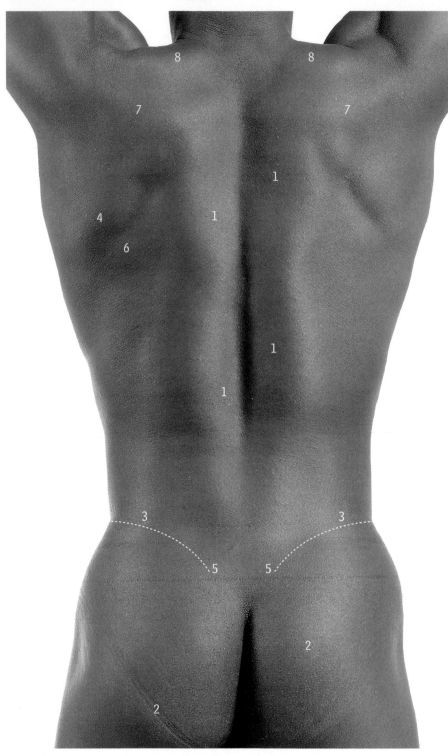

1   Erector spinae
2   Gluteus maximus
3   Iliac crest
4   Infraspinatus
5   Posterior superior
    iliac spine
6   Rhomboids
7   Spine of scapula
8   Trapezius

Back *superficial musculature*

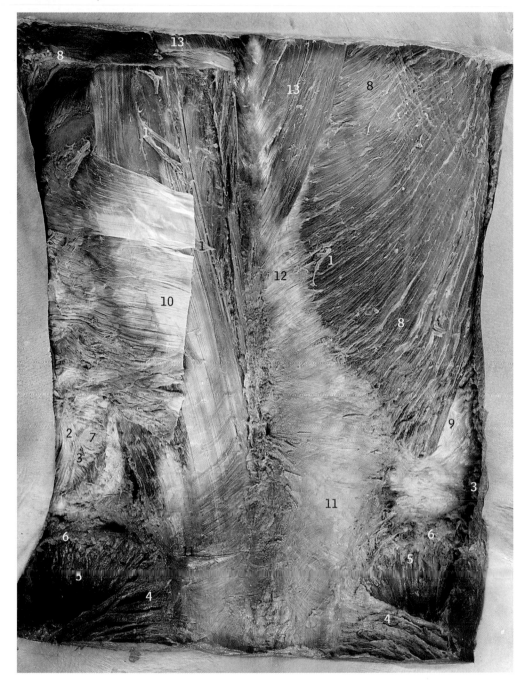

1 Branches of dorsal rami
   of thoracic nerves
2 External oblique
3 External oblique,
   free posterior border
4 Gluteus maximus
5 Gluteus medius
6 Iliac crest
7 Internal oblique
8 Latissimus dorsi
9 Latissimus dorsi,
   free lateral border
10 Serratus posterior inferior
11 Thoracolumbar fascia,
   lumbar part
12 Thoracolumbar fascia,
   thoracic part
13 Trapezius

The right side is a superficial dissection after removal of the skin and subcutaneous
fat of variable thickness to expose the thoracolumbar fascia and some posterior
shoulder girdle muscles. The left side is a deeper dissection in which the latissimus
dorsi and trapezius have been removed to expose the serratus posterior inferior.

Back *deep musculature*

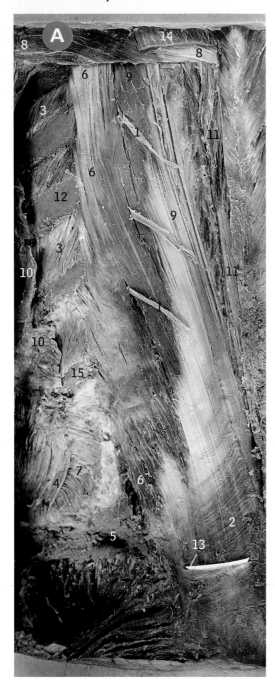

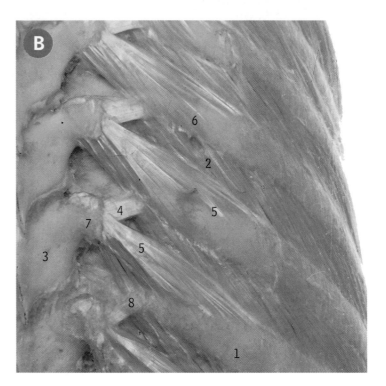

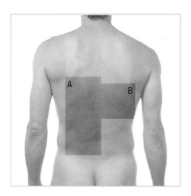

A Reflection of the serratus posterior inferior reveals the components of erector spinae and the posterior surface of the lowest ribs, left side

1 Dorsal rami, lower thoracic nerves
2 Erector spinae
3 External intercostal
4 External oblique, posterior (free) border
5 Iliac crest
6 Iliocostalis part of erector spinae
7 Internal oblique
8 Latissimus dorsi
9 Longissimus thoracic part of erector spinae
10 Serratus posterior inferior – cut
11 Spinalis thoracic part of erector spinae
12 Tenth rib
13 Thoracolumbar fascia, posterior part –
   white marker emerging from cut edge
14 Trapezius
15 Twelfth rib

In the upper lumbar region, erector spinae divides into three muscle masses: iliocostalis (6) laterally, an intermediate longissimus (9), and spinalis (11) medially.

B Removal of the erector spinae shows the deepest back muscles in the thoracic region, right side

1 Angle of ninth rib
2 External intercostal
3 Lamina of eighth thoracic vertebra
4 Lateral costotransverse ligament
5 Levator costae
6 Seventh rib
7 Transverse process of eighth thoracic vertebra
8 Tubercle of ninth rib

Upper cervical vertebrae

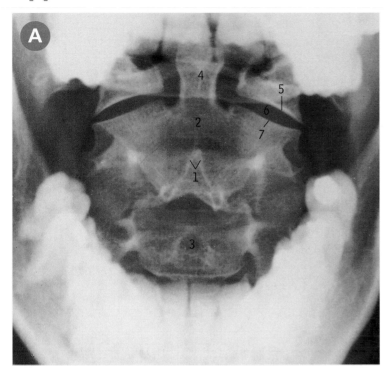

This is a standard radiographic view of the axis and its dens (4). The correct angle must be chosen with the mouth open to avoid overlying shadows of the teeth and jaws. The surfaces of the lateral atlanto-axial joints (5 and 7) do not appear congruent because the hyaline cartilage which covers the bony surfaces is not radio-opaque (this applies to any synovial joint). The outlines of the arches of the atlas are seen faintly between the sides of the shadow of the dens (4) and the lateral masses of the atlas (5).

1 Bifid spinous process of axis
2 Body of axis
3 Body of third cervical vertebra
4 Dens of axis
5 Inferior articular surface of lateral mass of atlas
6 Lateral atlanto-axial joint
7 Superior articular surface of axis

Lower cervical and upper thoracic vertebrae *from the front*

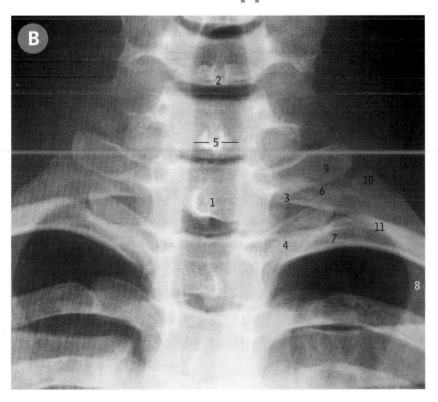

Note the tracheal shadow produced by the translucency of its contained air.

1 Body of first thoracic vertebra
2 Body of sixth cervical vertebra
3 Head of first rib
4 Head of second rib
5 Margin of tracheal shadow
6 Neck of first rib
7 Neck of second rib
8 Shaft of first rib
9 Transverse process of first thoracic vertebra
10 Tubercle of first rib
11 Tubercle of second rib

 Cervical spinal immobilization, see p. 115.

Spine

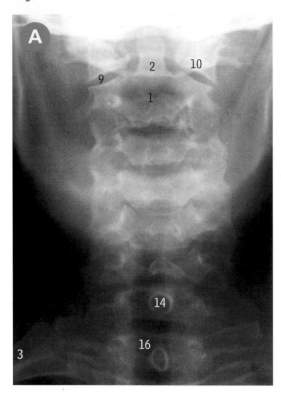

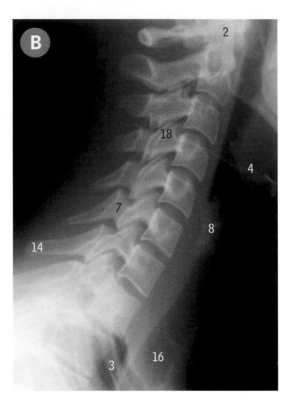

1 Body of axis
2 Dens of axis
3 First rib
4 Hyoid bone
5 Inferior articular process of first lumbar vertebra
6 Intervertebral disc space L2/3 level
7 Lamina of sixth cervical vertebra
8 Larynx
9 Lateral atlanto-axial joint
10 Lateral mass of atlas
11 Pars interarticularis of second lumbar vertebra
12 Pedicle of third lumbar vertebra
13 Spinous process of second lumbar vertebra
14 Spinous process of seventh cervical vertebra
15 Superior articular process of second lumbar vertebra
16 Trachea
17 Transverse process of third lumbar vertebra
18 Zygapophyseal joint

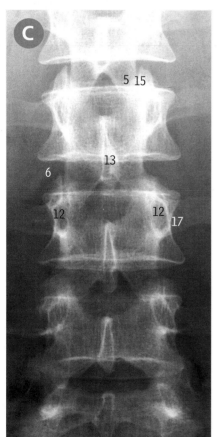

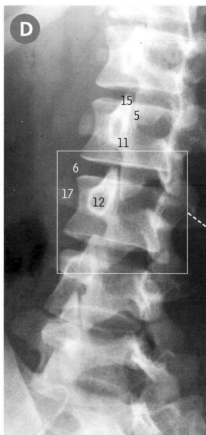

A cervical spine, anteroposterior projection

B cervical spine, lateral projection

C lumbar spine, anteroposterior projection

D lumbar spine, oblique projection

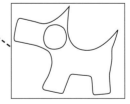

The Scottie dog is seen on the oblique projection lumbar spine. The nose (17) is the transverse process, the ear (15) is the superior articular process, the eye (12) is the pedicle and the neck (11) is the pars interarticularis which may be incomplete in spondylolysis.

Vertebral fractures, see p. 115.

Vertebral column and spinal cord
Clinical notes

Caudal anaesthesia is a special type of epidural (extradural) anaesthesia, the needle entering the epidural space via the sacral hiatus in the natal cleft for anaesthesia of the lower lumbar and sacral roots. (page 101)

Cervical spinal immobilization. Following actual or suspected injuries to the cervical spine it is extremely important to keep the spine immobile and under slight traction to prevent spinal cord compression and, therefore, paraplegia or quadriplegia while transporting the patient to hospital. (page 113)

Coccydynia is pain in the region of the coccyx commonly found in women after childbirth and is caused by stretching and possible fracture of coccygeal segments. It may also occur following a sudden fall directly onto the buttocks. (page 100)

Compression of a spinal nerve causes pain, anaesthesia and/or paralysis in its field of distribution. Common causes include a prolapsed intervertebral disc or, in the older patient, the impingement of an osteophyte making the intervertebral foramen too tight to allow free movement of the existing spinal nerve. (page 108)

Discectomy is a 'minimally invasive surgery' technique for disc disease in which, instead of removing the bony lamina, the operation is performed using a microscope to remove just that part of a protruding disc that is pressing against a nerve root and causing limb pain. (page 109)

Epidural anaesthesia is regional anaesthesia produced by pharmacological interruption of nerve transmission after placing an anaesthetic agent just outside the dura mater. It is usually carried out in the lower thoracic or lumbar regions by introduction of a needle in exactly the same fashion as a lumbar puncture, except that the needle tip is in the epidural (extradural) space. A small cannula is inserted just external to the thecal sac and the anaesthetic agent dripped in at that level. Tipping of the patient will enable the anaesthetic to reach different spinal levels by gravity. (page 107)

Herniated disc, known also as a 'slipped disc', is due to protrusion of the nucleus pulposus through the annulus fibrosus, most commonly seen in the lower lumbar region. (page 109)

Laminectomy is removal of vertebral laminae to treat disc protrusion but recently has been superseded by discectomy and microdiscectomy. A laminectomy may still be indicated for spinal stenosis. (page 98)

Lordosis. The cervical and lumbar regions of the normal spine have a natural lordosis (a concavity posteriorly). (page 106)

Lumbar puncture (spinal tap) is a procedure used to obtain cerebrospinal fluid (CSF) for diagnosis or to access the CSF for drug delivery. Entering the midline of the back in the space between the L4 and L5 vertebrae, the needle passes through the skin, subcutaneous tissue, supraspinous ligament and interspinous ligament between the ligamenta flava, and into the epidural space. It then passes through the tough dura mater into the subarachnoid space. (page 109)

Spinal anaesthesia uses the same technique as lumbar puncture to insert a needle into the CSF and then introduce anaesthetic agents into the spinal canal. Occasionally, in cases of spinal tumours, an anaesthetic/analgesic may be directly administered via a syringe driven pump system to control pain in the lower body. (page 107)

Spondylolisthesis is the anterior displacement or slipping of the body of one vertebra on another, usually in the lower lumbar region. (page 97)

Vertebral fractures may occur anywhere along the vertebral column. A common lumbar site, due to a congenital malformation in the pars interarticularis (spondylolysis), is best diagnosed by an oblique lumbar spine radiograph, which reveals a little Scottie dog profile with the fracture across the dog's collar. (opposite page)

Vertebral venous plexus (Batson's valveless plexus) is a multichannel set of veins that interconnects both inside and outside the spinal canal from the pelvis to the skull and serves as a transport system for metastases from the breast, prostate, ovary and uterus to the vertebral bodies and the cranial cavity. (page 108)

Upper limb

Upper limb

A *surface anatomy* **B** *muscles* **C** *bones*

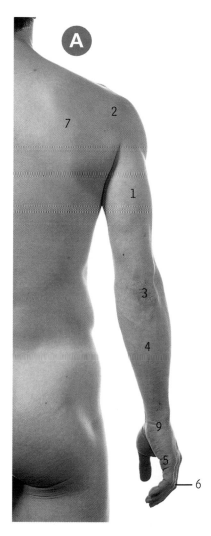

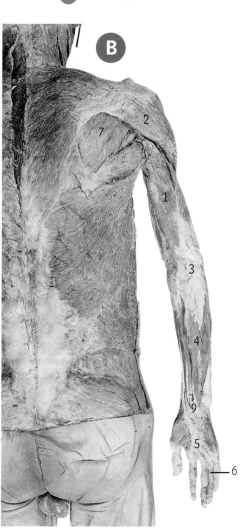

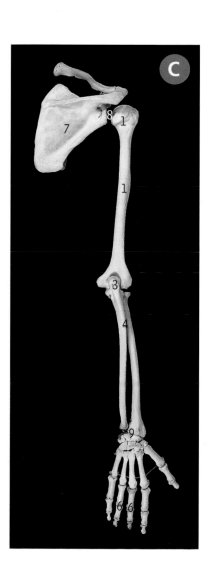

1	Arm	**6**	Interphalangeal joint
2	Deltoid	**7**	Scapula
3	Elbow joint	**8**	Shoulder joint
4	Forearm	**9**	Wrist joint
5	Hand		

Left scapula

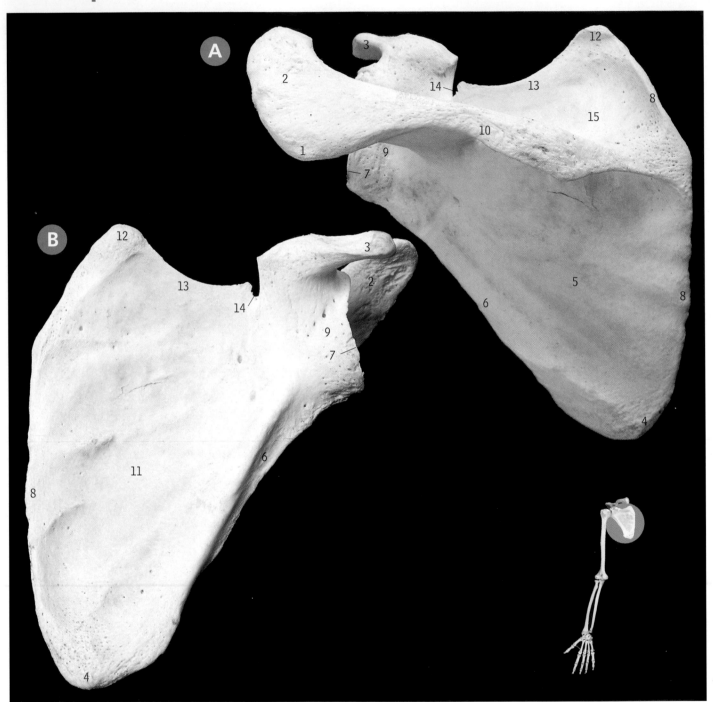

A dorsal surface

B costal surface

1 Acromial angle
2 Acromion
3 Coracoid process
4 Inferior angle
5 Infraspinous fossa
6 Lateral border
7 Margin of glenoid cavity
8 Medial border
9 Neck (and spinoglenoid notch on dorsal surface)
10 Spine
11 Subscapular fossa
12 Superior angle
13 Superior border
14 Suprascapular notch
15 Supraspinous fossa

Left scapula *attachments*

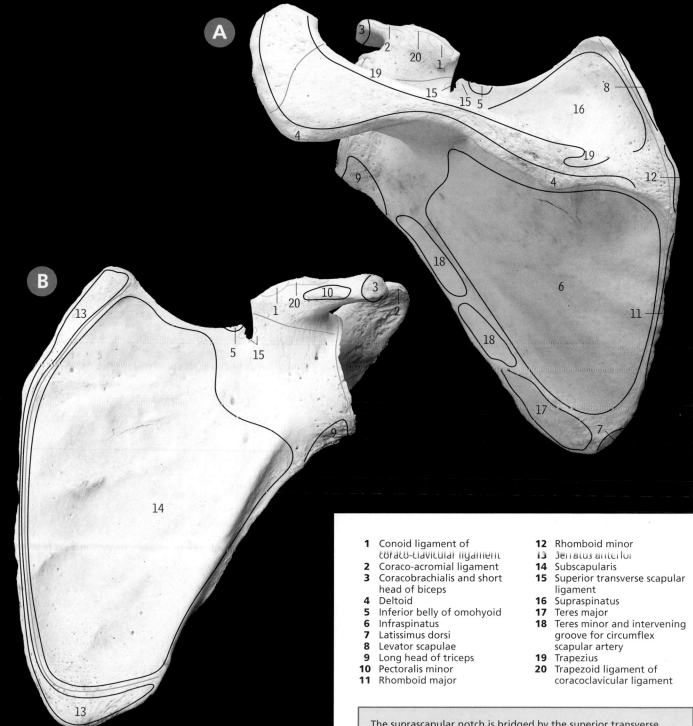

Blue lines = epiphysial lines; green lines = capsular attachments of shoulder joint; pale green lines = ligament attachments

1 Conoid ligament of coraco-clavicular ligament
2 Coraco-acromial ligament
3 Coracobrachialis and short head of biceps
4 Deltoid
5 Inferior belly of omohyoid
6 Infraspinatus
7 Latissimus dorsi
8 Levator scapulae
9 Long head of triceps
10 Pectoralis minor
11 Rhomboid major
12 Rhomboid minor
13 Serratus anterior
14 Subscapularis
15 Superior transverse scapular ligament
16 Supraspinatus
17 Teres major
18 Teres minor and intervening groove for circumflex scapular artery
19 Trapezius
20 Trapezoid ligament of coracoclavicular ligament

The suprascapular notch is bridged by the superior transverse scapular ligament (15).

The conoid (1) and trapezoid (20) ligaments together form the coracoclavicular ligament, which attaches the coracoid process of the scapula to the under-surface of the lateral end of the clavicle.

The coraco-acromial ligament (2) passes between the coracoid process and the acromion, forming with these bony processes an arch above the shoulder joint.

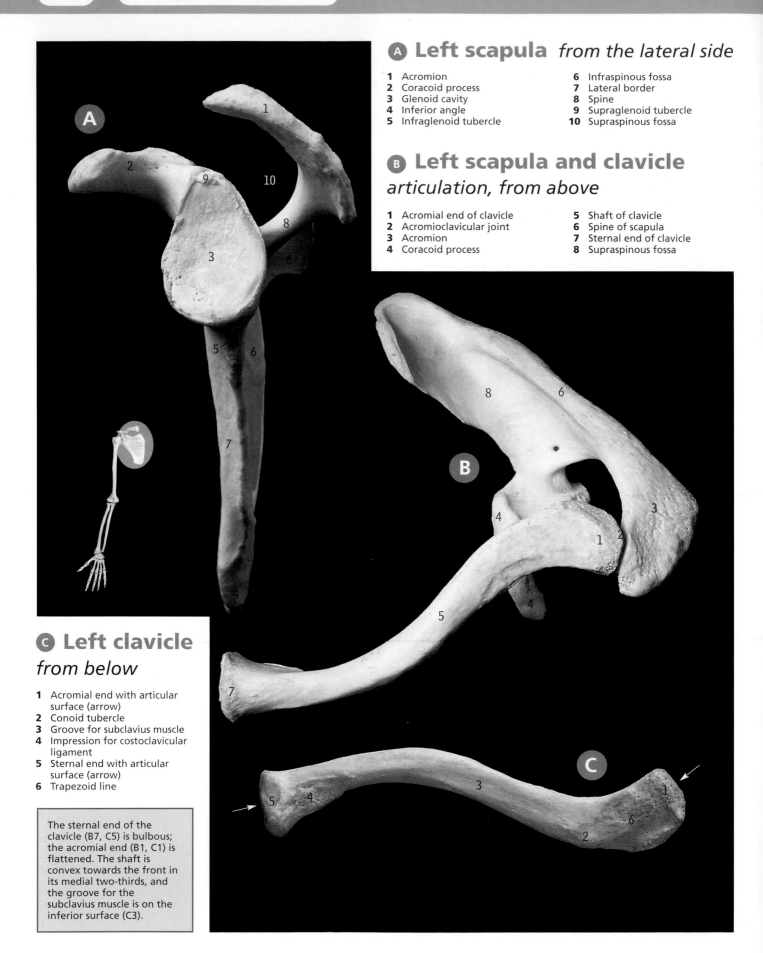

A Left scapula *from the lateral side*

1	Acromion	**6**	Infraspinous fossa
2	Coracoid process	**7**	Lateral border
3	Glenoid cavity	**8**	Spine
4	Inferior angle	**9**	Supraglenoid tubercle
5	Infraglenoid tubercle	**10**	Supraspinous fossa

B Left scapula and clavicle
articulation, from above

1	Acromial end of clavicle	**5**	Shaft of clavicle
2	Acromioclavicular joint	**6**	Spine of scapula
3	Acromion	**7**	Sternal end of clavicle
4	Coracoid process	**8**	Supraspinous fossa

C Left clavicle
from below

1 Acromial end with articular surface (arrow)
2 Conoid tubercle
3 Groove for subclavius muscle
4 Impression for costoclavicular ligament
5 Sternal end with articular surface (arrow)
6 Trapezoid line

The sternal end of the clavicle (B7, C5) is bulbous; the acromial end (B1, C1) is flattened. The shaft is convex towards the front in its medial two-thirds, and the groove for the subclavius muscle is on the inferior surface (C3).

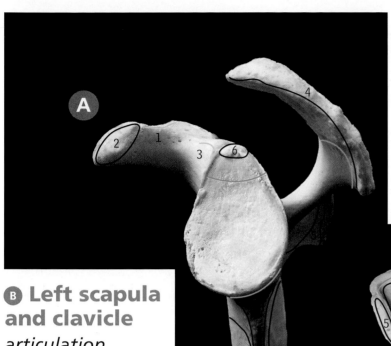

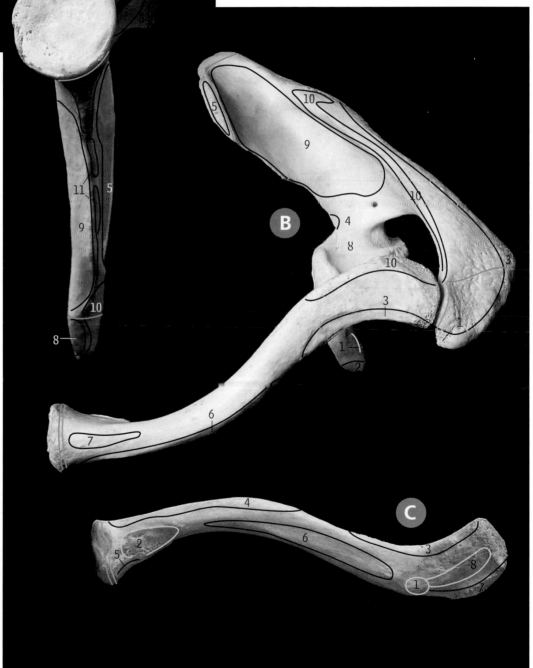

A Left scapula
attachments, from the lateral side

Blue lines = epiphysial lines; green lines = capsular attachments of shoulder joint; pale green lines = ligament attachments

1 Coraco-acromial ligament
2 Coracobrachialis and short head of biceps
3 Coracohumeral ligament
4 Deltoid
5 Infraspinatus
6 Long head of biceps
7 Long head of triceps
8 Serratus anterior
9 Subscapularis
10 Teres major
11 Teres minor (with intervening groove for circumflex scapular artery)

B Left scapula and clavicle
articulation, from above

Blue lines = epiphysial lines; green lines = capsular attachments of sternoclavicular and acromioclavicular joints; pale green lines = ligament attachments

1 Coraco-acromial ligament
2 Coracobrachialis and short head of biceps
3 Deltoid
4 Inferior belly of omohyoid
5 Levator scapulae
6 Pectoralis major
7 Sternocleidomastoid
8 Superior transverse scapular ligament
9 Supraspinatus
10 Trapezius

C Left clavicle
attachments, from below

Blue lines = epiphysial lines; green lines = capsular attachments of sternoclavicular and acromioclavicular joints; pale green lines = ligament attachments

1 Conoid ligament
2 Costoclavicular ligament
3 Deltoid
4 Pectoralis major
5 Sternohyoid
6 Subclavius and clavipectoral fascia
7 Trapezius
8 Trapezoid ligament

Right humerus *upper end*

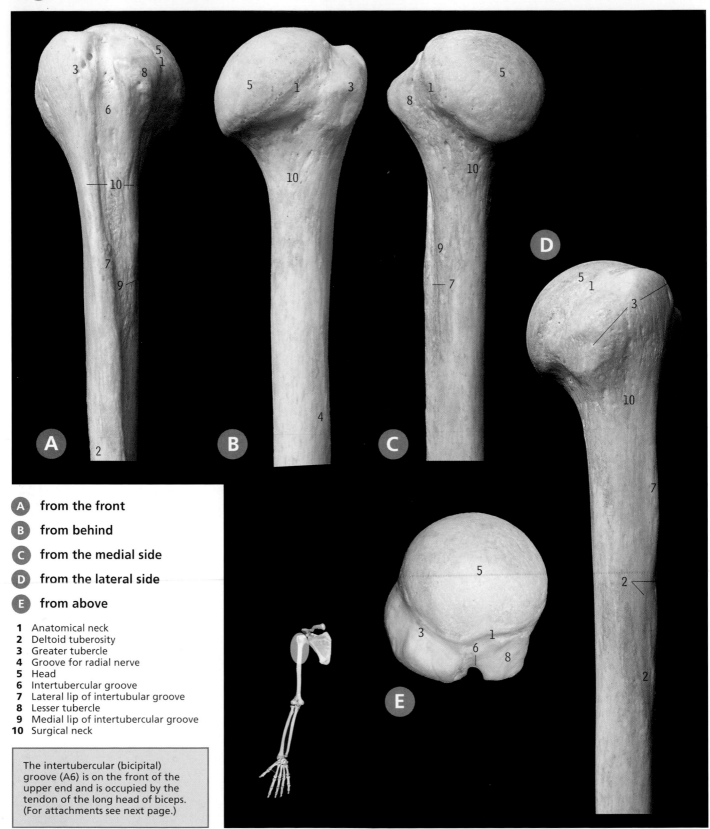

A   **from the front**

B   **from behind**

C   **from the medial side**

D   **from the lateral side**

E   **from above**

1   Anatomical neck
2   Deltoid tuberosity
3   Greater tubercle
4   Groove for radial nerve
5   Head
6   Intertubercular groove
7   Lateral lip of intertubular groove
8   Lesser tubercle
9   Medial lip of intertubercular groove
10   Surgical neck

The intertubercular (bicipital) groove (A6) is on the front of the upper end and is occupied by the tendon of the long head of biceps. (For attachments see next page.)

 Dislocation of the humerus, see p. 174.

Right humerus *attachments, upper end*

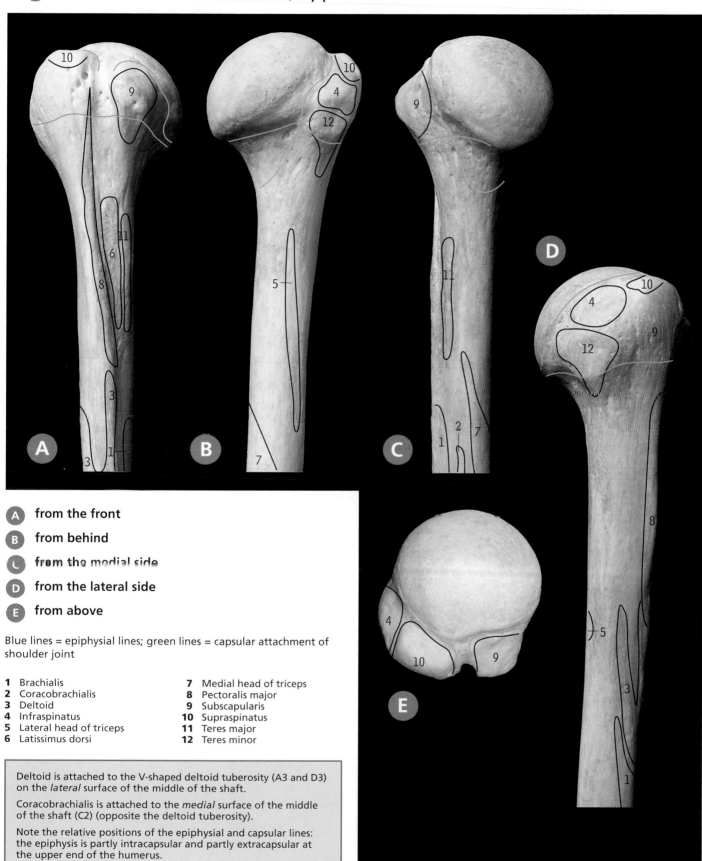

A from the front

B from behind

C from the medial side

D from the lateral side

E from above

Blue lines = epiphysial lines; green lines = capsular attachment of shoulder joint

1	Brachialis	**7**	Medial head of triceps
2	Coracobrachialis	**8**	Pectoralis major
3	Deltoid	**9**	Subscapularis
4	Infraspinatus	**10**	Supraspinatus
5	Lateral head of triceps	**11**	Teres major
6	Latissimus dorsi	**12**	Teres minor

Deltoid is attached to the V-shaped deltoid tuberosity (A3 and D3) on the *lateral* surface of the middle of the shaft.

Coracobrachialis is attached to the *medial* surface of the middle of the shaft (C2) (opposite the deltoid tuberosity).

Note the relative positions of the epiphysial and capsular lines: the epiphysis is partly intracapsular and partly extracapsular at the upper end of the humerus.

Right humerus *lower end*

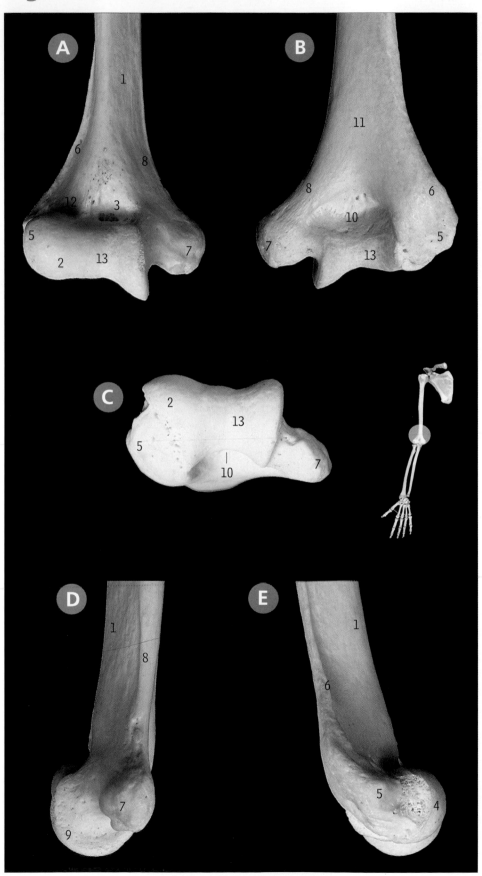

A from the front

B from behind

C from below

D from the medial side

E from the lateral side

1 Anterior surface
2 Capitulum
3 Coronoid fossa
4 Lateral edge of capitulum
5 Lateral epicondyle
6 Lateral supracondylar ridge
7 Medial epicondyle
8 Medial supracondylar ridge
9 Medial surface of trochlea
10 Olecranon fossa
11 Posterior surface
12 Radial fossa
13 Trochlea

The medial epicondyle (7) is more prominent than the lateral (5).

The medial part of the trochlea (13) is more prominent than the lateral part.

The olecranon fossa (10) on the posterior surface is deeper than the radial and coronoid fossae on the anterior surface (12 and 3).

Right humerus *attachments, lower end*

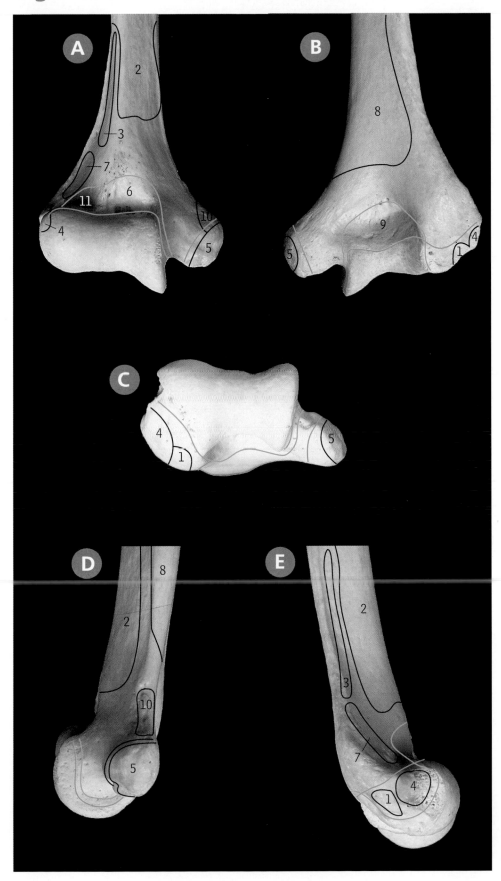

A from the front

B from behind

C from below

D from the medial side

E from the lateral side

Blue lines = epiphysial lines;
green lines = capsular attachment
of elbow joint

1 Anconeus
2 Brachialis
3 Brachioradialis
4 Common extensor origin
5 Common flexor origin
6 Coronoid fossa
7 Extensor carpi radialis longus
8 Medial head of triceps
9 Olecranon fossa
10 Pronator teres, humeral head
11 Radial fossa

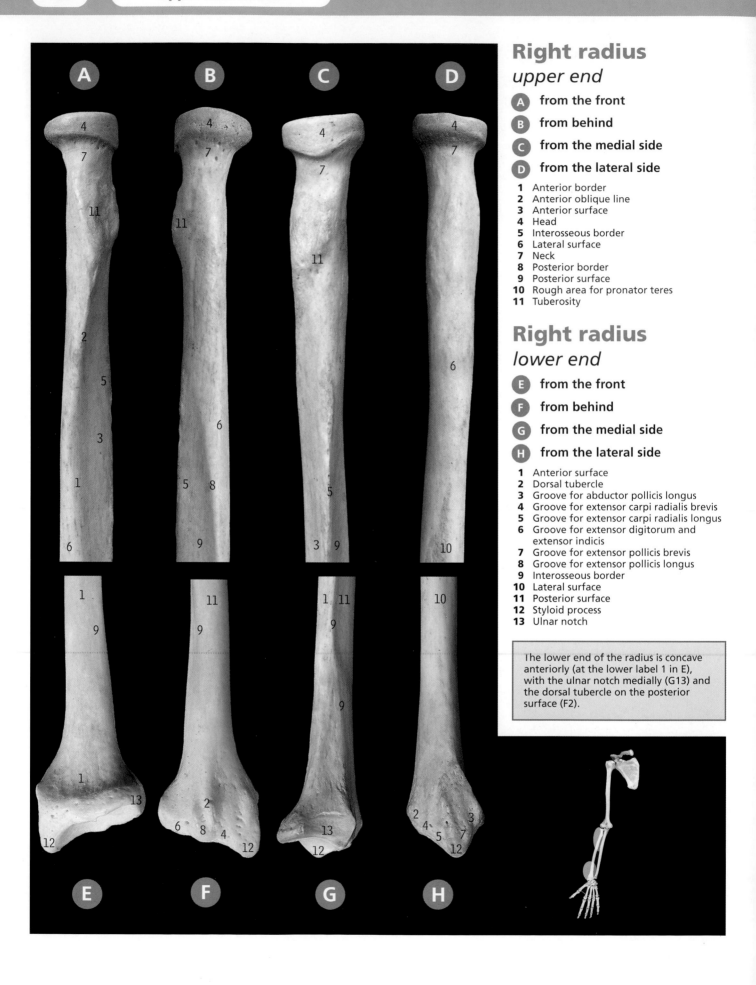

Right radius
upper end

A   from the front
B   from behind
C   from the medial side
D   from the lateral side

1 Anterior border
2 Anterior oblique line
3 Anterior surface
4 Head
5 Interosseous border
6 Lateral surface
7 Neck
8 Posterior border
9 Posterior surface
10 Rough area for pronator teres
11 Tuberosity

Right radius
lower end

E   from the front
F   from behind
G   from the medial side
H   from the lateral side

1 Anterior surface
2 Dorsal tubercle
3 Groove for abductor pollicis longus
4 Groove for extensor carpi radialis brevis
5 Groove for extensor carpi radialis longus
6 Groove for extensor digitorum and extensor indicis
7 Groove for extensor pollicis brevis
8 Groove for extensor pollicis longus
9 Interosseous border
10 Lateral surface
11 Posterior surface
12 Styloid process
13 Ulnar notch

The lower end of the radius is concave anteriorly (at the lower label 1 in E), with the ulnar notch medially (G13) and the dorsal tubercle on the posterior surface (F2).

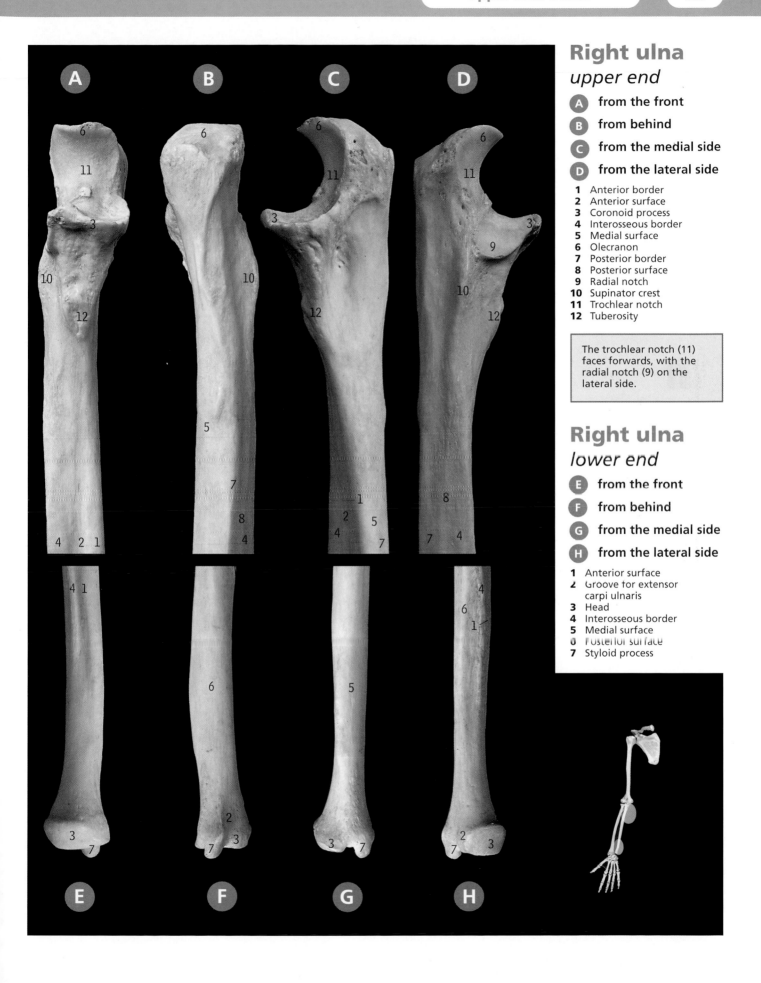

Right ulna
upper end

A from the front
B from behind
C from the medial side
D from the lateral side

1 Anterior border
2 Anterior surface
3 Coronoid process
4 Interosseous border
5 Medial surface
6 Olecranon
7 Posterior border
8 Posterior surface
9 Radial notch
10 Supinator crest
11 Trochlear notch
12 Tuberosity

The trochlear notch (11) faces forwards, with the radial notch (9) on the lateral side.

Right ulna
lower end

E from the front
F from behind
G from the medial side
H from the lateral side

1 Anterior surface
2 Groove for extensor carpi ulnaris
3 Head
4 Interosseous border
5 Medial surface
6 Posterior surface
7 Styloid process

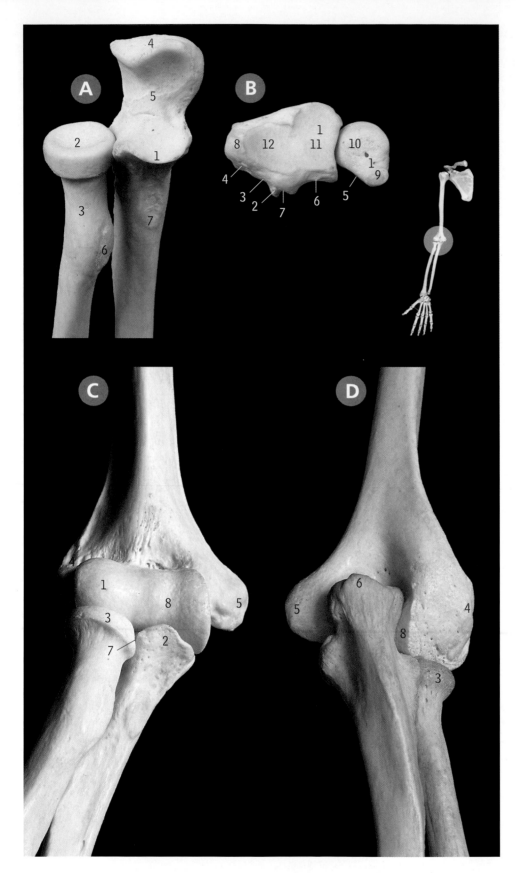

A Right radius and ulna

upper ends, from above and in front

1 Coronoid process of ulna
2 Head of radius
3 Neck of radius
4 Olecranon of ulna
5 Trochlear notch of ulna
6 Tuberosity of radius
7 Tuberosity of ulna

B Right radius and ulna

lower ends, from below

1 Attachment of articular disc
2 Dorsal tubercle
3 Groove for extensor carpi radialis brevis
4 Groove for extensor carpi radialis longus
5 Groove for extensor carpi ulnaris
6 Groove for extensor digitorum and extensor indicis
7 Groove for extensor pollicis longus
8 Styloid process of radius
9 Styloid process of ulna
10 Surface for disc
11 Surface for lunate
12 Surface for scaphoid

Right humerus, radius and ulna

articulation

C **from the front**

D **from behind**

1 Capitulum of humerus
2 Coronoid process of ulna
3 Head of radius
4 Lateral epicondyle of humerus
5 Medial epicondyle of humerus
6 Olecranon of ulna
7 Radial notch of ulna
8 Trochlea of humerus

The elbow joint and the proximal radio-ulnar joint share a common synovial cavity.

Supracondylar fracture of the humerus, see p. 175.

Right radius and ulna *attachments*

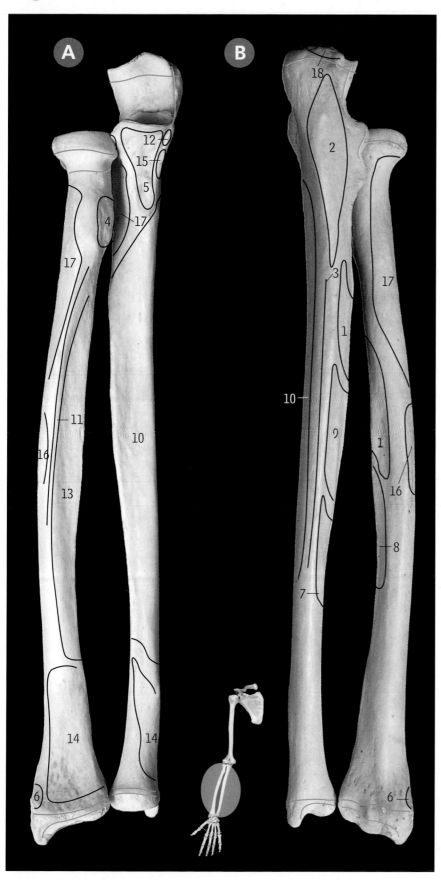

A from the front

B from behind

Blue lines = epiphysial lines; green lines = capsular attachments of elbow and wrist joints

1 Abductor pollicis longus
2 Anconeus
3 Aponeurotic attachment of flexor digitorum profundus, flexor carpi ulnaris and extensor carpi ulnaris
4 Biceps
5 Brachialis
6 Brachioradialis
7 Extensor indicis
8 Extensor pollicis brevis
9 Extensor pollicis longus
10 Flexor digitorum profundus
11 Flexor digitorum superficialis, radial head
12 Flexor digitorum superficialis, ulnar head
13 Flexor pollicis longus
14 Pronator quadratus
15 Pronator teres, ulnar head
16 Pronator teres
17 Supinator
18 Triceps

Abductor pollicis longus (1) and extensor pollicis brevis (8) are the only two muscles to have an origin from the posterior surface of the radius (although both extend on to the interosseous membrane and the abductor also has an origin from the posterior surface of the ulna). These muscles remain companions as they wind round the lateral side of the radius (page 157) and form the radial boundary of the anatomical snuffbox (page 158B).

In the young subject the radius sometimes fractures across the lower epiphysis following an injury to the wrist. In the adult the term 'Colles' fracture (pages 131, 174) refers to a transverse break across the lower radius within about 2.5 cm of the lower end of the bone. The ulnar styloid process is also often fractured.

Bones of the right hand

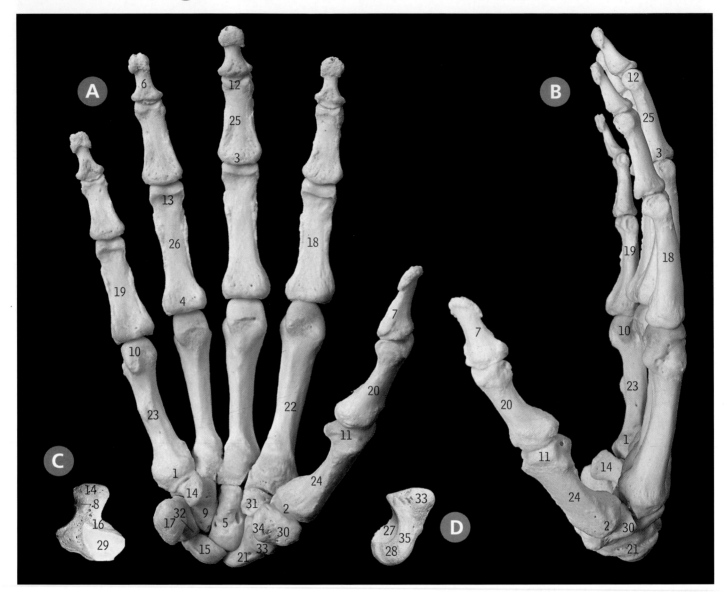

A palmar surface

B from the lateral side

C hamate from the medial side

D scaphoid, palmar surface

1   Base of fifth metacarpal
2   Base of first metacarpal
3   Base of middle phalanx of middle finger
4   Base of proximal phalanx of ring finger
5   Capitate
6   Distal phalanx of ring finger
7   Distal phalanx of thumb
8   Groove for deep branch of ulnar nerve
9   Hamate
10 Head of fifth metacarpal
11 Head of first metacarpal
12 Head of middle phalanx of middle finger
13 Head of proximal phalanx of ring finger
14 Hook of hamate
15 Lunate
16 Palmar surface, hamate

17 Pisiform
18 Proximal phalanx of index finger
19 Proximal phalanx of little finger
20 Proximal phalanx of thumb
21 Scaphoid
22 Shaft of second metacarpal
23 Shaft of fifth metacarpal
24 Shaft of first metacarpal
25 Shaft of middle phalanx of middle finger
26 Shaft of proximal phalanx of ring finger
27 Surface for capitate
28 Surface for lunate
29 Surface for triquetral
30 Trapezium
31 Trapezoid
32 Triquetral
33 Tubercle of scaphoid
34 Tubercle of trapezium
35 Waist of scaphoid

The scaphoid, lunate, triquetral and pisiform bones form the proximal row of carpal bones.

The trapezium, trapezoid, capitate and hamate bones form the distal row of carpal bones.

The tubercle (33) and waist (35) are the non-articular parts of the scaphoid and therefore contain nutrient foramina. A fracture across the waist may therefore interfere with the blood supply of the proximal pole of the bone and lead to avascular necrosis (see page 174). The waist of the scaphoid lies in the anatomical snuffbox; the tubercle may be palpated in front of the radial boundary of the snuffbox.

Bones of the right hand *dorsal surface*

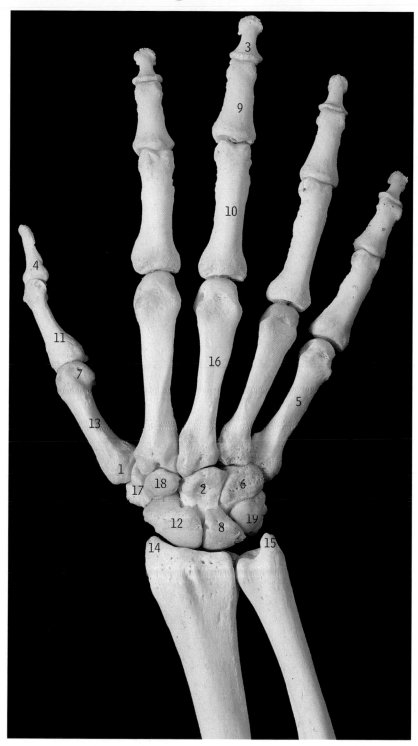

1 Base of first metacarpal
2 Capitate
3 Distal phalanx of middle finger
4 Distal phalanx of thumb
5 Fifth metacarpal
6 Hamate
7 Head of first metacarpal
8 Lunate
9 Middle phalanx of middle finger
10 Proximal phalanx of middle finger
11 Proximal phalanx of thumb
12 Scaphoid
13 Shaft of first metacarpal
14 Styloid process of radius
15 Styloid process of ulna
16 Third metacarpal
17 Trapezium
18 Trapezoid
19 Triquetral

The wrist joint (properly called the radiocarpal joint) is the joint between (proximally) the lower end of the radius and the interarticular disc which holds the lower ends of the radius and the ulna together, and (distally) the scaphoid, lunate and triquetral bones.

The midcarpal joint is the joint between the proximal and distal rows of carpal bones (see the note on page 130).

The carpometacarpal joint of the thumb is the joint between the trapezium and the base of the first metacarpal.

Colles' fracture, see p. 174.

Bones of the right hand *attachments*

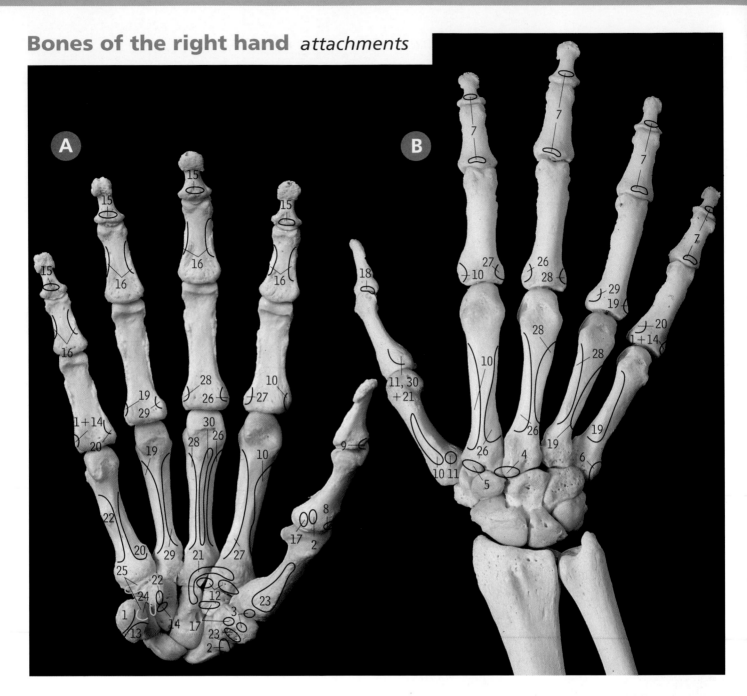

A palmar surface **B** dorsal surface

Pale green lines = ligament attachments

1	Abductor digiti minimi	**16**	Flexor digitorum superficialis
2	Abductor pollicis brevis	**17**	Flexor pollicis brevis
3	Abductor pollicis longus	**18**	Flexor pollicis longus
4	Extensor carpi radialis brevis	**19**	Fourth dorsal interosseous
5	Extensor carpi radialis longus	**20**	Fourth palmar interosseous
6	Extensor carpi ulnaris	**21**	Oblique head of adductor pollicis
7	Extensor expansion	**22**	Opponens digiti minimi
8	Extensor pollicis brevis	**23**	Opponens pollicis
9	Extensor pollicis longus	**24**	Pisohamate ligament
10	First dorsal interosseous	**25**	Pisometacarpal ligament
11	First palmar interosseous	**26**	Second dorsal interosseous
12	Flexor carpi radialis	**27**	Second palmar interosseous
13	Flexor carpi ulnaris	**28**	Third dorsal interosseous
14	Flexor digiti minimi brevis	**29**	Third palmar interosseous
15	Flexor digitorum profundus	**30**	Transverse head of adductor pollicis

The metacarpophalangeal joints are the joints between the heads of the metacarpals and the bases of the proximal phalanges.

The interphalangeal joints are the joints between the head of one phalanx and the base of the adjoining phalanx.

The pisiform is a sesamoid bone in the tendon of flexor carpi ulnaris and is anchored by the pisohamate and pisometacarpal ligaments (24 and 25).

Dorsal interossei arise from the sides of two adjacent metacarpal bones (as at 26, from the sides of the second and third metacarpals); palmar interossei arise only from the metacarpal of their own finger (as at 27, from the second metacarpal). Compare with dissection B on page 166 and note that when looking at the palm, parts of the dorsal interossei can be seen as well as the palmar interossei, but when looking at the dorsum of the hand (as on page 170A) only dorsal interossei are seen.

Right upper limb bones *secondary centres of ossification*

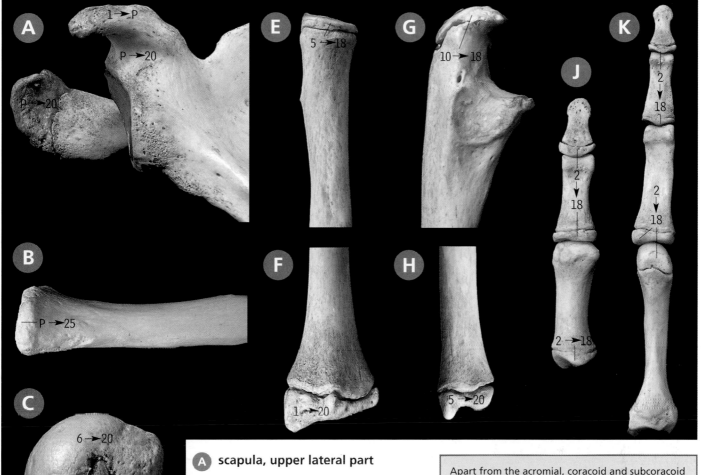

A scapula, upper lateral part

B clavicle, sternal end

C **D** humerus, upper and lower ends

E **F** radius, upper and lower ends

G **H** ulna, upper and lower ends

J first metacarpal and phalanges of thumb

K second metacarpal and phalanges of index finger

Figures in years after birth, commencement of ossification → fusion. (P = puberty)

The first figure indicates the approximate date when ossification begins in the secondary centre, and the second figure (beyond the arrowhead) when the centre finally becomes fused with the rest of the bone. Single average dates have been given (both here and for the lower limb bone centres on pages 314 and 315) and although there may be considerable individual variations, the 'growing end' of the bone (when fusion occurs last) is constant. The dates in females are often a year or more earlier than in males.

Apart from the acromial, coracoid and subcoracoid centres illustrated (A), the scapula usually has other centres for the inferior angle, medial border, and the lower part of the rim of the glenoid cavity (all P → 20; see pages 119 and 121).

The clavicle is the first bone in the body to start to ossify (fifth week of gestation). It ossifies in membrane, but the ends of the bone have a cartilaginous phase of ossification; a secondary centre appearing at the sternal end (B) unites with the body at about the twenty-fifth year.

The centre illustrated at the upper end of the humerus (C) is the result of the union at six years of centres for the head (one year), greater tubercle (three years) and lesser tubercle (five years).

At the lower end of the humerus (D) the centres for the capitulum, trochlea and lateral epicondyle fuse together before uniting with the shaft.

All the phalanges (as in K), and the first metacarpal (J) have a secondary centre at their proximal ends; the other metacarpals (as in K) have one at their distal ends.

All the carpal bones are cartilaginous at birth and none has a secondary centre. The largest, the capitate, is the first to begin to ossify (in the second month after birth), followed in a month or so by the hamate, with the triquetral at three years, lunate at four years, scaphoid, trapezoid and trapezium at five years and the pisiform last at nine years or later. There are often variations in the above common pattern.

Right shoulder

*surface markings,
from the front*

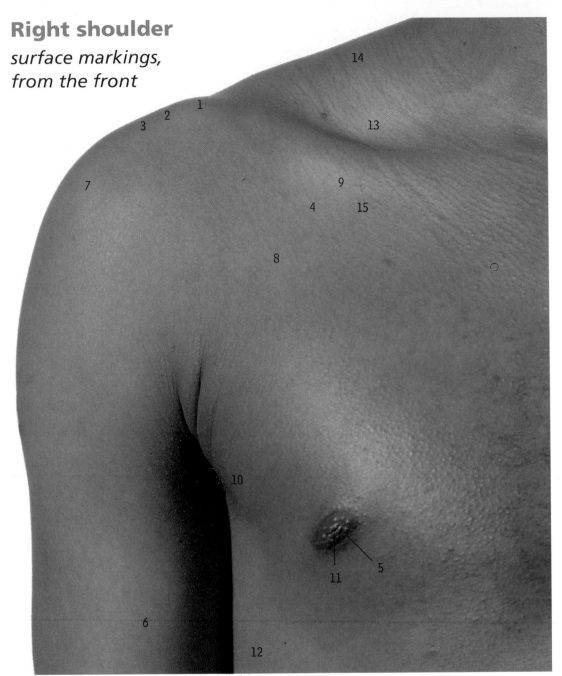

1	Acromial end of clavicle
2	Acromioclavicular joint
3	Acromion
4	Anterior margin of deltoid
5	Areola
6	Biceps
7	Deltoid overlying greater tubercle of humerus
8	Deltopectoral groove and cephalic vein
9	Infraclavicular fossa
10	Lower margin of pectoralis major
11	Nipple
12	Serratus anterior
13	Supraclavicular fossa
14	Trapezius
15	Upper margin of pectoralis major

The nipple in the male (11) normally lies at the level of the fourth intercostal space.

The lower border of pectoralis major (10) forms the anterior axillary fold.

Note that the most lateral bony point in the shoulder is the greater tubercle (7).

The clavicle is subcutaneous throughtout its length. Its acromial end (1) at the acromioclavicular joint (2) lies at a slightly higher level than the acromion of the scapula (3). At the most lateral part of the shoulder, the deltoid overlies the humerus; the acromion of the scapula does not extend so far laterally. Compare the positions of the features noted here with the dissection on the next page.

Reducing shoulder dislocations, see p. 175.

Right shoulder
*superficial
dissection*

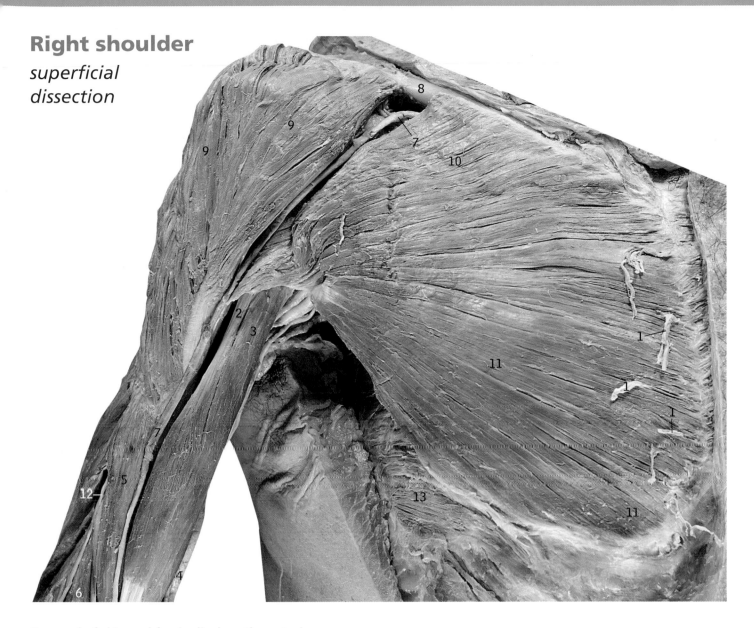

Removal of skin and fascia displays the anterior
musculature of the shoulder and thoracic wall.

1 Anterior perforating
  branches of intercostal
  neurovascular bundle
2 Biceps brachii, long head
3 Biceps brachii, short head
4 Brachial artery
5 Brachialis
6 Brachioradialis
7 Cephalic vein

8 Clavicle
9 Deltoid
10 Pectoralis major,
   clavicular head
11 Pectoralis major,
   sternal head
12 Radial nerve
13 Serratus anterior

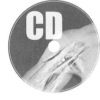

Right shoulder
superficial dissection, from the front

Removal of skin and fascia displays branches of the supraclavicular nerve (6) crossing the clavicle (9), and the cephalic vein (7) lying in the deltopectoral groove between deltoid (13) and pectoralis major (11).

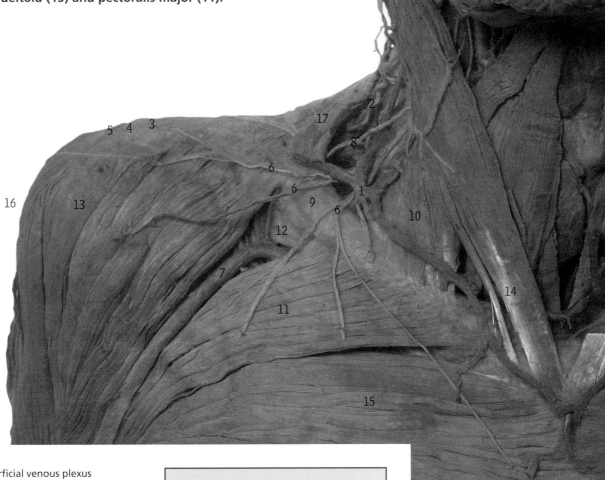

1 A superficial venous plexus
2 Accessory nerve
3 Acromial end of clavicle
4 Acromioclavicular joint
5 Acromion of scapula
6 Branches of supraclavicular nerves
7 Cephalic vein
8 Cervical nerve to trapezius
9 Clavicle
10 Clavicular head of sternocleidomastoid
11 Clavicular part of pectoralis major
12 Clavipectoral fascia
13 Deltoid
14 Sternal head of sternocleidomastoid
15 Sternocostal part of pectoralis major
16 Tip of shoulder
17 Trapezius

The position of the acromioclavicular joint (4) is indicated by the small 'step down' between the acromial end of the clavicle (3) and the acromion (5); compare with the surface feature 2 on page 134. This is the normal appearance; when the joint is dislocated, with the acromion being forced below the end of the clavicle, the 'step' is much exaggerated.

The cephalic vein (7) runs in the deltopectoral groove between deltoid (13) and pectoralis major (11) and pierces the clavipectoral fascia (12) to drain into the axillary vein.

Right shoulder *deeper dissection, from the front*

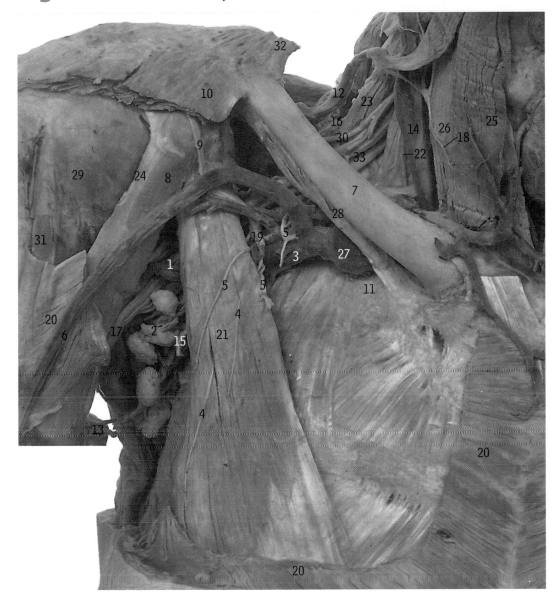

1 Anterior circumflex humeral artery and musculocutaneous nerve
2 Axillary lymph nodes
3 Axillary vein
4 Branch of medial pectoral nerve
5 Branches of lateral pectoral nerve
6 Cephalic vein
7 Clavicle
8 Coracobrachialis
9 Coracoid process and acromial branch of thoraco-acromial artery
10 Deltoid
11 First rib
12 Inferior belly of omohyoid (displaced upwards)
13 Intercostobrachial nerve
14 Internal jugular vein
15 Lateral thoracic artery
16 Long thoracic nerve (to serratus anterior)
17 Median nerve
18 Nerve to sternothyroid
19 Pectoral branch of thoraco-acromial artery
20 Pectoralis major
21 Pectoralis minor
22 Phrenic nerve overlying scalenus anterior
23 Scalenus medius
24 Short head of biceps
25 Sternohyoid
26 Sternothyroid
27 Subclavian vein
28 Subclavius
29 Subscapularis
30 Suprascapular nerve
31 Tendon of long head of biceps
32 Trapezius
33 Trunks of brachial plexus

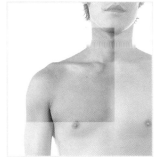

Most of deltoid (10) and pectoralis major (20) have been removed to show the underlying pectoralis minor (21) and its associated vessels and nerves. The clavipectoral fascia which passes between the clavicle (7) and the upper (medial) border of the pectoralis minor (21) has also been removed to show the axillary vein (3) receiving the cephalic vein (6) and continuing as the subclavian vein (27) as it crosses the first rib (11).

 Insertion of a central venous line, Klumpke's paralysis, see p. 175.

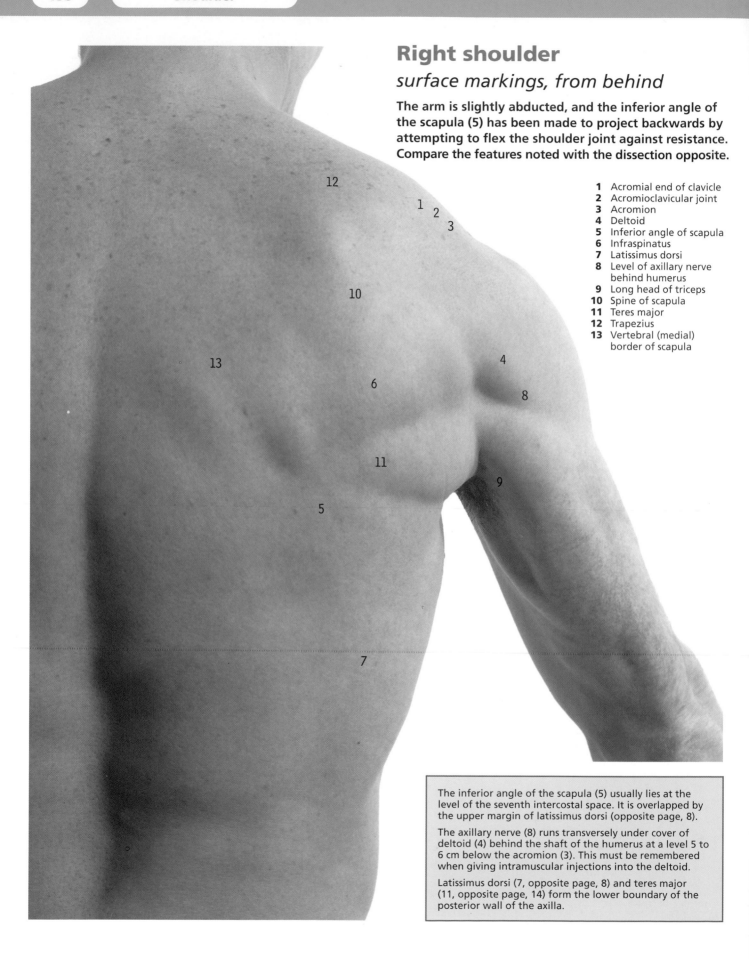

Right shoulder
surface markings, from behind

The arm is slightly abducted, and the inferior angle of the scapula (5) has been made to project backwards by attempting to flex the shoulder joint against resistance. Compare the features noted with the dissection opposite.

1 Acromial end of clavicle
2 Acromioclavicular joint
3 Acromion
4 Deltoid
5 Inferior angle of scapula
6 Infraspinatus
7 Latissimus dorsi
8 Level of axillary nerve behind humerus
9 Long head of triceps
10 Spine of scapula
11 Teres major
12 Trapezius
13 Vertebral (medial) border of scapula

The inferior angle of the scapula (5) usually lies at the level of the seventh intercostal space. It is overlapped by the upper margin of latissimus dorsi (opposite page, 8).

The axillary nerve (8) runs transversely under cover of deltoid (4) behind the shaft of the humerus at a level 5 to 6 cm below the acromion (3). This must be remembered when giving intramuscular injections into the deltoid.

Latissimus dorsi (7, opposite page, 8) and teres major (11, opposite page, 14) form the lower boundary of the posterior wall of the axilla.

Right shoulder *superficial dissection, from behind*

From above and below, trapezius (16) converges on to the spine of the scapula (13). The upper margin of latissimus dorsi (9) overlaps the inferior angle of the scapula and the lowest part of teres major (14). The long head of triceps (10) is seen emerging between teres minor (15) and teres major (14). As at the front, deltoid (5) covers the shoulder joint and upper part of the humerus.

The triangle of auscultation (17) is bounded by the trapezius, latissimus dorsi, and the medial border of the scapula; its floor is partly formed by rhomboid major. If the arms are brought forwards, the sixth intercostal space becomes available for auscultation.

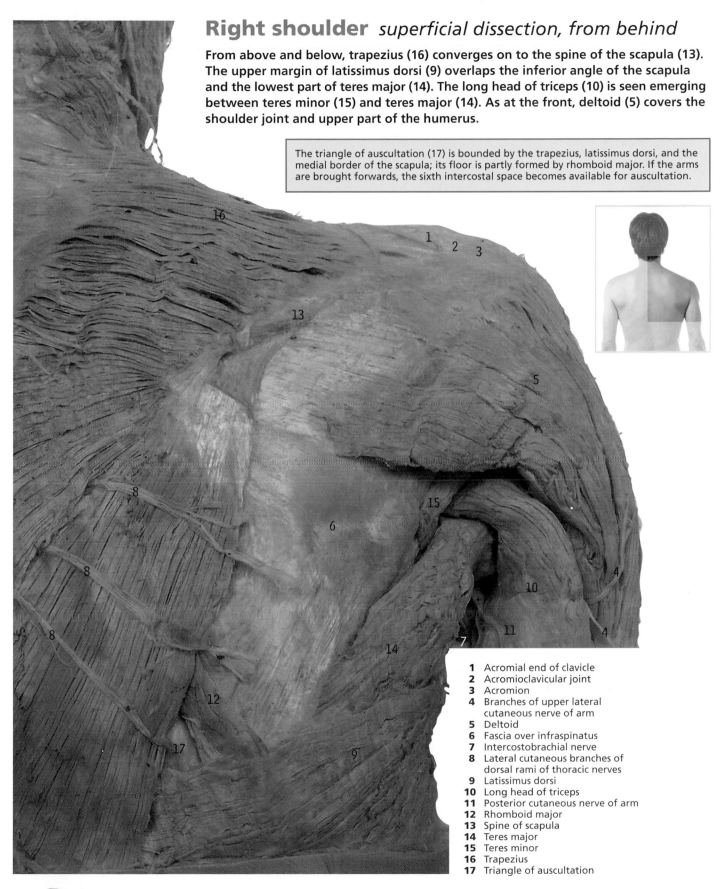

1 Acromial end of clavicle
2 Acromioclavicular joint
3 Acromion
4 Branches of upper lateral cutaneous nerve of arm
5 Deltoid
6 Fascia over infraspinatus
7 Intercostobrachial nerve
8 Lateral cutaneous branches of dorsal rami of thoracic nerves
9 Latissimus dorsi
10 Long head of triceps
11 Posterior cutaneous nerve of arm
12 Rhomboid major
13 Spine of scapula
14 Teres major
15 Teres minor
16 Trapezius
17 Triangle of auscultation

 Intramuscular injections, see p. 175.

Right shoulder *from behind*

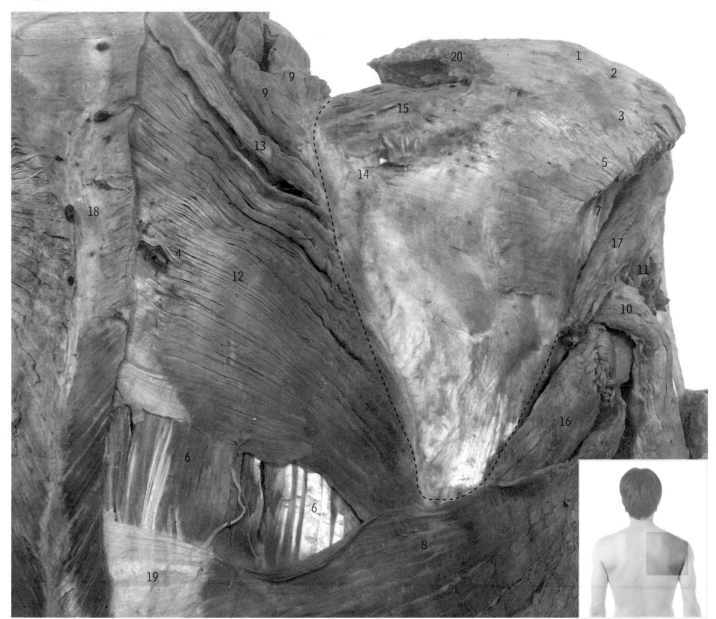

Interrupted line = outline of scapula

Most of trapezius (20) and deltoid (5) have been removed to show the underlying muscles. The medial cut edge of trapezius remains near the line of the thoracic spines (18). Levator scapulae (9), rhomboid minor (13) and rhomboid major (12) are seen converging on to the vertebral (medial) border of the scapula, and supraspinatus (15) lies above the spine of the scapula (14).

1	Acromial end of clavicle	12	Rhomboid major
2	Acromioclavicular joint	13	Rhomboid minor
3	Acromion	14	Spine of scapula
4	Branch of dorsal ramus	15	Supraspinatus
	of a thoracic nerve	16	Teres major
5	Deltoid	17	Teres minor
6	Erector spinae	18	Third thoracic spinous
7	Infraspinatus		process
8	Latissimus dorsi	19	Thoracic part of
9	Levator scapulae		thoracolumbar fascia
10	Long head of triceps	20	Trapezius
11	Posterior circumflex humeral		
	vessels and axillary nerve		

Ⓐ Right shoulder *from the right and behind*

The central parts of supraspinatus (13) and infraspinatus (5) have been removed to show the suprascapular nerve (12) which supplies both muscles. The removal of parts of infraspinatus and teres minor (15) displays the anastomosis between the circumflex scapular branch of the subscapular artery (3) and the suprascapular artery (11). Deltoid (4) has been reflected laterally to show the axillary nerve (2) and the posterior circumflex humeral vessels passing backwards through the quadrilateral space (see note below).

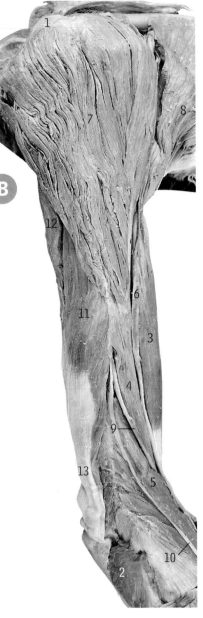

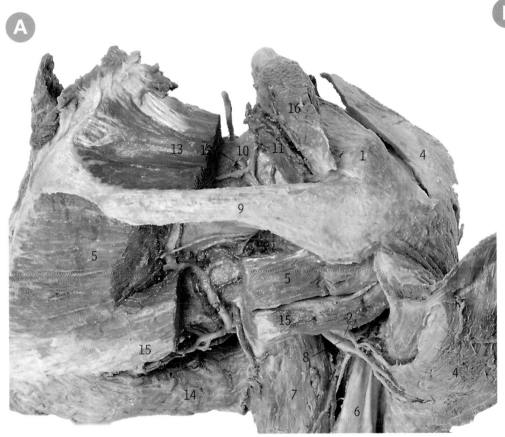

1	Acromioclavicular joint
2	Axillary nerve
3	Circumflex scapular artery
4	Deltoid
5	Infraspinatus
6	Lateral head of triceps
7	Long head of triceps
8	Posterior circumflex humeral artery
9	Spine of scapula
10	Superior transverse scapular (suprascapular) ligament
11	Suprascapular artery
12	Suprascapular nerve
13	Supraspinatus
14	Teres major
15	Teres minor
16	Trapezius

The axillary nerve (A2) and posterior circumflex humeral vessels (A8) pass backwards through the quadrilateral space which (viewed from behind) is bounded by teres minor (A15) above, below by teres major (A14), medially by the long head of triceps (A7), and laterally by the humerus. (Viewed from the front, the upper boundary of the space is subscapularis – see page 146, 23.)

Ⓑ Right shoulder and upper arm *from the right*

Deltoid (7) extends over the tip of the shoulder to its attachment halfway down the lateral side of the shaft of the humerus. Biceps (3) is on the front of the arm below pectoralis major (8) and triceps (11 and 12) is at the back.

1	Acromion	8	Pectoralis major
2	Anconeus	9	Radial nerve
3	Biceps brachii	10	Radial nerve, cutaneous branch
4	Brachialis	11	Triceps, lateral head
5	Brachioradialis	12	Triceps, long head
6	Cephalic vein	13	Triceps, tendon
7	Deltoid		

Right shoulder joint Ⓐ *horizontal section* Ⓑ *axial MR image*

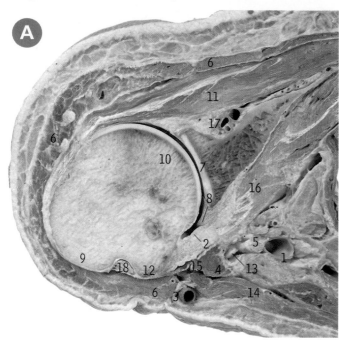

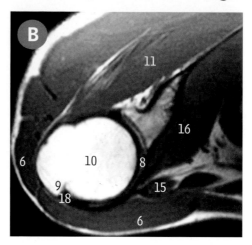

Viewed from above, this section shows the articulation of the head of the humerus (10) with the glenoid cavity of the scapula (7). The tendon of the long head of biceps (18) lies in the groove between the greater and lesser tubercles of the humerus (9 and 12). Subscapularis (16) passes immediately in front of the joint, and infraspinatus (11) behind it. Compare the MR image in B with features in A.

1	Axillary artery	11	Infraspinatus
2	Capsule	12	Lesser tubercle
3	Cephalic vein	13	Musculocutaneous
4	Coracobrachialis		nerve
5	Cords of brachial	14	Pectoralis major
	plexus	15	Short head of biceps
6	Deltoid	16	Subscapularis
7	Glenoid cavity	17	Suprascapular nerve
8	Glenoid labrum		and vessels
9	Greater tubercle	18	Tendon of long head of
10	Head of humerus		biceps in intertubercular
			groove

Right shoulder joint
from the front

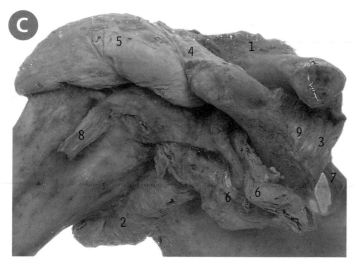

The synovial joint cavity inside the capsule (2) and the subacromial bursa (5) have been injected separately with green resin.

1 Acromioclavicular joint
2 Capsule of shoulder joint
3 Conoid ligament
4 Coraco-acromial ligament
5 Subacromial bursa
6 Subscapularis bursa
7 Superior transverse scapular (suprascapular) ligament
8 Tendon of long head of biceps
9 Trapezoid ligament

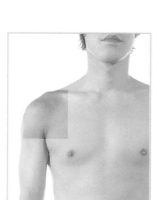

Shoulder *coronal MR arthrogram*

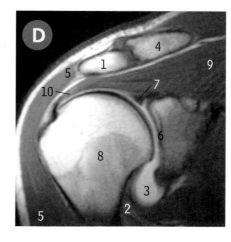

1 Acromion
2 Axillary nerve and circumflex humeral vessels
3 Axillary recess of shoulder joint
4 Clavicle
5 Deltoid
6 Glenoid cavity
7 Glenoid labrum
8 Humerus
9 Supraspinatus muscle
10 Supraspinatus tendon

Right shoulder joint *opened from behind*

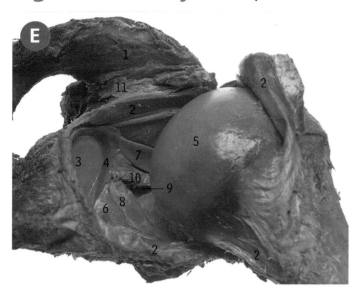

In this view, after removing all the posterior part of the capsule, the inner surface of the front of the capsule (2) is seen, with its reinforcing glenohumeral ligaments (6, 8 and 10).

1 Acromion
2 Capsule
3 Glenoid cavity
4 Glenoid labrum
5 Head of humerus
6 Inferior glenohumeral ligament

7 Long head of biceps
8 Middle glenohumeral ligament
9 Opening into subscapularis bursa
10 Superior glenohumeral ligament
11 Supraspinatus

The joint cavity communicates with the subscapularis bursa through an opening (9) between the superior (10) and middle (8) glenohumeral ligaments.

The tendon of the long head of biceps (7) is continuous with the glenoid labrum (4).

Shoulder *radiographs*

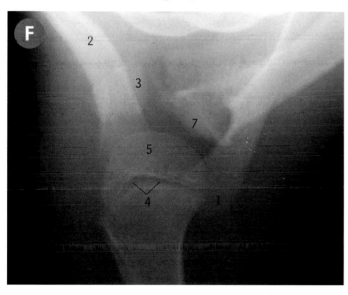

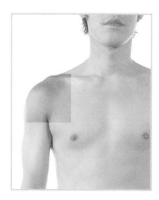

F axial projection in a six-year-old child

G anteroposterior projection in a nine-year-old child

In F the head of the humerus (5) lies against the glenoid cavity of the scapula (7), whose coracoid process (3) is seen end-on. In G note the epiphysial line (4) at the upper end of the humerus.

1 Acromion
2 Clavicle
3 Coracoid process
4 Epiphysial line

5 Head of humerus
6 Lateral border of scapula
7 Rim of glenoid cavity
8 Spine of scapula

The upper humeral epiphysis is a compound structure made up of epiphyses for the head, and greater and lesser tubercles. It rests on the spike-like upper humeral shaft, giving the appearance of an inverted V to the epiphysial line on the radiograph (G4). Compare with page 133, C.

 Supraspinatus tendon calcification, supraspinatus tendinitis, rotator cuff tears, bicipital tendinitis, see pp 174, 175.

Right axilla *anterior wall*

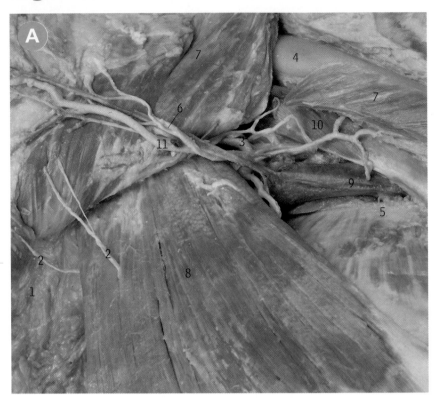

Pectoralis major (7) has been reflected upwards and laterally, and the clavipectoral fascia which passes from subclavius (10) to pectoralis minor (8) has been removed.

1   Axillary sheath
2   Branches of medial pectoral nerve
3   Cephalic vein
4   Clavicle
5   First rib
6   Lateral pectoral nerve
7   Pectoralis major
8   Pectoralis minor
9   Subclavian vein
10   Subclavius
11   Thoraco-acromial vessels

> The clavipectoral fascia (here removed, between subclavius, 10, and pectoralis minor, 8) is pierced by the cephalic vein (3), thoraco-acromial vessels (11), lateral pectoral nerve (6) and lymphatics.
>
> The axillary sheath (1) is the downward continuation of the prevertebral fascia of the neck and forms a dense covering for the axillary artery and the surrounding parts of the brachial plexus.
>
> The lateral pectoral nerve (6) is related to the medial (upper) border of pectoralis minor (8). The medial pectoral nerve (2) is related to the lateral (lower) border of pectoralis minor.

Right axilla and brachial plexus *from the front*

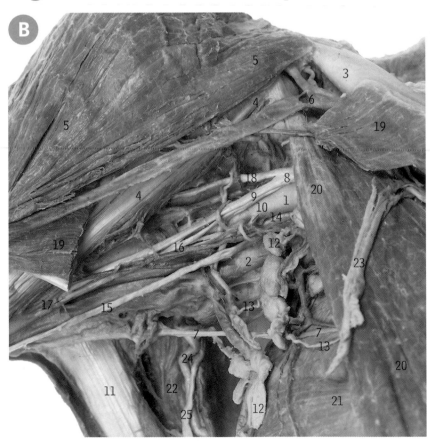

Pectoralis major (19) has been reflected and the clavipectoral fascia removed, together with the axillary sheath (A1) which surrounded the axillary artery and brachial plexus.

1   Axillary artery
2   Axillary vein
3   Clavicle
4   Coracobrachialis
5   Deltoid
6   Entry of cephalic vein into deltoid vein
7   Intercostobrachial nerve
8   Lateral cord of brachial plexus
9   Lateral root of median nerve
10   Lateral thoracic artery
11   Latissimus dorsi
12   Lymph nodes
13   Lymph vessels
14   Medial cord brachial plexus
15   Medial cutaneous nerve of arm
16   Medial root of median nerve
17   Median nerve
18   Musculocutaneous nerve
19   Pectoralis major
20   Pectoralis minor
21   Serratus anterior
22   Subscapularis
23   Thoraco-acromial vessels and lateral pectoral nerve
24   Thoracodorsal artery
25   Thoracodorsal nerve

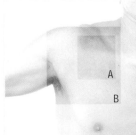

Right brachial plexus *from the front*

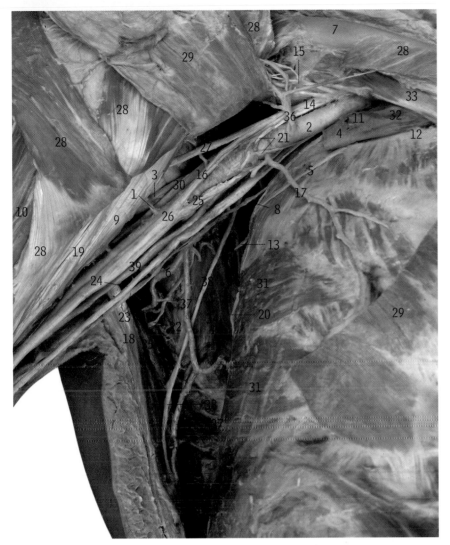

Pectoralis major and minor (28 and 29) have been reflected and the axillary sheath (page 144, A1) removed, together with most of the axillary vein (4) and its tributaries.

1 Anterior circumflex humeral artery
2 Axillary artery
3 Axillary nerve
4 Axillary vein
5 Branch from first thoracic nerve to intercostobrachial nerve
6 Circumflex scapular artery
7 Clavicle
8 Communication between 23 and 13
9 Coracobrachialis and short head of biceps
10 Deltoid
11 Entry of cephalic vein
12 First rib
13 Intercostobrachial nerve (cut end)
14 Lateral cord
15 Lateral pectoral nerve
16 Lateral root of median nerve
17 Lateral thoracic artery
18 Latissimus dorsi
19 Long head of biceps
20 Long thoracic nerve
21 Loop between medial and lateral pectoral nerves
22 Lower subscapular nerve
23 Medial cutaneous nerve of arm
24 Medial cutaneous nerve of forearm
25 Medial root of median nerve
26 Median nerve
27 Musculocutaneous nerve
28 Pectoralis major
29 Pectoralis minor
30 Radial nerve
31 Serratus anterior
32 Subclavian vein
33 Subclavius
34 Subscapularis
35 Teres major
36 Thoraco-acromial artery
37 Thoracodorsal artery
38 Thoracodorsal nerve
39 Ulnar nerve

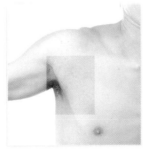

Erb's paralysis (Erb-Duchenne palsy), winging of the scapula, see pp 175, 176.

Right brachial plexus and branches

In this front view of the plexus, all the blood vessels have been removed to show the cords of the plexus and their branches more clearly. Note the 'capital M' pattern formed by the musculocutaneous nerve (18), the lateral root of the median nerve (8), the median nerve itself (17), the medial root of the median nerve (16) and the ulnar nerve (26). In this specimen the tendon of latissimus dorsi (9) is unusually broad and has become blended with the long head of triceps (10).

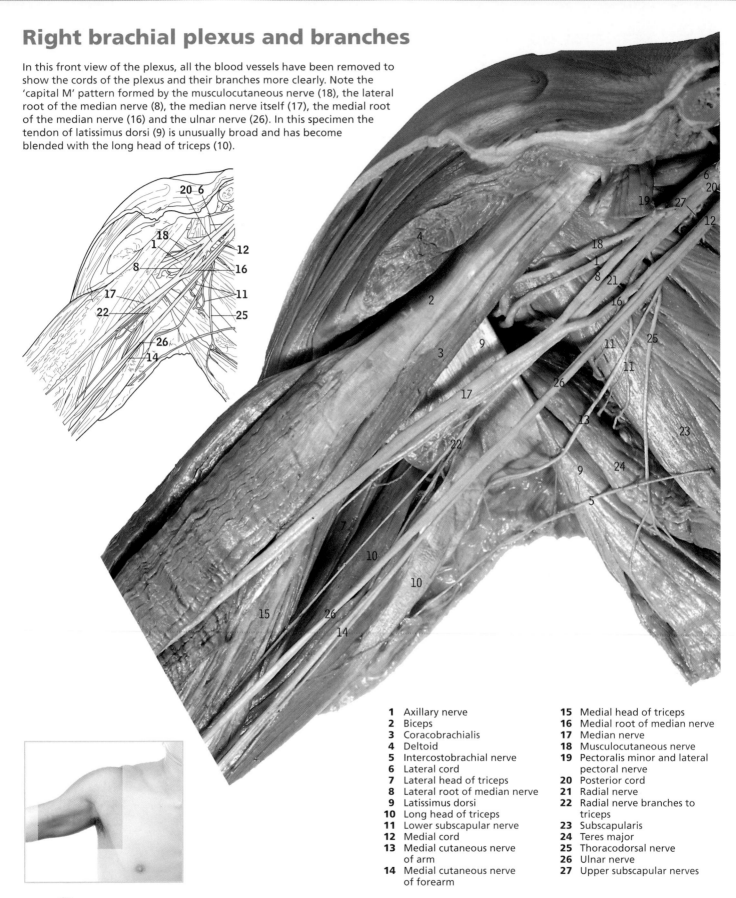

1 Axillary nerve	**15** Medial head of triceps
2 Biceps	**16** Medial root of median nerve
3 Coracobrachialis	**17** Median nerve
4 Deltoid	**18** Musculocutaneous nerve
5 Intercostobrachial nerve	**19** Pectoralis minor and lateral
6 Lateral cord	pectoral nerve
7 Lateral head of triceps	**20** Posterior cord
8 Lateral root of median nerve	**21** Radial nerve
9 Latissimus dorsi	**22** Radial nerve branches to
10 Long head of triceps	triceps
11 Lower subscapular nerve	**23** Subscapularis
12 Medial cord	**24** Teres major
13 Medial cutaneous nerve	**25** Thoracodorsal nerve
of arm	**26** Ulnar nerve
14 Medial cutaneous nerve	**27** Upper subscapular nerves
of forearm	

Axillary nerve paralysis, see p. 174.

Right arm *vessels and nerves, from the front*

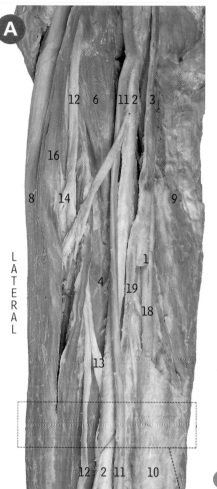

Biceps (16 and 8) has been turned laterally to show the musculocutaneous nerve (12) emerging from coracobrachialis (6), giving branches to biceps and brachialis (14 and 13) and becoming the lateral cutaneous nerve of the forearm (7) on the lateral side of the biceps tendon (17).

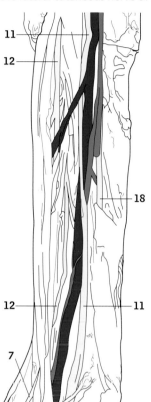

The median nerve (11) gradually crosses over in front of the brachial artery (2) from the lateral to the medial side. The ulnar nerve (18) passes behind the medial intermuscular septum (10), and the end of the basilic vein (1) is seen joining a vena comitans (19) of the brachial artery to form the brachial vein (3).

1	Basilic vein (cut end)	**11**	Median nerve
2	Brachial artery	**12**	Musculocutaneous nerve
3	Brachial vein	**13**	Nerve to brachialis
4	Brachialis	**14**	Nerve to short head of
5	Brachioradialis		biceps
6	Coracobrachialis	**15**	Pronator teres
7	Lateral cutaneous nerve	**16**	Short head of biceps
	of forearm	**17**	Tendon of biceps
8	Long head of biceps	**18**	Ulnar nerve
9	Long head of triceps	**19**	Vena comitans of
10	Medial intermuscular		brachial artery
	septum		

The musculocutaneous nerve (A12) supplies coracobrachialis (A6), biceps (A16 and 8) and brachialis (A4), and at the level where the muscle fibres of biceps become tendinous (A17) it pierces the deep fascia to become the lateral cutaneous nerve of the forearm (A7).

The median nerve does not give off any muscular branches in the arm.

The ulnar nerve (A18) leaves the anterior compartment of the arm by piercing the medial intermuscular septum (A10), and does not give off any muscular branches in the arm.

B Right arm *cross section, from below*

Looking from the elbow towards the shoulder, the section is taken through the middle of the arm. The musculocutaneous nerve (9) lies between brachialis (4) and biceps (2), and the median nerve (8) is on the medial side of the brachial artery (3) which has several venae comitantes adjacent (unlabelled). The ulnar nerve (13), with the superior ulnar collateral artery (11) beside it, is behind the median nerve (8) and the basilic vein (1). The radial nerve and the profunda brachii vessels (10) are in the posterior compartment at the lateral side of the humerus (6).

FRONT

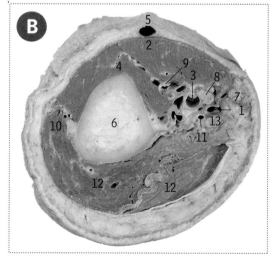

1	Basilic vein
2	Biceps
3	Brachial artery
4	Brachialis
5	Cephalic vein
6	Humerus
7	Medial cutaneous nerve of
	forearm
8	Median nerve
9	Musculocutaneous nerve
10	Radial nerve and profunda
	brachii vessels
11	Superior ulnar collateral artery
12	Triceps
13	Ulnar nerve

Right arm *posterior view*

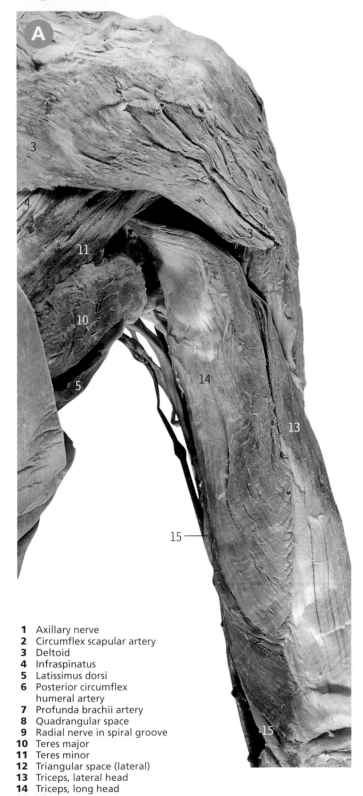

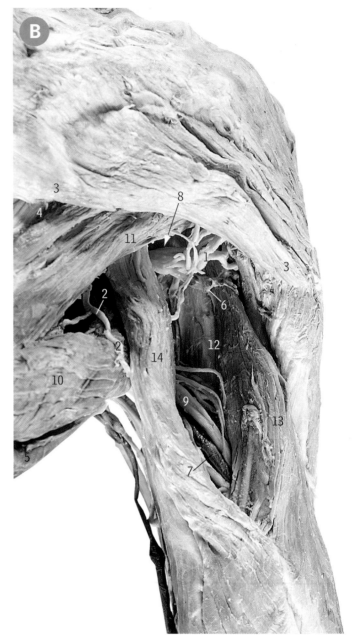

1 Axillary nerve
2 Circumflex scapular artery
3 Deltoid
4 Infraspinatus
5 Latissimus dorsi
6 Posterior circumflex
  humeral artery
7 Profunda brachii artery
8 Quadrangular space
9 Radial nerve in spiral groove
10 Teres major
11 Teres minor
12 Triangular space (lateral)
13 Triceps, lateral head
14 Triceps, long head
15 Ulnar nerve

Ⓐ after removal of skin and
  subcutaneous fat

Ⓑ after muscle separation
  to demonstrate spaces
  and neurovascular bundle

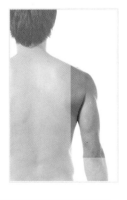

 Radial nerve paralysis, see p. 175.

Left elbow

C *surface markings, from behind* **D** *superficial dissection, from behind*

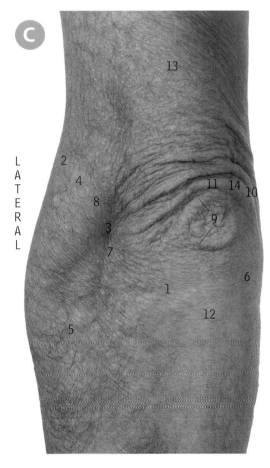

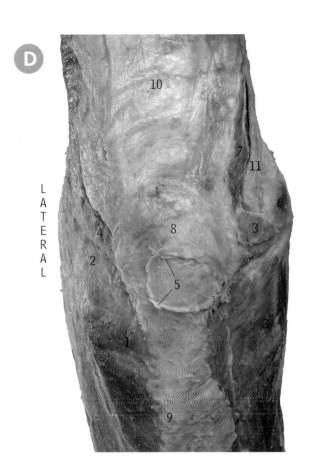

With the elbow fully extended, the extensor muscles (5, 4) form a bulge on the lateral side. In the adjacent hollow can be felt the head of the radius (7) and the capitulum of the humerus (3) which indicate the line of the humeroradial part of the elbow joint. The lateral and medial epicondyles of the humerus (8 and 10) are palpable on each side. Wrinkled skin lies at the back of the prominent olecranon of the ulna (11), and in this arm the margin of the olecranon bursa (9) is outlined. The most important structure in this region is the ulnar nerve (14) which is palpable as it lies in contact with the humerus behind the medial epicondyle (10). The posterior border of the ulna (12) is subcutaneous throughout its whole length.

1 Anconeus	**9** Margin of olecranon bursa
2 Brachioradialis	**10** Medial epicondyle of humerus
3 Capitulum of humerus	**11** Olecranon of ulna
4 Extensor carpi radialis longus	**12** Posterior border of ulna
5 Extensor muscles	**13** Triceps
6 Flexor carpi ulnaris	**14** Ulnar nerve
7 Head of radius	
8 Lateral epicondyle of humerus	

Skin and subcutaneous tissue and some deep fascia have been removed, but the margin of the olecranon bursa (5) has been preserved. The ulnar nerve (11) is behind the medial epicondyle (6) and passes downwards under cover of flexor carpi ulnaris (3).

1 Anconeus
2 Common extensor origin
3 Flexor carpi ulnaris
4 Lateral epicondyle of humerus
5 Margin of olecranon bursa
6 Medial epicondyle of humerus
7 Medial head of triceps
8 Olecranon of ulna
9 Posterior border of ulna
10 Triceps tendon
11 Ulnar nerve

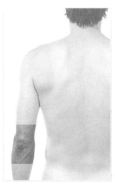

 Olecranon bursitis, triceps tendon reflex, ulnar nerve paralysis, see pp 175, 176.

Left elbow joint and proximal radio-ulnar joint

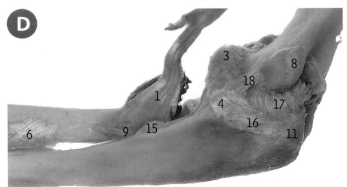

A

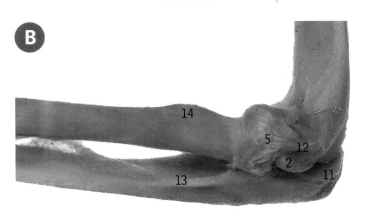

B

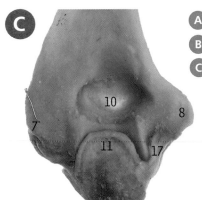

C

Right elbow joint and proximal radio-ulnar joint

D

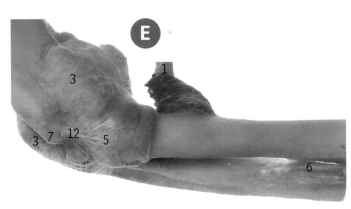

E

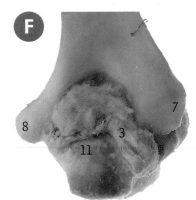

F

A   from the medial side
B   from the lateral side
C   from behind

D   from the medial side
E   from the lateral side
F   from behind

In A, B and C the forearm is flexed to a right angle. In D, E and F the forearm is partially flexed, and the synovial cavity within the capsule (3) and the bursa beneath the biceps tendon (1) have been injected with green resin.

1   Biceps tendon and underlying bursa
2   Capitulum
3   Capsule (distended)
4   Coronoid process of ulna
5   Head and neck of radius covered by annular ligament
6   Interosseous membrane
7   Lateral epicondyle
8   Medial epicondyle
9   Oblique cord
10   Olecranon fossa
11   Olecranon process of ulna
12   Radial collateral ligament
13   Supinator crest of ulna
14   Tuberosity of radius
15   Tuberosity of ulna
16   Ulnar collateral ligament: oblique band
17   Ulnar collateral ligament: posterior band
18   Ulnar collateral ligament: upper band

The synovial cavity of the proximal radio-ulnar joint is continuous with that of the elbow joint (the synovial cavity of the distal radio-ulnar joint is *not* continuous with that of the wrist joint).

The main ligaments of the elbow and proximal radio-ulnar joints are the capsule (3), the ulnar and radial collateral ligaments (16 to 18 and 12) and the annular ligament (5).

Dislocation of the radial head, see p. 175.

Left elbow joint

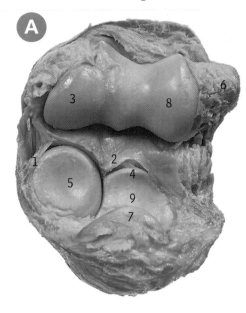

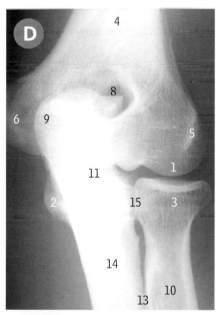

A **opened from behind**

The joint has been 'forced open' from behind: the capitulum (3) and trochlea (8) of the lower end of the humerus are seen from below with the forearm in forced flexion to show the upper ends of the radius and ulna (5 and 9) from above.

1 Annular ligament
2 Anterior part of capsule
3 Capitulum of humerus
4 Coronoid process of ulna
5 Head of radius
6 Medial epicondyle of humerus
7 Olecranon process of ulna
8 Trochlea of humerus
9 Trochlear notch of ulna

Elbow *radiograph*

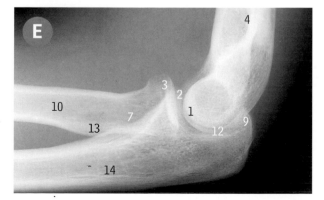

D **anterior projection**

E **lateral projection**

1 Capitulum of humerus
2 Coronoid process of ulna
3 Head of radius
4 Humerus
5 Lateral epicondyle of humerus
6 Medial epicondyle of humerus
7 Neck of radius
8 Olecranon fossa of humerus
9 Olecranon process of ulna
10 Radius
11 Trochlea of humerus
12 Trochlear notch of ulna
13 Tuberosity of radius
14 Ulna
15 Radioulnar joint

Left elbow

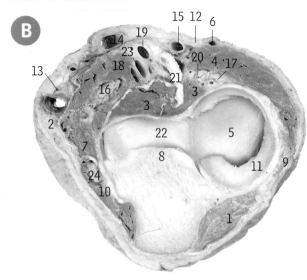

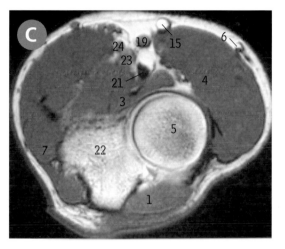

B **cross-section**   **C** **axial MR image**

The section is viewed from below, looking towards the shoulder, and is just below the point where the brachial artery has divided into radial and ulnar arteries (19 and 23). The cut has passed immediately below the trochlea (22) and capitulum (5) of the humerus, and has gone through the coronoid process of the ulna (8). The radial nerve (20) and its posterior interosseous branch (17) lie between brachioradialis (4) and brachialis (3). The median nerve (16) is under the main part of pronator teres (18), and the ulnar nerve (24) is passing under flexor carpi ulnaris (10).

1 Anconeus
2 Basilic vein
3 Brachialis
4 Brachioradialis
5 Capitulum of humerus
6 Cephalic vein
7 Common flexor origin
8 Coronoid process of ulna
9 Extensor carpi radialis longus and brevis
10 Flexor carpi ulnaris
11 Fringe of synovial membrane
12 Lateral cutaneous nerve of forearm
13 Medial cutaneous nerve of forearm
14 Median basilic vein
15 Median cephalic vein
16 Median nerve
17 Posterior interosseous nerve
18 Pronator teres
19 Radial artery
20 Radial nerve
21 Tendon of biceps
22 Trochlea of humerus
23 Ulnar artery
24 Ulnar nerve

Left cubital fossa
A *surface markings* **B** *superficial veins*

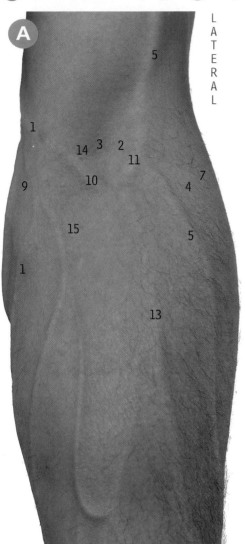

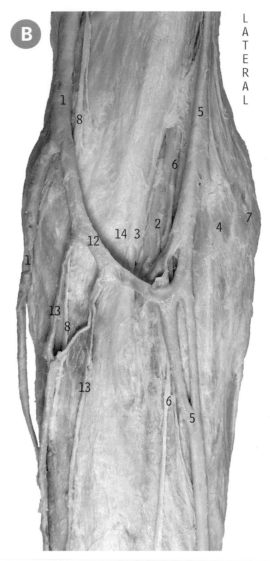

1 Basilic vein
2 Biceps tendon
3 Brachial artery
4 Brachioradialis
5 Cephalic vein
6 Lateral cutaneous nerve
   of forearm
7 Lateral epicondyle
8 Medial cutaneous nerve
   of forearm
9 Medial epicondyle
10 Median basilic vein
11 Median cephalic vein
12 Median cubital vein
13 Median forearm vein
14 Median nerve
15 Pronator teres

The superficial veins on the front of the elbow such as the cephalic (5) and basilic (1) and their intercommunicating tributaries are those most commonly used for intravenous injections and obtaining specimens of venous blood. The pattern of veins is typically M-shaped (as in A) or H-shaped (as in B), but there is much variation and it is not always possible or necessary to name every vessel.

The order of the structures in the cubital fossa from lateral to medial is: biceps tendon (2), brachial artery (3) and median nerve (14).

In A there is an M-shaped pattern of superficial veins (see notes). In B the cephalic (5) and basilic (1) veins are joined by a median cubital vein (12) into which drain two small median forearm veins (13). In C (page 153) the deep fascia has been removed but the bicipital aponeurosis (C2) is preserved; it runs downwards and medially from the biceps tendon (B2), crossing the brachial artery (C3) and the median nerve (C9). The musculocutaneous nerve becomes the lateral cutaneous nerve of the forearm (B6, C8) at the lateral border of biceps where the muscle becomes tendinous. Brachioradialis (A4, B4, C5) forms the lateral boundary and pronator teres (A15, C12) the medial boundary of the cubital fossa. The brachial arteriogram in D (page 153) outlines the main arteries (D2, 5 and 7).

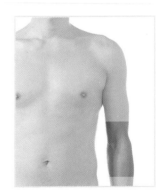

Auscultation of the brachial pulse, biceps tendon reflex, golfer's elbow, tennis elbow, see pp 174, 175, 176.

Left elbow and upper forearm

C *from the front* **D** *brachial arteriogram*

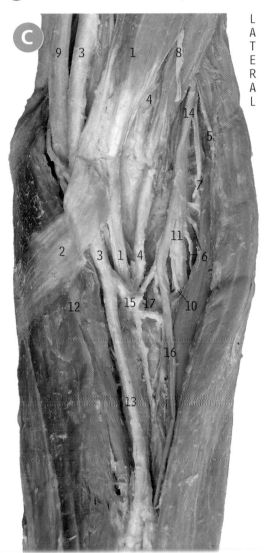

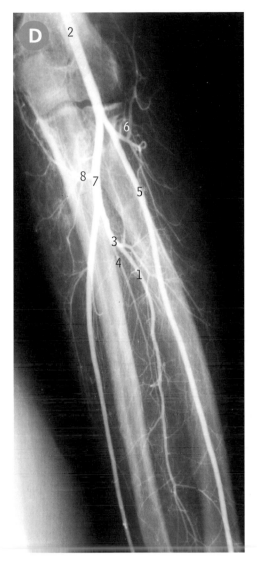

Brachioradialis (5) and extensor carpi radialis longus (7) have been displaced laterally to show the radial nerve (14) giving off branches to those muscles and then dividing into the superficial (cutaneous) branch (16) and the deep (posterior interosseous) branch (11) which enters supinator.

1 Anterior interosseous artery	**5** Radial artery
2 Brachial artery	**6** Radial recurrent artery
3 Common interosseous artery	**7** Ulnar artery
4 Posterior interosseous artery	**8** Ulnar recurrent artery

1 Biceps	**9** Median nerve
2 Bicipital aponeurosis	**10** Nerve to supinator
3 Brachial artery	**11** Posterior interosseous nerve
4 Brachialis	**12** Pronator teres
5 Brachioradialis and nerve	**13** Radial artery
6 Branches to extensor carpi radialis brevis	**14** Radial nerve
	15 Radial recurrent artery
7 Extensor carpi radialis longus and nerve	**16** Superficial branch of radial nerve
8 Lateral cutaneous nerve of forearm	**17** Supinator

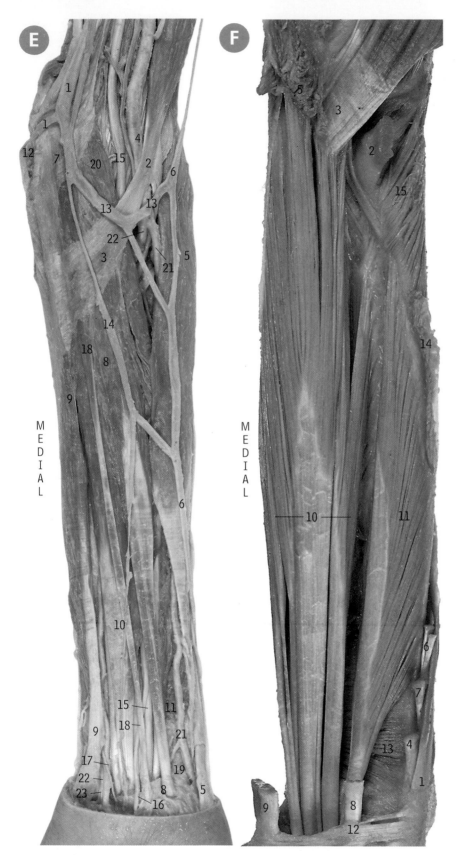

E Left forearm

superficial muscles, from the front

Skin and fascia have been removed, but the larger superficial veins (1, 6 and 13) have been preserved. On the lateral side the radial artery (21) is largely covered by brachioradialis (5). At the wrist the tendon of flexor carpi radialis (8) has the radial artery (21) on its lateral side; on its medial side is the median nerve (15), slightly overlapped from the medial side by the tendon of palmaris longus (18) (if present; it is absent in 13 per cent of arms).

1 Basilic vein	**12** Medial epicondyle
2 Biceps tendon	**13** Median cubital vein
3 Bicipital aponeurosis	**14** Median forearm vein
4 Brachial artery	**15** Median nerve
5 Brachioradialis	**16** Palmar branch of median nerve
6 Cephalic vein	**17** Palmar branch of ulnar nerve
7 Common flexor origin	**18** Palmaris longus
8 Flexor carpi radialis	**19** Pronator quadratus
9 Flexor carpi ulnaris	**20** Pronator teres
10 Flexor digitorum superficialis	**21** Radial artery
11 Flexor pollicis longus	**22** Ulnar artery
	23 Ulnar nerve

F Left forearm

deep muscles, from the front

All vessels and nerves have been removed, together with the superficial muscles, to show the deep flexor group – flexor digitorum profundus (10), flexor pollicis longus (11) and pronator quadratus (13).

1 Abductor pollicis longus	
2 Biceps	
3 Brachialis	
4 Brachioradialis	
5 Common flexor origin	
6 Extensor carpi radialis brevis	
7 Extensor carpi radialis longus	
8 Flexor carpi radialis	
9 Flexor carpi ulnaris	
10 Flexor digitorum profundus	
11 Flexor pollicis longus	
12 Flexor retinaculum	
13 Pronator quadratus	
14 Pronator teres	
15 Supinator	

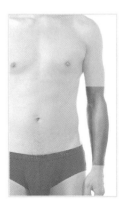

 Venous cutdown, venepuncture of the upper limb, see p. 176.

Ⓐ Right cubital fossa and forearm *arteries*

The arteries have been injected, and after removal of most of the superficial muscles the brachial artery (4) is seen dividing into the radial artery (18) and the ulnar artery (20). The radial artery gives off the radial recurrent (19) which runs upwards in front of supinator, giving branches to the carpal extensor muscles (10 and 9). The ulnar artery gives off the anterior and posterior ulnar recurrent vessels (2 and 15), and its common interosseous branch (8) is seen giving off the anterior interosseous (1) which passes down in front of the interosseous membrane between flexor pollicis longus (13) and flexor digitorum profundus (12).

1   Anterior interosseous artery overlying interosseous membrane
2   Anterior ulnar recurrent artery
3   Biceps tendon
4   Brachial artery
5   Brachialis
6   Brachioradialis
7   Common flexor origin
8   Common interosseous artery
9   Extensor carpi radialis brevis
10   Extensor carpi radialis longus
11   Flexor carpi ulnaris
12   Flexor digitorum profundus
13   Flexor pollicis longus
14   Medial epicondyle of humerus
15   Posterior ulnar recurrent artery
16   Pronator quadratus
17   Pronator teres
18   Radial artery
19   Radial recurrent artery overlying supinator
20   Ulnar artery

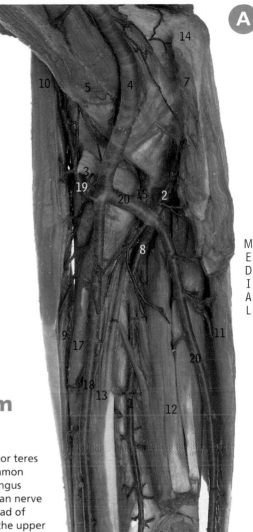

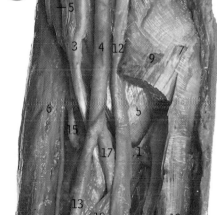

Ⓑ Right cubital fossa and forearm

arteries and nerves

Most of the humeral origins of pronator teres and flexor carpi radialis (from the common flexor origin, 9 and 7) and palmaris longus have been removed to show the median nerve (12) passing superficial to the deep head of pronator teres (18) and then deep to the upper border of the radial head of flexor digitorum superficialis (14).

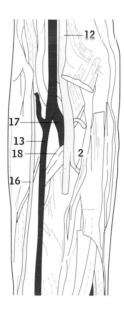

1   A muscular branch of median nerve
2   Anterior interosseous nerve
3   Biceps
4   Brachial artery
5   Brachialis
6   Brachioradialis (displaced laterally)
7   Common flexor origin
8   Flexor carpi ulnaris (displaced medially)
9   Humeral head of pronator teres
10   Humero-ulnar head of flexor digitorum superficialis
11   Lateral cutaneous nerve of forearm
12   Median nerve
13   Radial artery
14   Radial head of flexor digitorum superficialis
15   Radial recurrent artery
16   Superficial terminal branch of radial nerve overlying extensor carpi radialis longus
17   Ulnar artery
18   Ulnar head of pronator teres
19   Ulnar nerve and artery

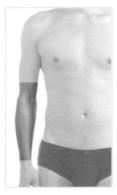

 Anterior interosseous nerve entrapment, Volkmann's contracture, see pp 174, 176.

ⒶLeft elbow

from the lateral side

With the forearm in midpronation and seen from the lateral side so that the radius (7) lies in front of the ulna, all muscles have been removed except supinator (8) to show its humeral and ulnar origins (see notes).

1 Annular ligament
2 Capitulum of humerus
3 Interosseous membrane
4 Lateral epicondyle
5 Posterior interosseous nerve
6 Radial collateral ligament
7 Radius
8 Supinator
9 Supinator crest of ulna

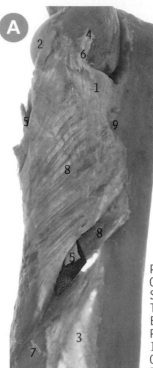

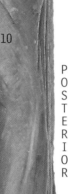

ⒷLeft forearm

deep muscles, from the lateral side

1 Abductor pollicis longus	**6** Extensor pollicis brevis
2 Biceps	**7** Extensor pollicis longus
3 Extensor carpi radialis brevis	**8** Extensor retinaculum
4 Extensor carpi radialis longus (double)	**9** Flexor pollicis longus
5 Extensor indicis	**10** Pronator teres
	11 Supinator

ⒸLeft forearm

posterior interosseous nerve, from behind

1 Abductor pollicis longus	**7** Extensor indicis
2 Branch of posterior interosseous artery	**8** Extensor pollicis brevis
	9 Extensor pollicis longus
3 Extensor carpi radialis brevis	**10** Extensor retinaculum
4 Extensor carpi radialis longus	**11** Posterior interosseous nerve
5 Extensor carpi ulnaris	**12** Supinator
6 Extensor digitorum	

The fibres of the interosseous membrane (A3) pass obliquely downwards from the radius (A7) to the ulna, so transmitting weight from the hand and radius to the ulna.

The supinator muscle (A8) arises from the lateral epicondyle of the humerus (A4), radial collateral ligament (A6), annular ligament (A1), supinator crest of the ulna (A9) and bone in front of the crest (page 127, D10), and an aponeurosis overlying the muscle. From these origins the fibres wrap themselves round the upper end of the radius above the pronator teres attachment, to be attached to the lateral surface of the radius and extending anteriorly and posteriorly as far as the tuberosity of the radius.

Posterior interosseous nerve entrapment, see p. 175.

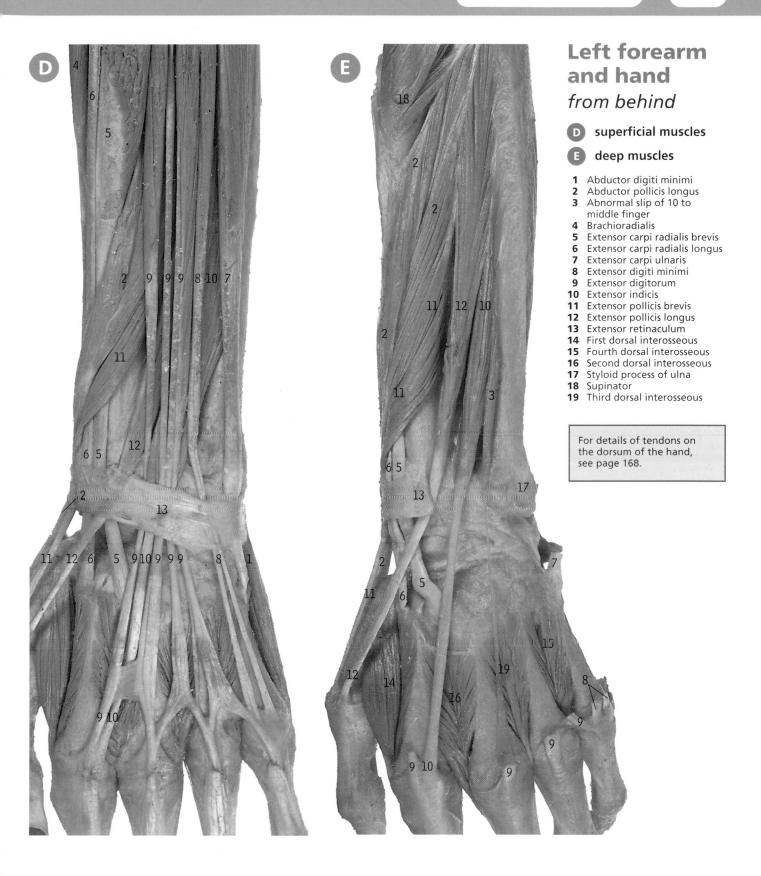

Left forearm and hand
from behind

D superficial muscles

E deep muscles

1 Abductor digiti minimi
2 Abductor pollicis longus
3 Abnormal slip of 10 to middle finger
4 Brachioradialis
5 Extensor carpi radialis brevis
6 Extensor carpi radialis longus
7 Extensor carpi ulnaris
8 Extensor digiti minimi
9 Extensor digitorum
10 Extensor indicis
11 Extensor pollicis brevis
12 Extensor pollicis longus
13 Extensor retinaculum
14 First dorsal interosseous
15 Fourth dorsal interosseous
16 Second dorsal interosseous
17 Styloid process of ulna
18 Supinator
19 Third dorsal interosseous

For details of tendons on the dorsum of the hand, see page 168.

De Quervain's disease, wrist drop, see pp 174, 176.

Ⓐ Palm of the left hand

Interrupted lines = radial and ulnar arteries and palmar arches

The surface markings of various structures within the wrist and hand are indicated; not all of them are palpable, e.g. the superficial and deep palmar arches (13 and 12), but their relative positions are important.

1	Abductor digiti minimi	**14**	Longitudinal crease
2	Abductor pollicis brevis	**15**	Median nerve
3	Adductor pollicis	**16**	Middle wrist crease
4	Distal transverse crease	**17**	Palmaris brevis
5	Distal wrist crease	**18**	Palmaris longus
6	Flexor carpi radialis	**19**	Pisiform
7	Flexor carpi ulnaris	**20**	Proximal transverse
8	Flexor digiti minimi brevis		crease
9	Flexor pollicis brevis	**21**	Proximal wrist
10	Head of metacarpal		crease
11	Hook of hamate	**22**	Radial artery
12	Level of deep palmar arch	**23**	Thenar eminence
13	Level of superficial palmar arch	**24**	Ulnar artery and nerve

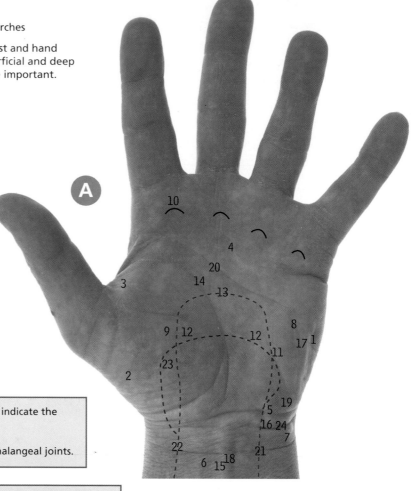

> The middle crease at the wrist indicates the level of the wrist joint.
>
> The radial artery at the wrist (A22) is the commonest site for feeling the pulse. The vessel is on the radial side of the tendon of flexor carpi radialis (A6) and can be compressed against the lower end of the radius.

> The curved lines (A10) proximal to the bases of the fingers indicate the ends of the heads of the metacarpals and the level of the metacarpophalangeal joints.
>
> The creases on the fingers indicate the level of the interphalangeal joints.

> The median nerve at the wrist (A15) lies on the ulnar side of the tendon of flexor carpi radialis (A6) and is slightly overlapped from the ulnar side by the tendon of palmaris longus (A18) (although this muscle is absent in 13 per cent of limbs).
>
> The ulnar nerve and artery at the wrist (A24) are on the radial side of the tendon of flexor carpi ulnaris (A7) and the pisiform bone (A19). The artery is on the radial side of the nerve and its pulsation can be felt, though less easily than that of the radial artery (A22).
>
> Abductor pollicis brevis (A2) and flexor pollicis brevis (A9), together with the underlying opponens pollicis, are the muscles which form the thenar eminence, the 'bulge' at the base of the thumb. Abductor digiti minimi (A1) and flexor digiti minimi brevis (A8), together with the underlying opponens digiti minimi, form the muscles of the hypothenar eminence, the less prominent bulge on the ulnar side of the palm where palmaris brevis (A17) lies subcutaneously.

Ⓑ Dorsum of the left hand

The fingers are extended at the metacarpophalangeal joints, causing the extensor tendons of the fingers (2, 3 and 4) to stand out, and partially flexed at the interphalangeal joints. The thumb is extended at the carpometacarpal joint and partially flexed at the metacarpophalangeal and interphalangeal joints. The lines proximal to the bases of the fingers indicate the ends of the heads of the metacarpals and the level of the metacarpophalangeal joints. The anatomical snuffbox (1) is the hollow between the tendons of abductor pollicis longus and extensor pollicis brevis (5) laterally and extensor pollicis longus (6) medially.

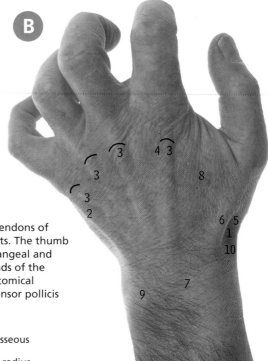

1	Anatomical snuffbox	**5**	Extensor pollicis brevis and
2	Extensor digiti minimi		abductor pollicis longus
3	Extensor digitorum	**6**	Extensor pollicis longus
4	Extensor indicis	**7**	Extensor retinaculum

8	First dorsal interosseous
9	Head of ulna
10	Styloid process of radius

Fingers *movements*

A flexion of the metacarpophalangeal joints and flexion of the interphalangeal joints

B extension of the metacarpophalangeal joints and flexion of the interphalangeal joints

C extension of the metacarpophalangeal and interphalangeal joints

When 'making a fist' with all finger joints flexed (A), the heads of the metacarpals (6) form the knuckles. To extend the metacarpophalangeal joints (B9) requires the activity of the long extensor tendons of the fingers, but to extend the interphalangeal joints (C10 and 5) as well requires the activity of the interossei and lumbricals, pulling on the dorsal extensor expansions (page 170). Only if the metacarpophalangeal joints remain flexed can the long extensors extend the interphalangeal joints.

1 Base of distal phalanx	**7** Head of middle phalanx
2 Base of metacarpal	**8** Head of proximal phalanx
3 Base of middle phalanx	**9** Metacarpophalangeal joint
4 Base of proximal phalanx	**10** Proximal interphalangeal
5 Distal interphalangeal joint	joint
6 Head of metacarpal	

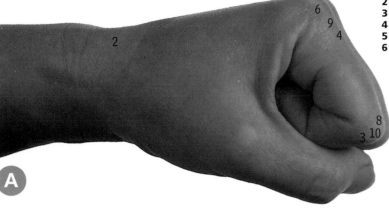

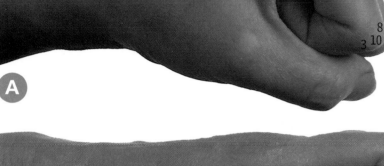

A Muscles producing movements at the metacarpophalangeal joints

Flexion: flexor digitorum profundus, flexor digitorum superficialis, lumbricals, interossei, with flexor digiti minimi brevis for the little finger and flexor pollicis longus, flexor pollicis brevis and the first palmar interosseous for the thumb.

Extension: extensor digitorum, extensor indicis (index finger) and extensor digiti minimi (little finger), with extensor pollicis longus and extensor pollicis brevis for the thumb.

Adduction: palmar interossei; when flexed, the long flexors assist.

Abduction: dorsal interossei and the long extensors, with abductor digiti minimi for the little finger.

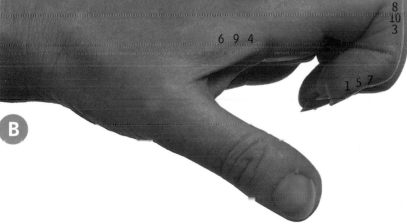

B Muscles producing movements at the interphalangeal joints

Flexion: at the proximal joints, flexor digitorum superficialis and flexor digitorum profundus; at the distal joints, flexor digitorum profundus. For the thumb, flexor pollicis longus.

Extension: with the metacarpophalangeal joints flexed, extensor digitorum, extensor indicis and extensor digiti minimi; with the metacarpophalangeal joints extended, interossei and lumbricals. For the thumb, extensor pollicis longus.

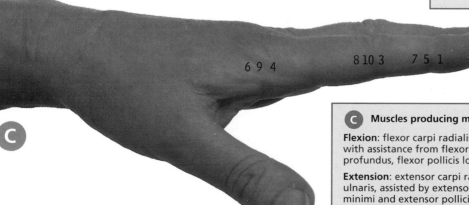

C Muscles producing movements at the wrist joint

Flexion: flexor carpi radialis, flexor carpi ulnaris, palmaris longus, with assistance from flexor digitorum superficialis, flexor digitorum profundus, flexor pollicis longus and abductor pollicis longus.

Extension: extensor carpi radialis longus and brevis, extensor carpi ulnaris, assisted by extensor digitorum, extensor indicis, extensor digiti minimi and extensor pollicis longus.

Abduction: flexor carpi radialis, extensor carpi radialis longus and brevis, abductor pollicis longus and extensor pollicis brevis.

Adduction: flexor carpi ulnaris, extensor carpi ulnaris.

Thumb *movements*

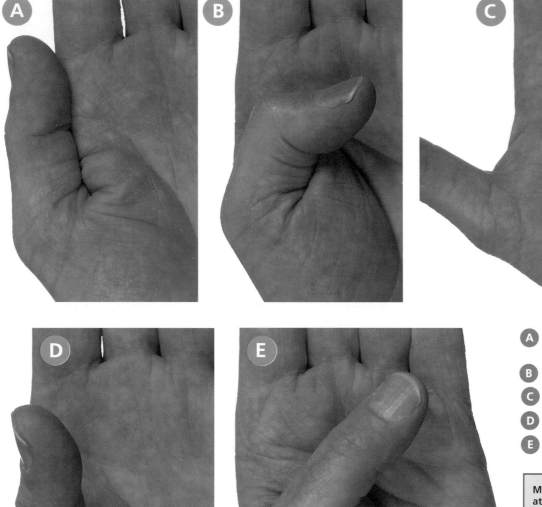

A   in the anatomical position

B   in flexion

C   in extension

D   in abduction

E   in opposition

Muscles producing movements at the carpometacarpal joint of the thumb

Flexion: flexor pollicis brevis, opponens pollicis, and (when the other thumb joints are flexed) flexor pollicis longus.

Extension: abductor pollicis longus, extensor pollicis longus, extensor pollicis brevis.

Abduction: abductor pollicis brevis, abductor pollicis longus.

Adduction: adductor pollicis.

Opposition: opponens pollicis, flexor pollicis brevis, reinforced by adductor pollicis and flexor pollicis longus.

With the thumb in the anatomical position (A), the thumb nail is at right angles to the fingers because the first metacarpal is at right angles to the others (page 130). This is a rather artificial position; in the normal position of rest the thumb makes an angle of about 60° with the plane of the palm (i.e. it is partially abducted). Flexion (B) means bending the thumb across the palm, keeping the phalanges at right angles to the palm. Extension (C) is the opposite movement, away from the palm. In abduction (D) the thumb is lifted forwards from the plane of the palm, and continuation of this movement inevitably leads to opposition (E), with rotation of the first metacarpal, twisting the whole digit so that the pulp of the thumb can be brought towards the palm at the base of the little finger (or more commonly in everyday use, to contact or overlap any of the flexed fingers). Opposition is a combination of abduction with flexion and medial rotation at the carpometacarpal joint; it is not necessarily accompanied by flexion at the other thumb joints.

Wrist drop, see p. 176.

Palm of the left hand

A *palmar aponeurosis*

Removal of the palmar skin reveals the palmar aponeurosis.

B *after removal of palmar aponeurosis*

Deeper dissection of the palm reveals the flexor retinaculum, the palmar branches of the median and ulnar nerves and the superficial palmar arch, flanked by the muscles of the thenar and hypothenar eminences.

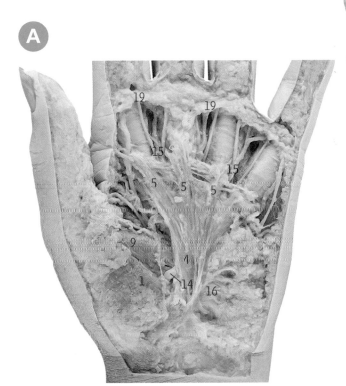

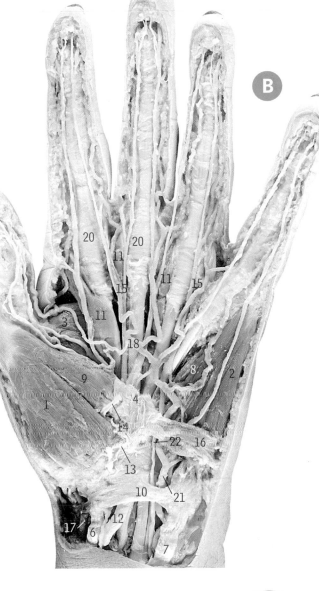

1	Abductor pollicis brevis	**9**	Flexor pollicis brevis
2	Abductor digiti minimi	**10**	Flexor retinaculum
3	Adductor pollicis	**11**	Lumbrical
4	Aponeurosis, central part	**12**	Median nerve
5	Aponeurosis, digital slips	**13**	Median nerve, palmar branch
6	Flexor carpi radialis	**14**	Median nerve, recurrent branch
7	Flexor carpi ulnaris	**15**	Palmar digital vessels and nerves
8	Flexor digiti minimi brevis	**16**	Palmaris brevis

17	Radial artery
18	Superficial palmar arch
19	Superficial transverse metacarpal ligaments
20	Synovial sheaths of flexor tendons
21	Ulnar artery
22	Ulnar nerve

Dupuytren's contracture, see p. 175.

Left wrist and hand

Ⓐ *palmar surface* **Ⓑ** *axial MR image*

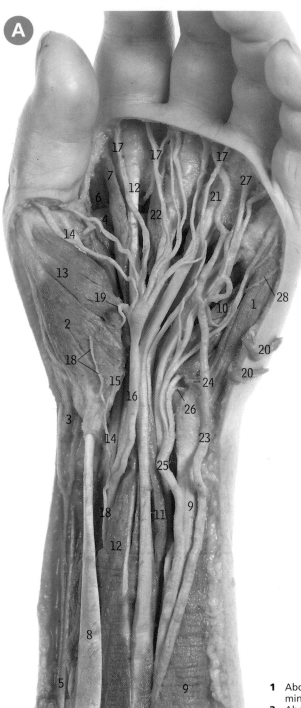

Parts of the fibrous flexor sheaths of the fingers (A21) have also been excised to show the contained tendons of flexor digitorum superficialis (A12) and flexor digitorum profundus (A11). In the palm the lumbrical muscles (A7 and 22) arise from the profundus tendons. Compare features in the MR image with the dissection.

1	Abductor digiti minimi	16	Median nerve
2	Abductor pollicis brevis	17	Median nerve, digital branch
3	Abductor pollicis longus	18	Median nerve, palmar cutaneous branch
4	Adductor pollicis		
5	Brachioradialis	19	Median nerve, recurrent branch
6	First dorsal interosseous	20	Palmaris brevis
7	First lumbrical	21	Remaining parts of fibrous flexor sheath
8	Flexor carpi radialis		
9	Flexor carpi ulnaris	22	Second lumbrical
10	Flexor digiti minimi brevis	23	Ulnar artery
11	Flexor digitorum profundus	24	Ulnar artery, deep branch
12	Flexor digitorum superficialis	25	Ulnar nerve
13	Flexor pollicis brevis	26	Ulnar nerve, deep branch
14	Flexor pollicis longus	27	Ulnar nerve, digital branch
15	Flexor retinaculum	28	Ulnar nerve, muscular branch

The lumbrical muscles have no bony attachments. They arise from the tendons of flexor digitorum profundus (A11) – the first and second (A7 and A22) from the tendons of the index and middle fingers respectively, and the third and fourth from adjacent sides of the middle and ring, and ring and little fingers respectively. Each is attached distally to the radial side of the dorsal digital expansion of each finger (page 170).

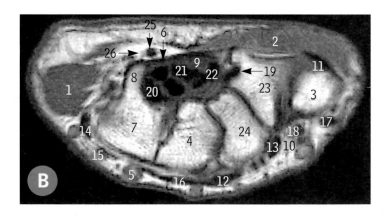

1	Abductor digiti minimi muscle	12	Tendon of extensor carpi radialis brevis muscle	19	Tendon of flexor carpi radialis muscle
2	Abductor pollicis brevis muscle	13	Tendon of extensor carpi radialis longus muscle	20	Tendon of flexor digitorum profundus muscle
3	Base of first metacarpal	14	Tendon of extensor carpi ulnaris muscle		
4	Capitate			21	Tendon of flexor digitorum superficialis muscle
5	Dorsal venous arch	15	Tendon of extensor digiti minimi muscle		
6	Flexor retinaculum	16	Tendon of extensor digitorum muscle	22	Tendon of flexor pollicis longus muscle
7	Hamate			23	Trapezium
8	Hook of hamate	17	Tendon of extensor pollicis brevis muscle	24	Trapezoid
9	Median nerve			25	Ulnar artery
10	Radial artery	18	Tendon of extensor pollicis longus muscle	26	Ulnar nerve
11	Tendon of abductor pollicis longus muscle				

Superficial palmar arch

A *incomplete in the left hand*

B *complete in the right hand*

In two-thirds of hands the superficial palmar arch is not complete (as in A29). In the other third it is usually completed by the superficial palmar branch of the radial artery (B30).

In the palm the superficial arterial arch (29) and its branches (as at 1) lie superficial to the common palmar digital nerves (22 and 7), but on the fingers the palmar digital nerves (as at 3) lie superficial (anterior) to the palmar digital arteries (as at 2).

1 A common palmar digital artery
2 A palmar digital artery
3 A palmar digital nerve
4 Abductor digiti minimi
5 Abductor pollicis brevis
6 Abductor pollicis longus
7 Common palmar digital branch of ulnar nerve
8 Common stem of 28 and 26
9 Deep branch of ulnar artery
10 Deep branch of ulnar nerve
11 Deep palmar arch
12 First lumbrical
13 Flexor carpi radialis
14 Flexor carpi ulnaris and pisiform
15 Flexor digitorum profundus
16 Flexor digitorum superficialis
17 Flexor pollicis brevis
18 Flexor pollicis longus
19 Flexor retinaculum
20 Fourth lumbrical
21 Median nerve
22 Median nerve dividing into common palmar digital branches
23 Muscular (recurrent) branch of median nerve
24 Opponens digiti minimi
25 Palmaris brevis
26 Princeps pollicis artery
27 Radial artery
28 Radialis indicis artery
29 Superficial palmar arch
30 Superficial palmar branch of radial artery
31 Ulnar artery
32 Ulnar nerve

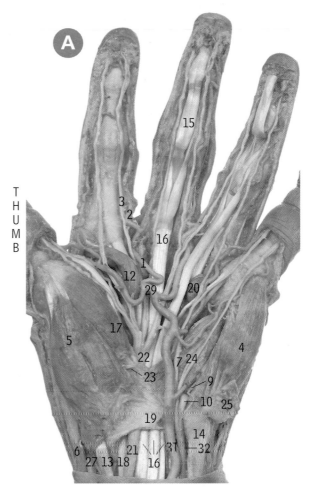

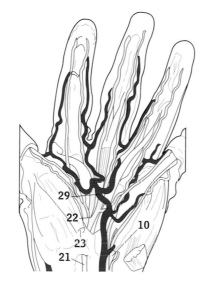

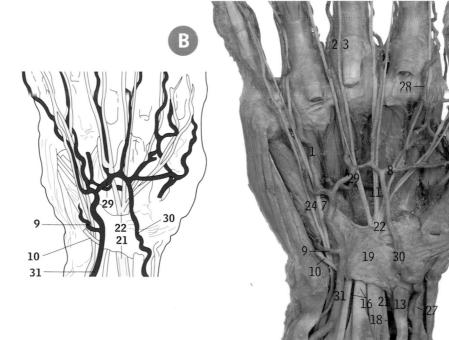

Arterial cutdown, carpal tunnel syndrome, see p. 174.

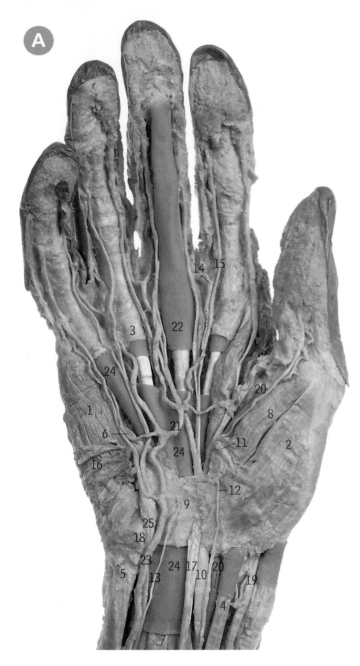

A Palm of the right hand
with synovial sheaths

The synovial sheaths of the wrist and fingers have been emphasized by blue tissue. On the middle finger the fibrous flexor sheath has been removed (but retained on the other fingers, as at 3) to show the whole length of the synovial sheath (22). On the index and ring fingers the synovial sheath projects slightly proximal to the fibrous sheath. The synovial sheath of the little finger is continuous with the sheath surrounding the finger flexor tendons under the flexor retinaculum (the ulnar bursa, 24), and the sheath of flexor pollicis longus is the radial bursa (20), which also continues under the retinaculum (9).

1	Abductor digiti minimi	13	Palmar branch of ulnar nerve
2	Abductor pollicis brevis	14	Palmar digital artery
3	Fibrous flexor sheath	15	Palmar digital nerve
4	Flexor carpi radialis	16	Palmaris brevis
5	Flexor carpi ulnaris	17	Palmaris longus
6	Flexor digiti minimi brevis	18	Pisiform bone
7	Flexor digitorum superficialis	19	Radial artery
8	Flexor pollicis brevis	20	Radial bursa and flexor
9	Flexor retinaculum		pollicis longus
10	Median nerve	21	Superficial palmar arch
11	Muscular (recurrent) branch	22	Synovial sheath
	of median nerve	23	Ulnar artery
12	Palmar branch of median	24	Ulnar bursa
	nerve	25	Ulnar nerve

In the carpal tunnel (beneath the flexor retinaculum), one synovial sheath envelops the eight tendons of flexor digitorum superficialis and profundus (A24), another envelops the flexor pollicis longus tendon (A20), and flexor carpi radialis (in its own compartment of the flexor retinaculum) has its own sheath also (A4). The synovial sheaths for flexor carpi radialis and flexor pollicis longus extend as far as the tendon insertions.

The sheath of the long finger flexors is continuous with the digital synovial sheath of the little finger, but is *not* continuous with the digital synovial sheaths of the ring, middle or index fingers; these fingers have their own synovial sheaths whose proximal ends project slightly beyond the *fibrous* sheaths within which the digital *synovial* sheaths lie.

The muscular (recurrent) branch (A11) of the median nerve usually supplies abductor pollicis brevis, flexor pollicis brevis and opponens pollicis, but of all the muscles in the body flexor pollicis brevis (A8) is the one most likely to have an anomalous supply: in about one-third of hands by the median nerve, in another third by the ulnar nerve, and in the rest by both the median and ulnar nerves.

B Right middle finger
long flexor tendons and vincula

The fibrous and synovial sheaths have been removed, and the flexor tendons (1 and 2) have been pulled anteriorly to show the vincula (3 and 6), which are small fibrous bands carrying blood vessels from the sheaths to the tendons.

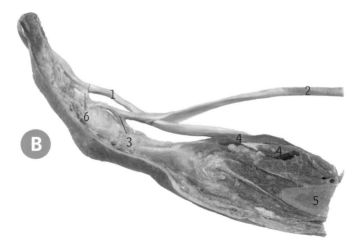

1	Flexor digitorum profundus	4	Lumbrical muscles
2	Flexor digitorum superficialis	5	Metacarpal bone
3	Long vinculum of superficialis	6	Short vinculum of profundus
	tendon		tendon

Palm of the right hand

C *deep palmar arch* **D** *arteriogram of palmar arteries*

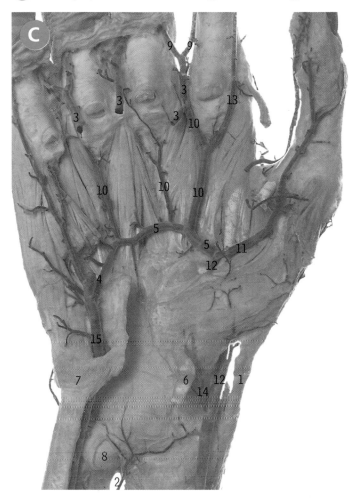

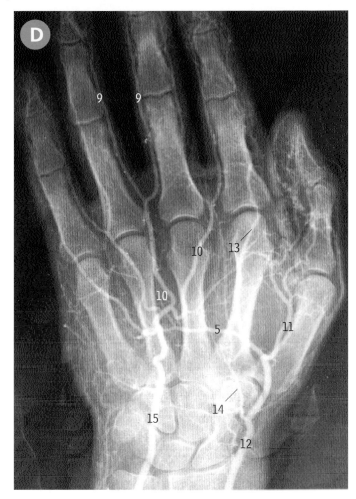

Most muscles and tendons have been removed and the arteries have been distended by injection. The deep palmar arch (5) is seen giving off the palmar metacarpal arteries (10) which join the common palmar digital arteries (3) from the superficial arch. Compare C with the vessels in the arteriogram.

1	Abductor pollicis longus	**9**	Palmar digital arteries
2	Branch of anterior interosseous artery to anterior carpal arch	**10**	Palmar metacarpal arteries
		11	Princeps pollicis artery
3	Common palmar digital arteries (from superficial arch)	**12**	Radial artery
		13	Radialis indicis artery (anomalous origin)
4	Deep branch of ulnar artery	**14**	Superficial palmar branch of radial artery
5	Deep palmar arch		
6	Flexor carpi radialis	**15**	Ulnar artery
7	Flexor carpi ulnaris and pisiform		
8	Head of ulna		

Arterial punctures, trigger finger, see pp 174, 176.

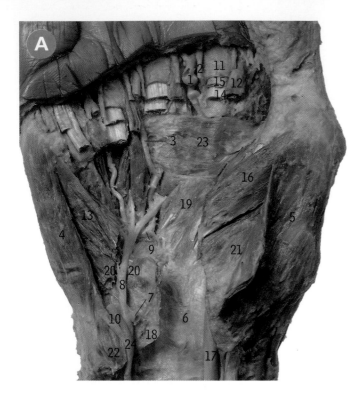

Ⓐ Palm of the right hand
deep branch of the ulnar nerve

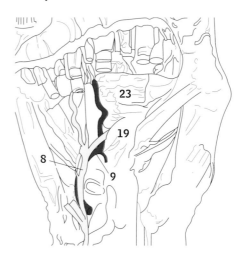

The long flexor tendons (15 and 14) and lumbricals (12) have been cut off near the heads of the metacarpals, and parts of the hypothenar muscles removed to show the deep branches of the ulnar nerve and artery (8 and 7) running into the palm and curling laterally to pass between the transverse and oblique heads of adductor pollicis (23 and 19).

1	A common palmar digital artery	13	Flexor digiti minimi brevis
2	A palmar digital nerve	14	Flexor digitorum profundus
3	A palmar metacarpal artery	15	Flexor digitorum superficialis
4	Abductor digiti minimi	16	Flexor pollicis brevis
5	Abductor pollicis brevis	17	Flexor pollicis longus
6	Carpal tunnel	18	Flexor retinaculum (cut edge)
7	Deep branch of ulnar artery	19	Oblique head of adductor pollicis
8	Deep branch of ulnar nerve	20	Opponens digiti minimi
9	Deep palmar arch	21	Opponens pollicis
10	Digital branches of ulnar nerve	22	Pisiform
11	Fibrous flexor sheath	23	Transverse head of adductor pollicis
12	First lumbrical	24	Ulnar nerve

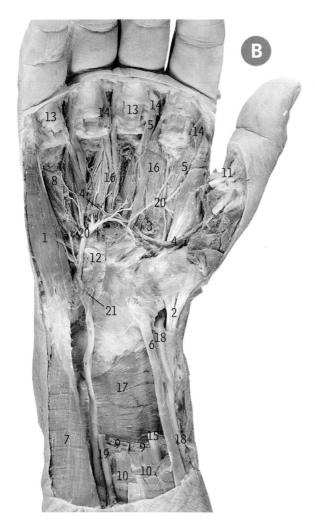

Ⓑ Palm of the right hand
deep dissection

Deep to the adductor pollicis and the flexor tendons lie the pronator quadratus proximally and the extensive deep palmar branches of the ulnar nerve and deep palmar arch distally.

1	Abductor digiti minimi	13	Flexor tendon sheaths
2	Abductor pollicis longus	14	Lumbrical – cut
3	Adductor pollicis – cut	15	Median nerve – cut
4	Deep palmar arch	16	Palmar interossei
5	Dorsal interossei	17	Pronator quadratus
6	Flexor carpi radialis	18	Radial artery
7	Flexor carpi ulnaris	19	Ulnar artery – cut
8	Flexor digiti minimi – cut	20	Ulnar nerve, deep branches to intrinsic hand muscles
9	Flexor digitorum profundus – cut		
10	Flexor digitorum superficialis – cut	21	Ulnar nerve, superficial branch (cut at wrist)
11	Flexor pollicis longus		
12	Flexor retinaculum – cut		

C Palm of the right hand
ligaments and joints

The capsule of the carpometacarpal joint of the thumb (between the base of the first metacarpal and the trapezium) has been removed, to show the saddle-shaped joint surfaces which allow the unique movement of opposition of the thumb to occur. The palmar and lateral ligaments (11 and 8) of the joint remain intact. The capsule of the distal radio-ulnar joint has also been removed to show the articular disc, but the wrist joint, the ulnar part of which lies distal to the disc, has not been opened.

1 Articular disc of distal radio-ulnar joint
2 Base of first metacarpal
3 Collateral ligament of interphalangeal joint
4 Deep transverse metacarpal ligament
5 Head of capitate
6 Hook of hamate
7 Interosseous metacarpal ligament
8 Lateral ligament of carpometacarpal joint of thumb
9 Lunate
10 Marker in groove on trapezium for flexor carpi radialis tendon
11 Palmar ligament of carpometacarpal joint of thumb
12 Palmar ligament of metacarpophalangeal joint with groove for flexor tendon
13 Palmar radiocarpal ligament
14 Palmar ulnocarpal ligament
15 Pisiform
16 Pisohamate ligament
17 Pisometacarpal ligament
18 Sacciform recess of capsule of distal radio-ulnar joint
19 Sesamoid bones of flexor pollicis brevis tendons (with adductor pollicis on ulnar side)
20 Trapezium
21 Tubercle of scaphoid
22 Tubercle of trapezium
23 Ulnar collateral ligament of wrist joint

The collateral ligaments of the metacarpophalangeal and interphalangeal joints (D2, C3) pass obliquely forwards from the posterior part of the side of the head of the proximal bone to the anterior part of the side of the base of the distal bone.

Opposition of the thumb is a combination of flexion and abduction with medial rotation of the first metacarpal (page 160). The saddle-shape of the joint between the base of the first metacarpal and the trapezium, together with the way that the capsule and its reinforcing ligaments are attached to the bones, ensures that when flexor pollicis brevis and opponens pollicis contract they produce the necessary metacarpal rotation.

The articular disc (1) holds the lower ends of the radius and ulna together, and separates the distal radio-ulnar joint from the wrist joint, so that the cavities of these joints are not continuous (unlike those of the elbow and proximal radio-ulnar joints, which have one continuous cavity – page 150).

DIP = distal interphalangeal joint
PIP = proximal interphalangeal joint
MP = metacarpophalangeal joint

D Right index finger
metacarpophalangeal (MP) joint, from the radial side

Part of the capsule has been removed to define the collateral ligament (2).

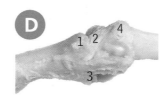

1 Base of proximal phalanx
2 Collateral ligament
3 Fibrous flexor sheath
4 Head of second metacarpal

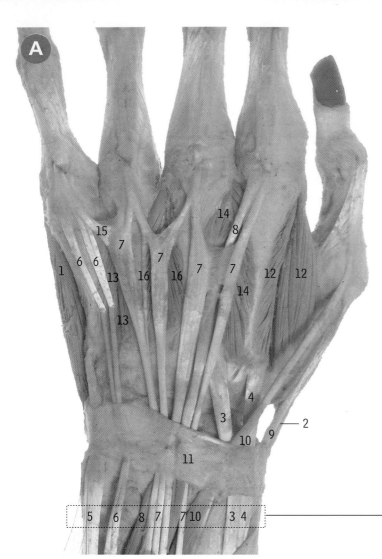

A Dorsum of the left hand
muscles and tendons

All vessels, nerves and fascia have been removed to show the long tendons passing under the extensor retinaculum (11). See the notes below for the identification of finger tendons.

1 Abductor digiti minimi	10 Extensor pollicis longus
2 Abductor pollicis longus	11 Extensor retinaculum
3 Extensor carpi radialis brevis	12 First dorsal interosseous
4 Extensor carpi radialis longus	13 Fourth dorsal interosseous
5 Extensor carpi ulnaris	14 Second dorsal interosseous
6 Extensor digiti minimi	15 Slip from extensor
7 Extensor digitorum	digitorum to little finger
8 Extensor indicis	16 Third dorsal interosseous
9 Extensor pollicis brevis	17 Tubercle of radius (Lister)

It is normal for the tendon of extensor digiti minimi (A6) to be double. In this specimen the extensor digitorum tendon (A7) to the ring finger is also double, with a slip passing to the middle finger.

The 'tendon' of extensor digitorum (A15) to the little finger normally consists, as here, of a slip from the digitorum tendon (A7) to the ring finger, joining the digiti minimi tendon (A6) just proximal to the metacarpophalangeal joint. Similar slips may joint adjacent digitorum tendons on other fingers, as here between the ring and middle fingers.

B Wrist *axial MR image*

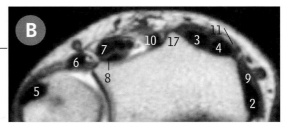

C Dorsum of the right wrist and hand
synovial sheaths

Fascia and cutaneous branches of the ulnar nerve have been removed; the extensor reticulum (13) and the radial nerve (2) have been preserved and the synovial sheaths have been emphasized by blue tissue. From the radial to the ulnar side, the six compartments of the extensor retinaculum contain the tendons of: a, abductor pollicis longus and extensor pollicis brevis (1 and 11); b, extensor carpi radialis longus and brevis (6 and 5); c, extensor pollicis longus (12); d, extensor digitorum and extensor indicis (9 and 10); e, extensor digiti minimi (8); f, extensor carpi ulnaris (7).

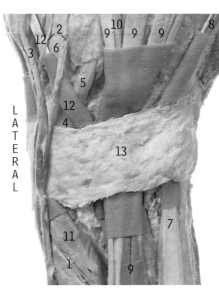

1 Abductor pollicis longus
2 Branches of radial nerve
3 Cephalic vein
4 Common sheath for 5 and 6
5 Extensor carpi radialis brevis
6 Extensor carpi radialis longus
7 Extensor carpi ulnaris
8 Extensor digiti minimi
9 Extensor digitorum
10 Extensor indicis
11 Extensor pollicis brevis
12 Extensor pollicis longus
13 Extensor retinaculum

Wrist ganglion, see p. 176.

Dorsum of the right hand
muscles and tendons

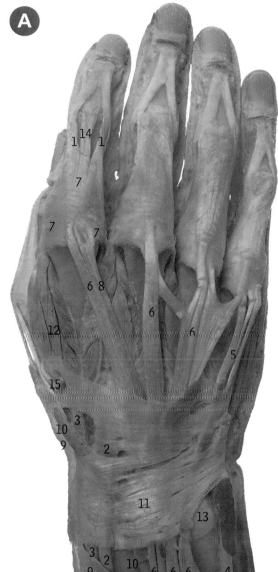

A

1 Collateral slip of
   expansion to distal
   phalanx
2 Extensor carpi radialis
   brevis
3 Extensor carpi radialis
   longus
4 Extensor carpi ulnaris
5 Extensor digiti minimi
6 Extensor digitorum
7 Extensor expansion
8 Extensor indicis
9 Extensor pollicis brevis
10 Extensor pollicis longus
11 Extensor retinaculum
12 First dorsal interosseous
13 Head of ulna
14 Intermediate part of
   expansion to middle
   phalanx
15 Radial artery

Right hand *from the radial side,*
muscles and tendons

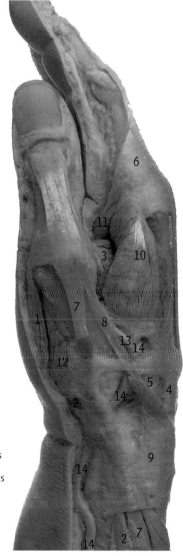

B

1 Abductor
   pollicis brevis
2 Abductor
   pollicis longus
3 Adductor pollicis
4 Extensor carpi
   radialis brevis
5 Extensor carpi
   radialis longus
6 Extensor
   expansion
7 Extensor
   pollicis brevis
8 Extensor
   pollicis longus
9 Extensor
   retinaculum
10 First dorsal
   interosseous
11 First lumbrical
12 Opponens pollicis
13 Princeps pollicis
   artery (unusual
   origin)
14 Radial artery

All vessels and nerves (except the radial artery, 15) have been removed; the extensor retinaculum (11) is preserved, together with some fascia distal to it to give some support to synovial sheaths which have been partially injected with green resin (compare with page 168, C). The margins of the distal parts of the extensor digital expansions (as at 7 and 1) have been emphasized by removal of the intervening connective tissue.

This is the specimen seen in A, now rotated to show muscles and tendons on the radial (lateral) side. The synovial sheaths of extensor pollicis brevis (7) and extensor pollicis longus (8) show some injected resin. Between the thumb and index finger the first dorsal interosseous (10) passes to the expansion (6), with the first lumbrical (11) running into the expansion just beyond the interosseous. Adductor pollicis (3) passes through to the proximal phalanx of the thumb.

In A the extensor digitorum tendon to the ring finger (6) is double, as well as giving a slip to the digiti minimi tendon (5), and to the extensor tendon of the middle finger. Some fascia distal to the extensor retinaculum (11) is preserved.

At the lateral side of the wrist the radial artery (B14) lies in the 'anatomical snuffbox', which is bounded laterally by the tendons of abductor pollicis longus and extensor pollicis brevis (B2 and B7) and medially by the tendon of extensor pollicis longus (B8).

The princeps pollicis artery (B13) has a more proximal origin than usual; it normally arises from the radial artery after that artery has passed through the first dorsal interosseous muscle (B10) to enter the palm.

The radial artery (B14, and A15 on page 170) enters the palm by passing through the first dorsal interosseous muscle (B10, and A13 on page 170), in B just after giving off the princeps pollicis artery (B13), and in A on page 170 after giving off the first dorsal metacarpal artery (A13).

A Dorsum of the right hand *arteries*

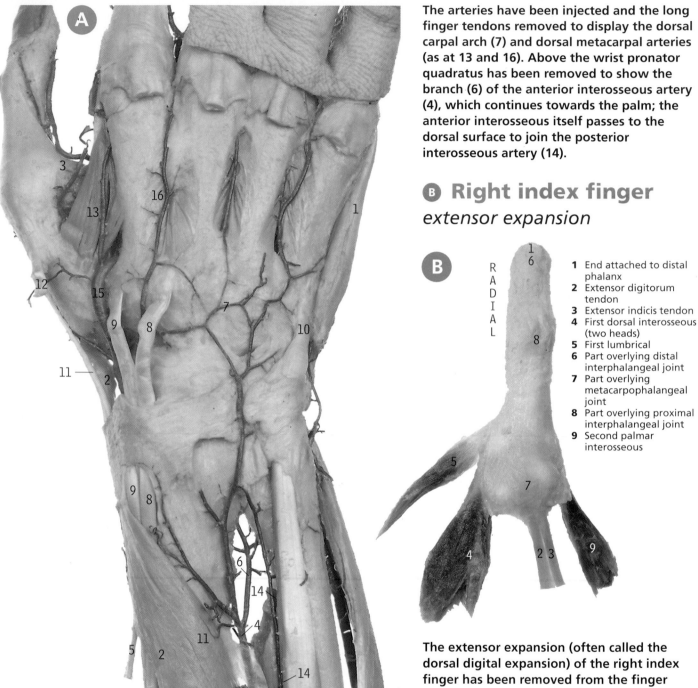

The arteries have been injected and the long finger tendons removed to display the dorsal carpal arch (7) and dorsal metacarpal arteries (as at 13 and 16). Above the wrist pronator quadratus has been removed to show the branch (6) of the anterior interosseous artery (4), which continues towards the palm; the anterior interosseous itself passes to the dorsal surface to join the posterior interosseous artery (14).

B Right index finger *extensor expansion*

RADIAL

1 End attached to distal phalanx
2 Extensor digitorum tendon
3 Extensor indicis tendon
4 First dorsal interosseous (two heads)
5 First lumbrical
6 Part overlying distal interphalangeal joint
7 Part overlying metacarpophalangeal joint
8 Part overlying proximal interphalangeal joint
9 Second palmar interosseous

The extensor expansion (often called the dorsal digital expansion) of the right index finger has been removed from the finger with its attached lumbrical (5) and interosseous muscles (4 and 9) and extensor tendons (2 and 3), and is seen from the dorsal surface but with the lower 'angles' somewhat spread out.

1 Abductor digiti minimi	9 Extensor carpi radialis longus
2 Abductor pollicis longus	10 Extensor carpi ulnaris
3 Adductor pollicis and branch of princeps pollicis artery	11 Extensor pollicis brevis
4 Anterior interosseous artery	12 Extensor pollicis longus
5 Brachioradialis	13 First dorsal interosseous and first dorsal metacarpal artery
6 Branch of anterior interosseous artery to anterior carpal arch	14 Posterior interosseous artery
7 Dorsal carpal arch	15 Radial artery
8 Extensor carpi radialis brevis	16 Second dorsal interosseous and second dorsal metacarpal artery

Three tendons pass to different levels of the thumb: abductor pollicis longus (A2) to the base of the first metacarpal, extensor pollicis brevis (A11) to the base of the proximal phalanx, and extensor pollicis longus (A12) to the base of the distal phalanx.

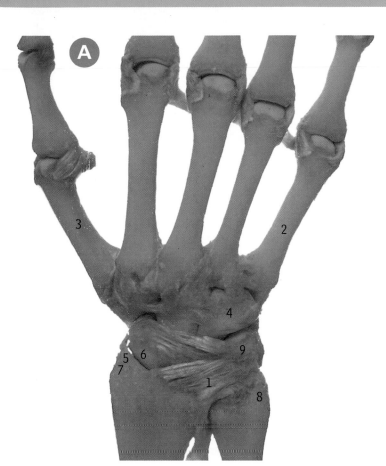

A Dorsum of the right hand
ligaments and joints

Most joint capsules have been removed, including the radial parts of the wrist joint capsule, thus showing the articulation between the scaphoid (6) and the lower end of the radius (7).

1 Dorsal radiocarpal ligament
2 Fifth metacarpal
3 First metacarpal
4 Hamate
5 Radial collateral ligament of wrist joint
6 Scaphoid
7 Styloid process of radius
8 Styloid process of ulna
9 Triquetral

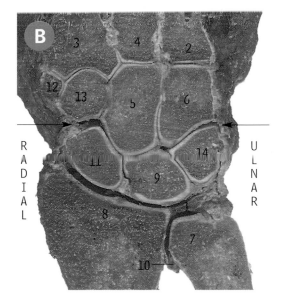

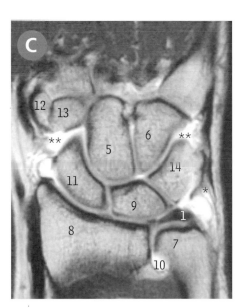

Right wrist
coronal section

B dissection

C coronal MR arthrogram

1 Articular disc (triangular fibrocartilage)
2 Base of fourth metacarpal
3 Base of second metacarpal
4 Base of third metacarpal
5 Capitate
6 Hamate
7 Head of ulna
8 Lower end of radius
9 Lunate
10 Sacciform recess of distal radio-ulnar joint
11 Scaphoid
12 Trapezium
13 Trapezoid
14 Triquetral

* Tiny perforation in fibrocartilage – normal variation
** Contrast in midcarpal and radiocarpal joints

Viewed from the dorsal surface, the section has passed through the wrist near this surface, and the first and fifth metacarpals have not been included in the cut. The arrows between the two rows of carpal bones indicate the line of the midcarpal joint. Compare the MR image with the section.

 Dislocation of the lunate, avascular necrosis of the scaphoid, see p. 174.

Right midcarpal and wrist joints

Ⓐ *midcarpal joint, opened up in forced flexion*

Ⓑ *wrist joint, opened up in forced extension*

BACK OF RIGHT THUMB EDGE

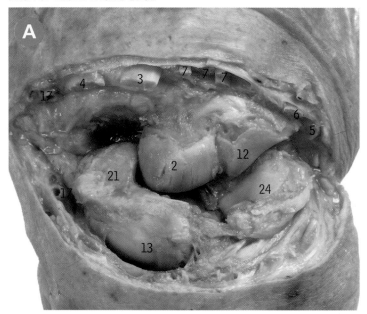

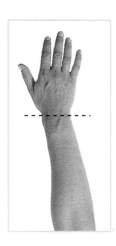

1 Articular disc
2 Capitate
3 Extensor carpi radialis brevis
4 Extensor carpi radialis longus
5 Extensor carpi ulnaris
6 Extensor digiti minimi
7 Extensor digitorum
8 Flexor carpi radialis tendon
9 Flexor carpi ulnaris tendon
10 Flexor digitorum profundus tendon
11 Flexor digitorum superficialis tendon
12 Hamate
13 Lunate
14 Median nerve
15 Palmar arch vein
16 Palmaris longus tendon
17 Radial artery
18 Radial artery, palmar arch branch
19 Radial surface for lunate
20 Radial surface for scaphoid
21 Scaphoid
22 Styloid process of radius
23 Styloid process of ulna
24 Triquetral
25 Ulnar artery

FRONT OF RIGHT THUMB EDGE

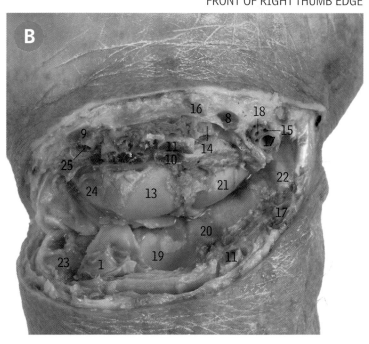

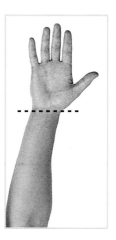

Both joints have been opened up (far beyond the normal range of movement) in order to demonstrate the bones of the joint surfaces. The wrist joint in B has been forced open in flexion, since flexion takes place mostly at this joint, and the midcarpal joint in A has been forced open in extension, since extension takes place mostly at this joint. The proximal (wrist joint) surfaces of the scaphoid (21), lunate (13) and triquetral (24) are seen in B, and their distal (midcarpal joint) surfaces in A.

Wrist and hand *radiographs*

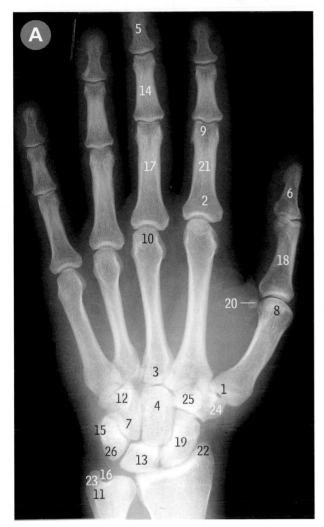

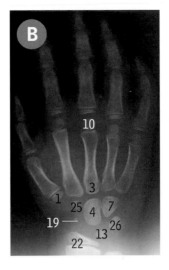

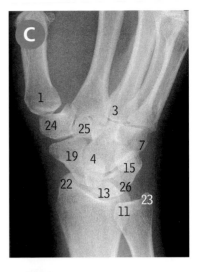

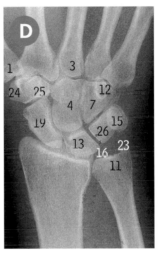

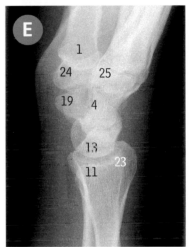

A dorsopalmar projection

P of a four-year-old child

C oblique projection

D posteroanterior projection

E lateral projection

The epiphysis at the lower end of the radius appears on a radiograph at 2 years and in the ulna at 6 years. The first carpal bone to appear is the capitate at 1 year.

Compare the epiphyses of the metacarpals and phalanges seen in B with the bony specimens in J and K on page 133

1	Base of first metacarpal	15	Pisiform
2	Base of phalanx	16	Position of articular disc (triangular
3	Base of third metacarpal		fibrocartilage) of distal radio-ulnar joint
4	Capitate	17	Proximal phalanx of middle finger
5	Distal phalanx of middle finger	18	Proximal phalanx of thumb
6	Distal phalanx of thumb	19	Scaphoid
7	Hamate	20	Sesamoid bone in flexor pollicis brevis
8	Head of first metacarpal	21	Shaft of phalanx
9	Head of phalanx	22	Styloid process at lower end of radius
10	Head of third metacarpal	23	Styloid process of ulna
11	Head of ulna	24	Trapezium
12	Hook of hamate	25	Trapezoid
13	Lunate	26	Triquetral
14	Middle phalanx of middle finger		

Scaphoid fracture, see p. 175.

Upper limb
Clinical notes

Anterior interosseous nerve entrapment. The deep branch of the median nerve, the anterior interosseous, may be trapped around the elbow following a fracture. The result is weakness in the flexor pollicis longus or flexor profundus muscles of the index and middle finger, making it impossible to flex the distal phalanx. (page 155)

Arterial cutdown, performed when repeated arterial blood sampling is required in a seriously ill patient, is performed on the radial artery in the non-dominant hand. Before proceeding it is important to confirm the patency of the deep palmar arch by occluding the radial artery and checking the ulnar arterial pulse (Allen's test). (page 163)

Arterial punctures. Two common sites for obtaining arterial blood in the upper limb are the brachial artery in the cubital fossa and the radial artery at the wrist. The site for the brachial artery is just medial and superior to the bicipital aponeurosis (i.e. the same point at which the blood pressure is taken). The radial artery is easily palpable just proximal to the wrist joint and lateral to the tendon of flexor carpi radialis. It is important when doing a radial arterial puncture to check that there is an ulnar artery pulse to allow for anastomosis should any damage or spasm following the radial puncture (Allen's test). (page 165)

Auscultation of the brachial pulse. The arterial blood pressure is usually taken from the brachial artery using a sphygmomanometer. The artery is first palpated in the cubital fossa anterior to the medial epicondyle and just superomedial to the bicipital aponeurosis, which may be felt as a strong band across the elbow. A cuff with pressure gauge placed proximally on the arm is inflated above the suspected systolic blood pressure and slowly deflated until the arterial pressure waves are heard through the stethoscope at the cubital fossa; this is the systolic blood pressure. Further release of the air from the cuff makes the beats disappear; this happens at the diastolic blood pressure. The pressure waves are normally heard at around the levels of 120 mmHg for systolic pressure and 70–80 mmHg for diastolic pressure. (page 152)

Avascular necrosis of the scaphoid. Following a fracture of the waist of the scaphoid, avascular necrosis may occur in the proximal fragment. This is because the arterial supply to this bone goes from distal to proximal and, therefore, the proximal fragment becomes avascular. The condition is often not diagnosed until 6 to 8 weeks after injury; the X-ray may then show an apparent increase in the density of the avascular fragment. Later there may be osseous collapse and removal of this segment may be necessary if immobilization has not occurred at the time of injury. (page 171)

Axillary nerve paralysis often occurs after shoulder dislocations or fractures of the humeral neck. The sensory loss is over the lateral upper part of the arm and the motor loss of the deltoid muscle makes it extremely difficult to abduct the arm or put one's hand into the trouser pocket. (page 146)

Biceps tendon reflex is elicited by tapping with a hammer the end of the thumb held against the biceps tendon. The reflex (mainly through C6) causes the biceps muscle to contract and the elbow to flex. (page 152)

Bicipital tendinitis. The long head of biceps muscle in the bicipital groove may become frayed and rupture. The presenting symptoms include pain on supination against resistance and, if there is rupture, a noticeable bulge appears on the anterior surface of the arm when the elbow is flexed. (page 143)

Carpal tunnel syndrome is a constellation of symptoms due to compression of the median nerve in the carpal tunnel beneath the flexor retinaculum. The sensory loss is usually in the radial two and a half fingers and the thumb, and the presenting symptom may be pain along the radial side of the hand. The muscles affected are the three small thenar muscles (abductor pollicis brevis, flexor pollicis brevis and opponens pollicis). If the condition is long standing there may be a noticeable loss of muscle bulk in the thenar eminence. Treatment usually involves division of the flexor retinaculum distal to the wrist. (page 163)

Colles' fracture is named after Abraham Colles, a Dublin surgeon. This fracture of the lower end of the radius with posterior displacement is commonly due to a fall on to an outstretched hand. Complications include median nerve irritation, rupture of the extensor pollicis longus tendon, and subluxation of the distal radio-ulnar joint. (page 131)

De Quervain's disease is a chronic inflammatory thickening of the tendon sheath usually seen in the abductor pollicis longus and extensor pollicis brevis muscles as they run across the lower end of the radius near the radial styloid. There is a palpable thickening of the tendon sheath and pain on movements of the thumb. (page 157)

Dislocation of the humerus. Dislocation of the humeral head at the shoulder joint is a relatively common injury and is in an inferior (no muscle support) or anterior (rotator cuff tear) direction, risking injury to the axillary nerve. An anterior dislocation is usually associated with a capsular or labral injury. (page 122)

Dislocation of the lunate. Severe forced dorsiflexion of the wrist may occasionally cause the capitate or lunate to become dislocated. When the wrist then returns to the neutral position the lunate is displaced anteriorly, causing pressure on the median nerve (paraesthesia in the thumb and index fingers). Manipulative reduction consists of pulling on the wrist, which is then palmar flexed slowly while pressure is applied on the lunate itself. (page 171)

Dislocation of the radial head, seen in young children usually before the age of 5 (also known as a 'pulled elbow'), is due to subluxation of the radial head from the annular ligament. The conical adult shape of the radial head and neck develop late and their cylindrical shape in childhood reduces retention by the annular ligament. (page 150)

Dupuytren's contracture is a deformity of the hand due to thickening of the palmar aponeurosis (of unknown aetiology) with resultant fibrosis and eventual contracture of the fingers. Presenting as a small hard nodule in the base of the ring finger, it tends to affect the ring and little finger as puckering and adherence of the palmar aponeurosis to the skin. Eventually the metacarpophalangeal and proximal interphalangeal joints become permanently flexed. (page 161)

Erb's paralysis (Erb-Duchenne palsy) is a brachial plexus injury to the upper roots, often an obstetric injury during a difficult delivery when traction is applied to the baby's head when it is in lateral flexion and the shoulder of the opposite side is pulled downwards. This most common of obstetric brachial plexus injuries involves the fifth and sixth cervical nerve roots. After delivery the baby's arm may be in a 'waiter's tip' position with the shoulder adducted, the elbow extended and the wrist pronated and flexed. It is usually evident at birth and may improve during the first year of the child's life. (page 145)

Golfer's elbow. Similar to tennis elbow, this relatively uncommon problem presents as pain over the medial epicondyle and is aggravated by extension of the elbow in a supinated forearm. It is due to repetitive strain from any of the common flexor origin muscles. (page 152)

Klumpke's paralysis is a brachial plexus lesion most commonly due to an abduction strain at the time of childbirth causing injury to the C8 and T1 roots of the brachial plexus, resulting in a claw hand deformity due to the paralysis of the intrinsic hand muscles (T1 myotome). The sympathetic trunk may also be affected, causing constriction of the pupil and a Horner's syndrome. The injury may not be diagnosed at birth becoming obvious only when the baby fails to grasp objects normally. (page 137)

Insertion of a central venous line. A central venous line may be introduced via either the subclavian or internal jugular veins. Occasionally, the brachiocephalic vein on the right is used to enter the great veins of the neck. From here the catheter is threaded into the superior vena cava and the right atrium. Central venous access is used to deliver chemotherapy, parenteral nutrition or antibiotics, or to measure the central venous pressure. (page 137)

Intramuscular injections are most commonly performed in the centre or anterior part of the deltoid muscle because injecting the posterior deltoid may endanger the axillary nerve as it exits the quadrangular (quadrilateral) space. (page 139)

Olecranon bursitis is inflammation of the bursa overlying the olecranon process of the ulna, associated with prolonged pressure at this point. (page 149)

Posterior interosseous nerve entrapment occurs where this branch of the radial nerve passes through two planes of fibres within the supinator muscle, often following elbow trauma or a fibrous band within the supinator. There is no sensory loss if the posterior interosseous nerve alone is damaged but there is an inability to extend the fingers using the extensor digitorum muscle. Extension of the distal interphalangeal joints of the fingers is possible through the action of the ulnar-innervated interossei. If the radial nerve itself is damaged there is a more pronounced wrist drop. (page 156)

Radial nerve paralysis, commonly known as a 'crutch' palsy or 'Saturday night' palsy, is usually caused by compression of the radial nerve in the axilla (crutches fitting poorly into the armpit or a drunken stupor in which arms are flopped over an armchair are common causes). The injury affects both elbow and wrist extension but the sensory loss is minimal: normally only a small area of skin superficial to the first dorsal interosseous muscle on the back of the hand. (page 148)

Reducing shoulder dislocations. Usually under general anaesthetic the arm is fully externally rotated, adducted across the body and, still in adduction, swung into internal rotation (Kocher's method). In another method (Hippocratic) an unbooted foot is placed in the patient's axilla and, with slight traction on the hand, the humerus is gently levered back into the glenoid fossa. Both before and after reduction it is important to check for axillary nerve damage. (page 134)

Rotator cuff tears often follow dislocation of the shoulder and can be in any of the rotator cuff muscles (supraspinatus, infraspinatus, teres minor and subscapularis). (page 143)

Scaphoid fracture often occurs at the waist of the scaphoid and initially may be extremely difficult to diagnose. There is acute tenderness in the anatomical snuffbox which is bounded by the tendons of extensor pollicis longus and abductor pollicis longus. Owing to the proximal segment's loss of blood supply, avascular necrosis is a known complication of this fracture and osteoarthritis may be severe if not treated. (page 173)

Supracondylar fracture of the humerus is usually seen in young children following a fall on the outstretched hand, producing a posterior displacement of the distal fragment. The structures at risk are the brachial artery and the median nerve and in a postero-lateral displacement, the radial nerve. If the artery has a fragment of bone against it, ischaemic changes may occur in the forearm and hand which will lead to a Volkmann's ischaemic contracture. (page 128)

Supraspinatus tendon calcification, calcium deposits within the supraspinatus tendon near its insertion, is of unknown aetiology and may cause eventual attrition and rupture of the tendon. (page 143)

Supraspinatus tendinitis. Deep to the acromion and the deltoid muscle, the subacromial bursa allows the supraspinatus tendon below it to glide freely in abduction. Injury or inflammatory change in the bursa can cause a painful arc on abduction, particularly when the greater tuberosity comes in contact with the acromion. On abduction the pain will be relieved when the acromion no longer touches the supraspinatus muscle. This painful 'arc' is fairly diagnostic of the condition. (page 143)

Tennis elbow, tenderness over the lateral epicondyle at the elbow, is caused by any repetitive movement (tennis serves, computer entries) which involves the extensor group of muscles. (page 152)

Triceps tendon reflex, elicited by tapping with a hammer the triceps tendon just above the olecranon, extends the elbow. This pathway is mainly through C7. Diminished or exaggerated reflex responses indicate abnormality of function. A cut nerve, for example, will give no reflex, whereas exaggerated reflexes are characteristic of an upper motor neurone lesion because the responsiveness of the anterior horn cells has been enhanced by elimination of the normal inhibition from higher centres. (page 149)

Trigger finger, a form of digital tenosynovitis (a chronic inflammatory thickening of the tendon sheath), often affects the synovial sheaths of the fingers at the level of the metacarpal head. The patient presents with a clicking sensation and tenderness on the affected digit. The condition is known as trigger thumb when it affects the thumb. (page 165)

Ulnar nerve paralysis commonly results from damage to the nerve behind the medial epicondyle of the humerus, producing impaired power of adduction of the wrist, an inability to spread the fingers and claw hand (paralysis of the interossei). There may also be an inability to adduct the thumb. The hypothenar muscles become wasted and sensation may be impaired in the ulnar one and a half fingers on both palmar and dorsal surfaces. (page 149)

Venous cutdown. If central venous cannulation is not available, the two major cutdown sites in the upper limb are the median cubital vein in the cubital fossa and the cephalic vein at the wrist over the radiocarpal joint. Both procedures involve aseptic technique and knowing the precise positions of these superficial veins. (page 154)

Venepuncture of the upper limb is a very common procedure carried out on most hospital admissions. The most common sites are the median cubital vein in the antecubital fossa and the cephalic vein just proximal to the wrist joint. In difficult patients the dorsal venous arch of the hand may also be used. A useful tip is that veins are more fixed at a branching 'tree of a tributary'. (page 154)

Volkmann's contracture is a deformity of the upper limb due to muscular ischaemia following injury to the brachial artery (supracondylar fracture of the humerus). An interruption of the blood supply of the upper limb musculature leads to necrosis and eventual fibrosis. Clinically, the finger flexors are usually the most severely affected, the patient being unable to extend the fingers when the wrist is flexed. (page 155)

Winging of the scapula, a scapula that sticks out from the posterior chest like an angel's wing, is noticeable when the hand is pushed against a wall or used to open a door. It is most commonly caused by a weakness of the serratus anterior or sometimes latissimus dorsi muscles. This may be due to muscular disease or nerve palsy. (page 145)

Wrist drop is a complication of radial nerve palsy due to loss of the forearm extensor muscles and may be associated with a loss of sensation over the first dorsal web space between the thumb and index finger. (page 160)

Wrist ganglion is a cystic swelling, usually arising from a herniation of synovial fluid, found at the wrist near the lower end of the radius and ulna. Although the condition normally requires no treatment, the treatment of old was to hit the ganglion with a heavy book to rupture the hernial sac. (page 168)

Thorax

5

Thorax Ⓐ *surface anatomy, from the front*

Ⓑ *axial skeleton, from behind*

Ⓒ *axial skeleton, from the front*
(skull, vertebral column and thoracic cage)

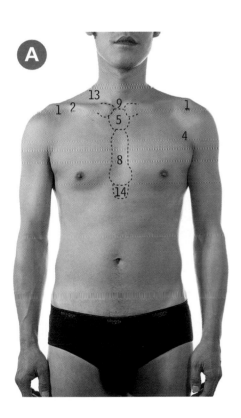

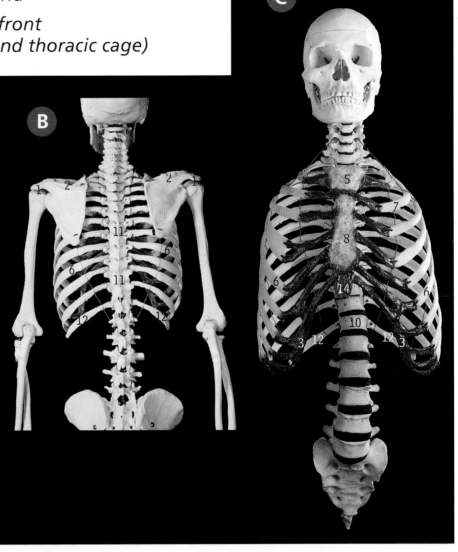

1 Acromion
2 Clavicle
3 Costal margin
4 Deltopectoral groove
5 Manubrium
6 Rib
7 Second rib
8 Sternal body
9 Suprasternal notch
10 Thoracic vertebra, body
11 Thoracic vertebra, spine
12 Twelfth rib
13 Trapezius
14 Xiphisternum

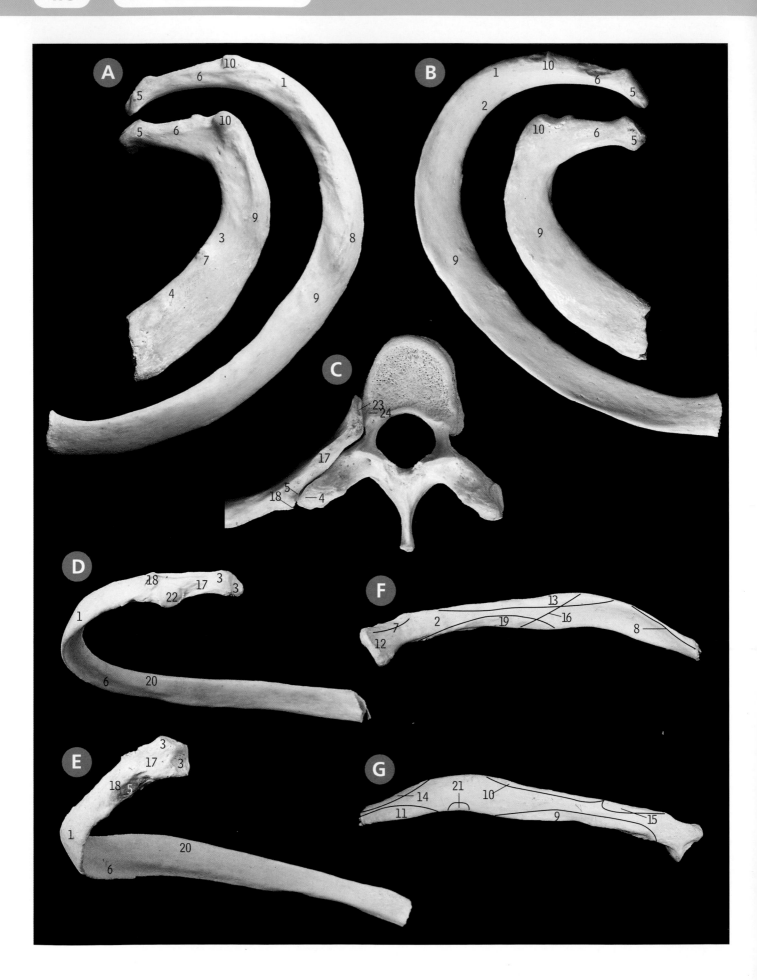

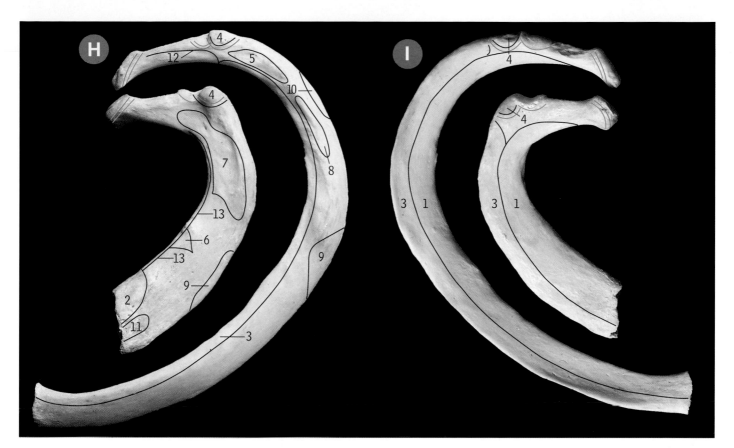

Left first rib (inner) and second rib (outer)

A from above

B from below

1 Angle
2 Costal groove
3 Groove for subclavian artery and first thoracic nerve
4 Groove for subclavian vein
5 Head
6 Neck
7 Scalene tubercle
8 Serratus anterior tuberosity
9 Shaft
10 Tubercle

The atypical ribs are the first, second, tenth, eleventh and twelfth.

The **first rib** has a head with one facet (A5), a prominent tubercle (A10), no angle and no costal groove. The shaft has superior and inferior surfaces.

The **second rib** has a head with two facets (B5), an angle (B1) near the tubercle (B10), a broad costal groove (B2) posteriorly, and an external surface facing upwards and outwards with the inner surface facing correspondingly downwards and inwards.

The **twelfth rib** has a head with one facet (F12) but there is no tubercle, no angle and no costal groove. The shaft tapers at its end (the ends of all other ribs widen slightly).

Ribs and relationships

C a typical rib and vertebra articulated, from above

D the left fifth rib from behind (a typical upper rib)

E the left seventh rib from behind (a typical lower rib)

F the left twelfth rib from the front, with attachments

G the left twelfth rib from behind, with attachments

1 Angle of rib
2 Area covered by pleura
3 Articular facet of head
4 Articular facet of transverse process
5 Articular part of tubercle
6 Costal groove
7 Costotransverse ligament
8 Diaphragm
9 Erector spinae
10 External intercostal
11 External oblique
12 Head
13 Internal intercostal
14 Latissimus dorsi
15 Levator costae
16 Line of pleural reflexion
17 Neck of rib
18 Non-articular part of tubercle
19 Quadratus lumborum
20 Shaft of rib
21 Serratus posterior inferior
22 Tubercle
23 Upper costal facet of head of rib
24 Upper costal facet of vertebral body

Left first rib (inner) and second rib (outer), attachments

H from above **I** from below

Blue lines = epiphysial lines; green lines = capsule attachments of costovertebral joints

1 Area covered by pleura
2 Costoclavicular ligament
3 Intercostal muscles and membranes
4 Lateral costotransverse ligament
5 Levator costae
6 Scalenus anterior
7 Scalenus medius
8 Scalenus posterior
9 Serratus anterior
10 Serratus posterior superior
11 Subclavius
12 Superior costotransverse ligament
13 Suprapleural membrane

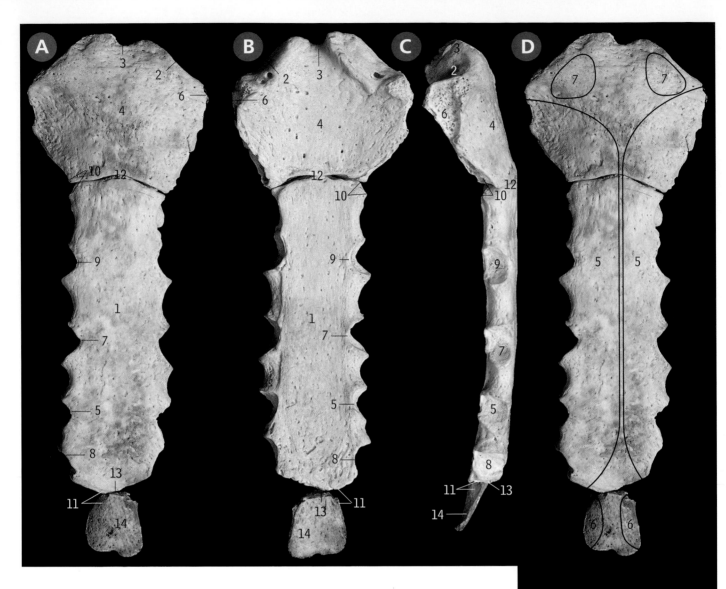

The sternum

A from the front

B from behind

C from the right

1 Body
2 Clavicular notch
3 Jugular notch
4 Manubrium
5 Notch for fifth costal cartilage
6 Notch for first costal cartilage
7 Notch for fourth costal cartilage
8 Notch for sixth costal cartilage
9 Notch for third costal cartilage
10 Notches for second costal cartilage
11 Notches for seventh costal cartilage
12 Sternal angle and manubriosternal joint
13 Xiphisternal joint
14 Xiphoid process

The sternum consists of the manubrium (4), body (1) and xiphoid process (14).

The body of the sternum (1) is formed by the fusion of four sternebrae, the sites of the fusion sometimes being indicated by three slight transverse ridges.

The manubrium (4) and body (1) are bony but the xiphoid process (14), which varies considerably in size and shape, is cartilaginous although it frequently shows some degree of ossification.

The manubriosternal and xiphisternal joints (12 and 13) are both symphyses, the surfaces being covered by hyaline cartilage and united by a fibrocartilaginous disc.

Bone marrow aspiration, see p. 218.

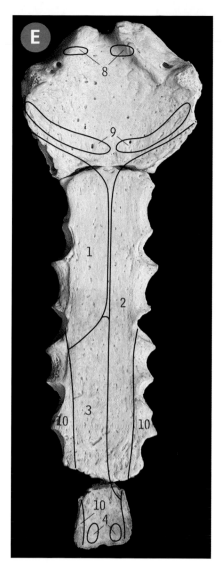

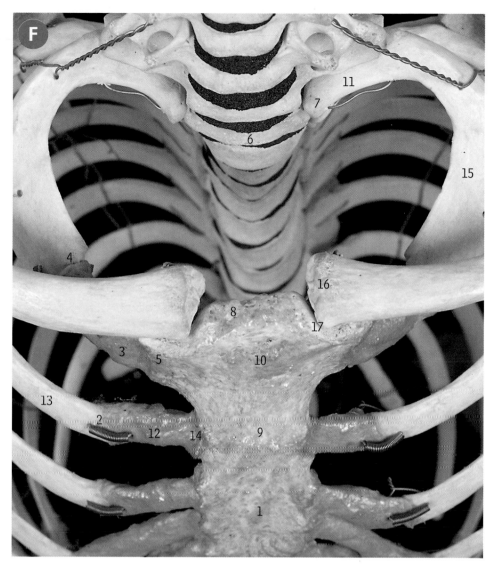

The sternum

attachments

D from the front

E from behind

1 Area covered by left pleura
2 Area covered by right pleura
3 Area in contact with pericardium
4 Diaphragm
5 Pectoralis major
6 Rectus abdominis
7 Sternocleidomastoid
8 Sternohyoid
9 Sternothyroid
10 Transversus thoracis

The two pleural sacs are in contact from the levels of the second to fourth costal cartilages (E2 and 1).

F Thoracic inlet *in an articulated skeleton, from above and in front*

The thoracic inlet or outlet (upper aperture of the thorax) is approximately the same size and shape as the outline of the kidney, and is bounded by the first thoracic vertebra (6), first ribs (15), and costal cartilages (3), and the upper border of the manubrium of the sternum (jugular notch, 8). It does not lie in a horizontal plane but slopes downwards and forwards.

The second costal cartilage (12) joins the manubrium and body of the sternum (10 and 1) at the level of the manubriosternal joint (9). This is an important landmark, since the joint line is palpable as a ridge at the slight angle between the manubrium and body, and the second costal cartilage and rib can be identified lateral to it. Other ribs can be identified by counting down from the second.

1 Body of sternum
2 Costochondral joint
3 First costal cartilage
4 First costochondral joint
5 First sternocostal joint
6 First thoracic vertebra
7 Head of first rib
8 Jugular notch
9 Manubriosternal joint
   (angle of Louis)
10 Manubrium of sternum
11 Neck of first rib
12 Second costal cartilage
13 Second rib
14 Second sternocostal joint
15 Shaft of first rib
16 Sternal end of clavicle
17 Sternoclavicular joint

 Costochondritis, rib/sternal fractures, see pp 218, 219.

Heart, left pleura and lung *surface markings, in the female*

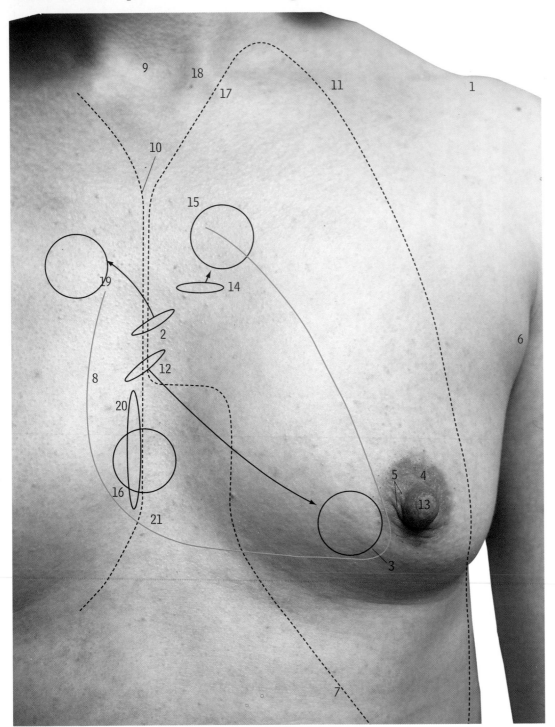

Blue line = heart; dotted lines = pleura

The positions of the four heart valves are indicated by ellipses, and the sites where the sounds of the corresponding valves are best heard with the stethoscope are indicated by the circles.

The manubriosternal joint (10) is palpable and a guide to identifying the second costal cartilage (15) which joins the sternum at this level (see page 181, F9, 14 and 12).

The pleura and lung extend into the neck for 2.5 cm above the medial third of the clavicle.

In the midclavicular line the lower limit of the *pleura* reaches the eighth costal cartilage, in the midaxillary line it reaches the tenth rib, and at the lateral border of the erector spinae muscle it crosses the twelfth rib. The lower border of the *lung* is about two ribs higher than the pleural reflexion.

Behind the sternum the pleural sacs are adjacent to one another in the midline from the level of the second to fourth costal cartilages, but then diverge owing to the mass of the heart on the left.

1 Acromioclavicular joint	**7** Costal margin (at eighth costal cartilage)	**12** Mitral valve	**18** Sternocleidomastoid
2 Aortic valve		**13** Nipple of breast	**19** Third costal cartilage
3 Apex of heart	**8** Fourth costal cartilage	**14** Pulmonary valve	**20** Tricuspid valve
4 Areola of breast	**9** Jugular notch	**15** Second costal cartilage	**21** Xiphisternal joint
5 Areolar glands of breast	**10** Manubriosternal joint	**16** Sixth costal cartilage	
6 Axillary tail of breast	**11** Midpoint of clavicle	**17** Sternoclavicular joint	

Heart sounds, see p. 218.

Female breast *mammary gland*

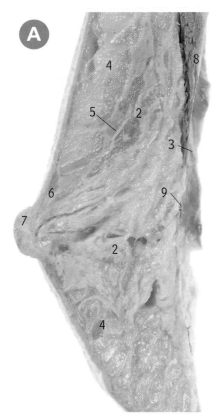

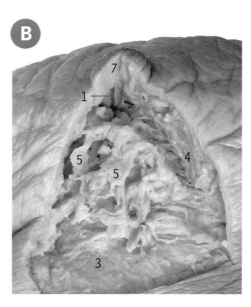

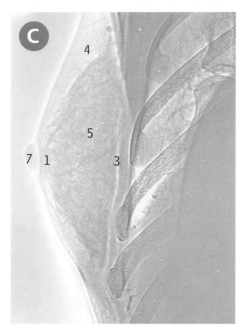

A **median sagittal section**

B **dissection of lower part, from the front and below**

C **xeromammogram**

1	Ampulla of lactiferous duct
2	Condensed glandular tissue
3	Fascia over pectoralis major
4	Fat
5	Fibrous septum
6	Lactiferous duct
7	Nipple
8	Pectoralis major
9	Retromammary space

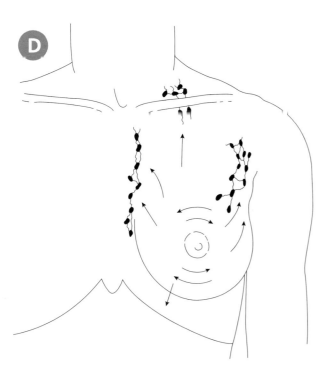

D Breast *lymph drainage*

There is a diffuse network of anastomosing lymphatic channels within the breast, including the overlying skin, and *lymph in any part may travel to any other part*. Larger channels drain most of the lymph to axillary nodes, but some from the medial part pass through the thoracic wall near the sternum to parasternal nodes adjacent to the internal thoracic vessels. These are the commonest and initial sites for cancerous spread, but other nodes may be involved (especially in the later spread of disease); these include infraclavicular and supraclavicular (deep cervical) nodes, nodes in the mediastinum, and nodes in the abdomen (via the diaphragm and rectus sheath). Spread to the opposite breast may also occur.

Breast examination, carcinoma of the breast, mastectomy, orange-peel skin, see pp 218, 219.

Ⓐ Right side of the thorax *from behind with the arm abducted*

With the arm fully abducted, the medial (vertebral) border of the scapula (5) comes to lie at an angle of about 60° to the vertical, and indicates approximately the line of the oblique fissure of the lung (interrupted line).

1 Deltoid
2 Fifth intercostal space
3 Inferior angle of scapula
4 Latissimus dorsi
5 Medial border of scapula
6 Spine of scapula
7 Spinous process of third thoracic vertebra
8 Teres major
9 Trapezius

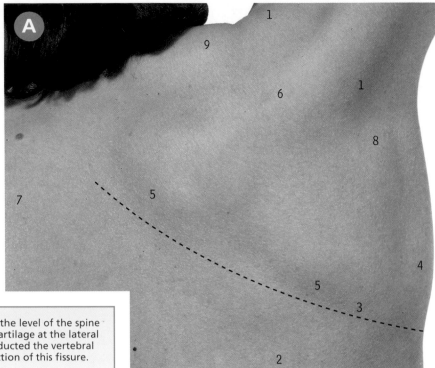

> The line of the oblique fissure of the lung runs from the level of the spine of the third thoracic vertebra (7) to the sixth costal cartilage at the lateral border of the sternum (see B). With the arm fully abducted the vertebral border of the scapula (5) is a good guide to the direction of this fissure.

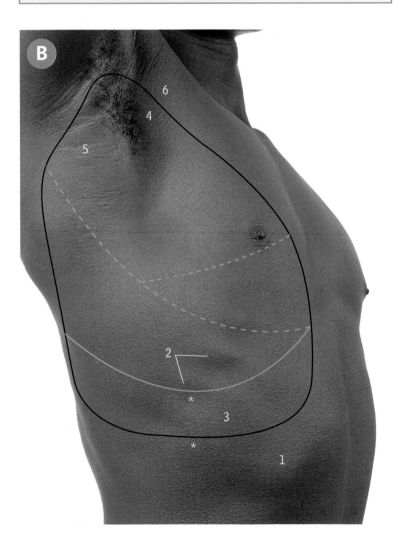

Ⓑ Right side of the thorax *surface markings, from the right, with the arm abducted*

The black line indicates the extent of the pleura, and the solid green line the lower limit of the lung; note the gap between the two at the lower part of the thorax, indicating the costodiaphragmatic recess of pleura, which does not contain any lung. The transverse and oblique fissures of the lung are represented by the interrupted green lines.

1 Costal margin
2 Digitations of serratus anterior
3 External oblique
4 Floor of axilla
5 Latissimus dorsi
6 Pectoralis major

> The transverse fissure of the right lung is represented by a line drawn horizontally backwards from the fourth costal cartilage until it meets the line of the oblique fissure (described in A) running forwards to the sixth costal cartilage. The triangle so outlined indicates the middle lobe of the lung, with the superior lobe above it and the inferior lobe below and behind it.
>
> On the left side where the lung has only two lobes, superior and inferior, there is no transverse fissure; the surface marking for the oblique fissure is similar to that on the right.
>
> * The asterisks represent the places where the lower edges of the lung and pleura cross the eighth and tenth ribs respectively in the midaxillary line.

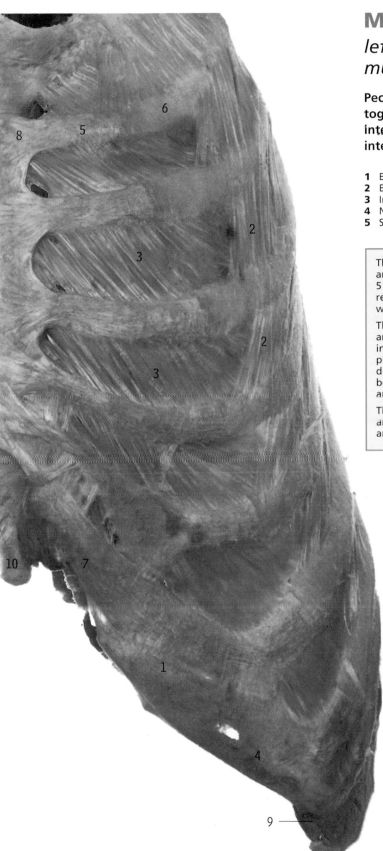

Muscles of the thorax
left external and internal intercostal muscles, from the front

Pectoral and abdominal muscles have been removed, together with all vessels and nerves and the anterior intercostal membranes, to show the external and internal intercostal muscles (as at 2 and 3).

1	Eighth costal cartilage	**6**	Second rib
2	External intercostal	**7**	Seventh costal cartilage
3	Internal intercostal	**8**	Sternal angle
4	Ninth costal cartilage	**9**	Tenth costal cartilage
5	Second costal cartilage	**10**	Xiphoid process

The fibres of the **external intercostal muscles** (2) run downwards and medially, and near the costochondral junctions (as between 5 and 6) give place to the anterior intercostal membrane (here removed); these are thin sheets of connective tissue through which the underlying internal intercostal muscles (3) can be seen.

The fibres of the **internal intercostal muscles** (3) run downwards and laterally. At the front they are covered by the anterior intercostal membranes, and at the back of the thorax they give place to the posterior intercostal membranes. The different directions of the muscle fibres enable the two muscle groups to be distinguished – down and medially for the externals (2), down and laterally for the internals (3).

The seventh costal cartilage (7) is the lowest to join the sternum and together with the eighth, ninth and tenth cartilages (1, 4 and 9) forms the costal margin.

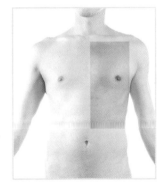

Flail chest, see p. 218.

Muscles of the thorax

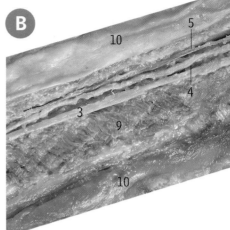

right intercostal muscles

A from the outside

B from the inside

1 Eighth rib
2 External intercostal
3 Fifth intercostal nerve
4 Fifth posterior intercostal artery
5 Fifth posterior intercostal vein
6 Fifth rib
7 Fourth rib
8 Innermost intercostal
9 Internal intercostal
10 Pleura
11 Seventh rib
12 Sixth intercostal nerve
13 Sixth rib

> The **internal intercostal muscles** are continuous posteriorly with the posterior intercostal membranes which are covered up by the medial ends of the external intercostals (as at 2).

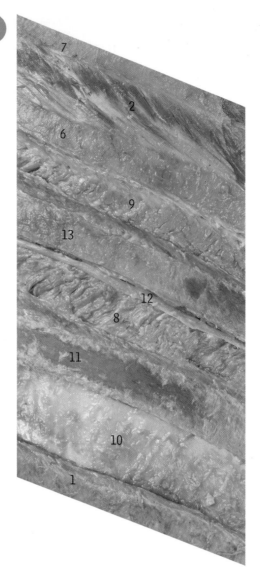

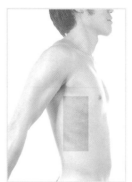

In A each intercostal space has been dissected to a different depth, showing from above downwards an external intercostal muscle (2), internal intercostal (9), innermost intercostal (8) and pleura (10). The main intercostal vessels and nerve lie between the internal and innermost muscles; the nerve (12) is seen in the sixth interspace immediately below the sixth rib (13) and lying on the outer surface of the innermost intercostal (8), but the artery and vein are under cover of the costal groove. The vessels as well as the nerve are seen in the fifth intercostal space when this is dissected from the inside of the thorax, as in B; here the pleura and innermost intercostal muscle have been removed, and the vessels (5 and 4) and fifth intercostal nerve (3) lie against the inner surface of the internal intercostal (9).

Clicking rib syndrome, intercostal nerve block, see pp 218, 219.

Muscles of the thorax

A *right transversus thoracis, from behind (inside view)*
B *left lower subcostal and innermost intercostal muscles*

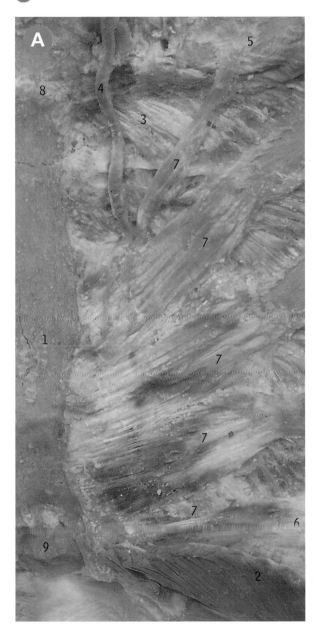

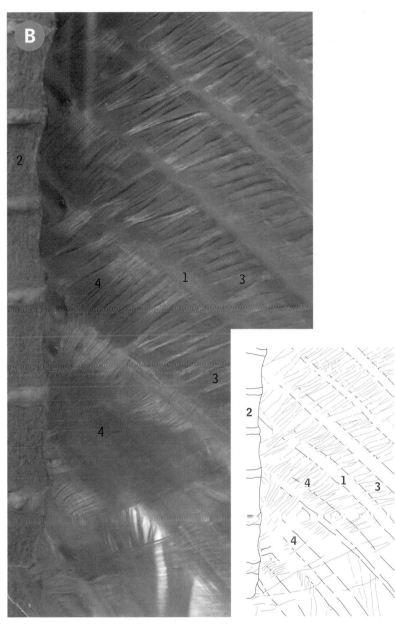

This view of the internal surface of the thoracic wall shows the posterior surface of the right half of the sternum and adjacent wall, with the pleura removed. The internal thoracic artery (4) is seen passing deep to the slips of transversus thoracis (7, previously called sternocostalis).

Transversus thoracis (A7) is in the same plane as the **innermost intercostal muscles** at the lateral side of the thoracic wall (B3) and the subcostal muscles on the posterior part (B4).

The **subcostal muscles** (B4) span more than one rib. They and the innermost intercostals (B3, intercostales intimi) are often poorly developed or absent in the upper part of the thorax.

This view of the lower left hemithorax is seen from the right and in front, with vertebral bodies (as at 2) sectioned and the pleura, vessels and nerves removed, and shows part of the innermost layer of thoracic wall muscles (3 and 4).

1	Body of sternum	6	Sixth rib
2	Diaphragm	7	Slips of transversus thoracis muscle
3	Internal intercostal		
4	Internal thoracic artery	8	Sternal angle
5	Second rib	9	Xiphoid process

1	Eighth rib	3	Innermost intercostal
2	Eighth thoracic vertebra	4	Subcostal

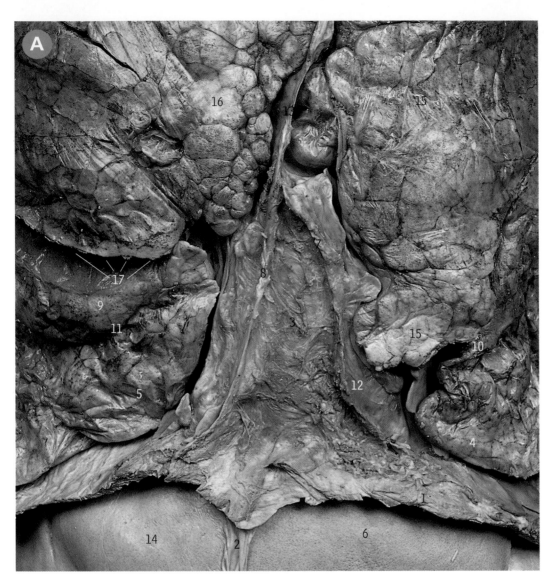

Ⓐ Lungs and pericardium
from the front

1 Diaphragm
2 Falciform ligament
3 Fibrous pericardium
4 Inferior lobe of left lung
5 Inferior lobe of right lung
6 Left lobe of liver
7 Line of reflexion of left pleura
8 Line of reflexion of right pleura
9 Middle lobe of right lung
10 Oblique fissure
11 Oblique fissure of right lung
12 Pleura overlying pericardium
13 Right and left parietal pleurae in contact
14 Right lobe of liver
15 Superior lobe of left lung
16 Superior lobe of right lung
17 Transverse fissure of right lung

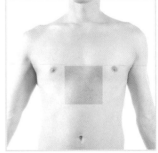

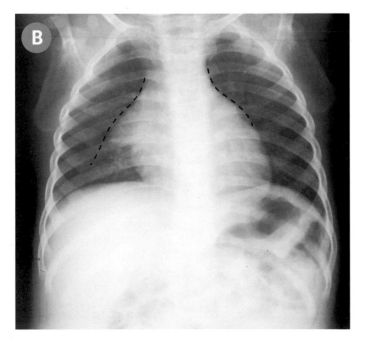

The anterior thoracic and abdominal walls have been removed. The cut edges of the two pleural sacs are seen lying adjacent to one another (13), but lower down over the front of the pericardium (3) they become separated (8 and 7).

The pleurae become separated at the level of the fourth costal cartilage (junction of 13, 8 and 7) owing to the leftward bulge of the heart, and therefore the central part of the fibrous pericardium (3) is not covered by pleura.

Ⓑ Chest *radiograph of a child*

The child's thymus can be seen on a plain chest radiograph, appearing as a spinnaker sail (sail sign), as outlined by the interrupted line.

Heart and pericardium

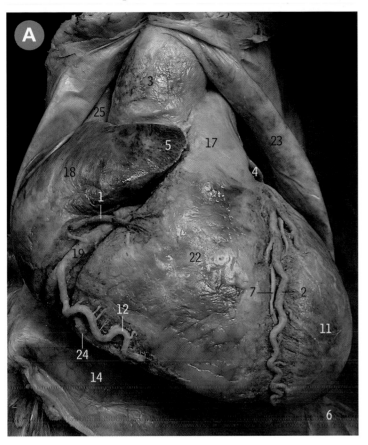

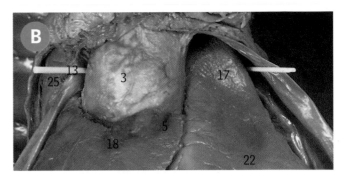

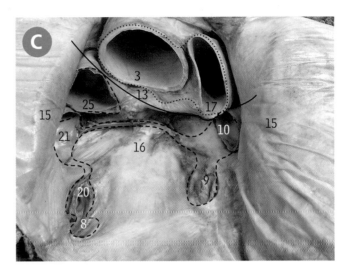

from the front

with marker in the transverse sinus

oblique sinus after removal of the heart

1	Anterior cardiac vein	**15**	Pericardium turned laterally over lung
2	Anterior interventricular branch of left coronary artery	**16**	Posterior wall of pericardial cavity and oblique sinus
3	Ascending aorta	**17**	Pulmonary trunk
4	Auricle of left atrium	**18**	Right atrium
5	Auricle of right atrium	**19**	Right coronary artery
6	Diaphragm	**20**	Right inferior pulmonary vein
7	Great cardiac vein	**21**	Right superior pulmonary vein
8	Inferior vena cava	**22**	Right ventricle
9	Left inferior pulmonary vein	**23**	Serous pericardium overlying fibrous pericardium (turned laterally)
10	Left superior pulmonary vein		
11	Left ventricle	**24**	Small cardiac vein
12	Marginal branch of right coronary artery	**25**	Superior vena cava
13	Marker in transverse sinus		
14	Pericardium fused with tendon of diaphragm		

The **right border of the heart** is formed by the right atrium (A18).

The **left border** is formed mostly by the left ventricle (A11) with at the top the uppermost part (infundibulum) of the right ventricle (A22) and the tip of the left auricle (A4).

The **inferior border** is formed by the right ventricle (A22) with a small part of the left ventricle at the apex (page 182, 2).

In A the pericardium has been incised and turned back (23) to display the anterior surface of the heart. The pulmonary trunk (17) leaves the right ventricle (22) in front and to the left of the ascending aorta (3), which is overlapped by the auricle (5) of the right atrium (18). The superior vena cava (25) is to the right to the aorta and still largely covered by pericardium. The anterior interventricular branch (2) of the left coronary artery and the great cardiac vein (7) lie in the interventricular groove between the right and left ventricles (22 and 11), and the right coronary artery (19) is in the atrioventricular groove between the right ventricle (22) and right atrium (18). In B only the upper part of another heart is shown, with a marker in the transverse sinus, the space behind the aorta (3) and pulmonary trunk (17). In C the heart has been removed from the pericardium, leaving the orifices of the great vessels. The dotted line indicates the attachment of the single sleeve of serous pericardium surrounding the aorta (3) and pulmonary trunk (17). The interrupted line indicates the attachment of another more complicated but still single sleeve of serous pericardium surrounding all the other six great vessels (the four pulmonary veins, 10, 9, 20 and 21, and the superior and inferior venae cavae, 25 and 8). The narrow interval between the two sleeves is the transverse sinus; the solid line in C indicates the path of the marker in B. The area of the pericardium (16) between the pulmonary veins and limited above by the reflexion of the serous pericardium on to the back of the heart is the oblique sinus.

 Cardiac tamponade, pericardial effusion, see pp 218, 219.

Heart *with blood vessels injected* **A** *from the front* **B** *from behind*

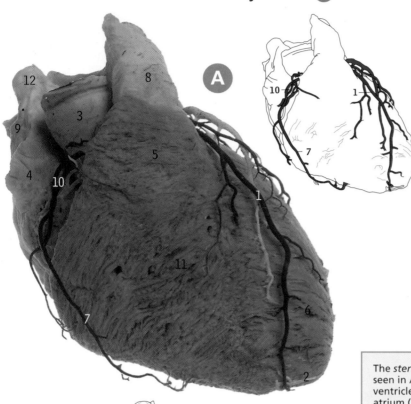

The coronary arteries have been injected with red latex and the cardiac veins with grey latex. The pulmonary trunk (8) passes upwards from the infundibulum (5) of the right ventricle (11), and at its commencement it is just in front and to the left of the ascending aorta (3).

1. Anterior interventricular branch of left coronary artery and great cardiac vein in interventricular groove
2. Apex
3. Ascending aorta
4. Auricle of right atrium (displaced laterally)
5. Infundibulum of right ventricle
6. Left ventricle
7. Marginal branch of right coronary artery
8. Pulmonary trunk
9. Right atrium
10. Right coronary artery in anterior atrioventricular groove
11. Right ventricle
12. Superior vena cava

The *sternocostal* surface of the heart is the *anterior* surface (as seen in A on page 189 and A above) formed mainly by the right ventricle (A11, D7), with parts of the left ventricle (A6) and right atrium (A9 and D10).

The *apex* of the heart (A2) is formed by the left ventricle.

The *base* of the heart is the *posterior* surface, formed mainly by the left atrium (B8) with a small part of the right atrium (B13).

The *inferior* surface is the *diaphragmatic* surface, formed by the two ventricles (mainly the left) (B10 and B15).

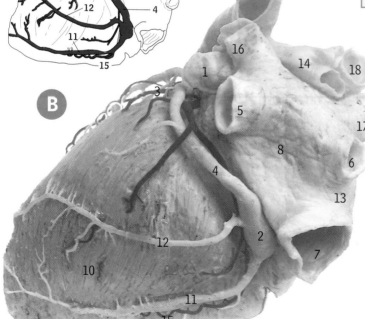

1. Auricle of left atrium
2. Coronary sinus in posterior atrioventricular groove
3. Great cardiac vein and anterior interventricular branch of left coronary artery
4. Great cardiac vein and circumflex branch of left coronary artery
5. Inferior left pulmonary vein
6. Inferior right pulmonary vein
7. Inferior vena cava
8. Left atrium
9. Left pulmonary artery
10. Left ventricle
11. Middle cardiac vein and posterior interventricular branch of right coronary artery in posterior interventricular groove
12. Posterior vein of left ventricle
13. Right atrium
14. Right pulmonary artery
15. Right ventricle
16. Superior left pulmonary vein
17. Superior right pulmonary vein
18. Superior vena cava

 Coronary bypass surgery, myocardial infarction, see pp 218, 219.

C Right atrium *from the front and right*

The anterior wall has been incised near its left margin and reflected to the right, showing on its internal surface the vertical crista terminalis (2) and horizontal pectinate muscles (7). The fossa ovalis (3) is on the interatrial septum, and the opening of the coronary sinus (6) is to the left of the inferior vena caval opening (4).

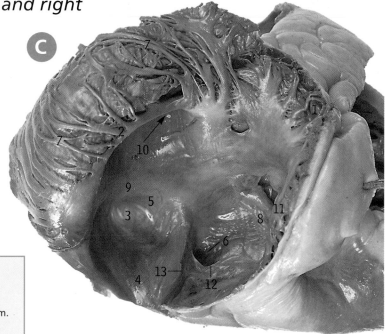

1	Auricle	7	Pectinate muscles
2	Crista terminalis	8	Position of atrioventricular node
3	Fossa ovalis	9	Position of intervenous tubercle
4	Inferior vena cava	10	Superior vena cava
5	Limbus	11	Tricuspid valve
6	Opening of	12	Valve of coronary sinus
	coronary sinus	13	Valve of inferior vena cava

The fossa ovalis (3) forms part of the interatrial septum, and is part of the embryonic primary septum.

The limbus (5), which forms the margin of the fossa ovalis (3), represents the lower margin of the embryonic secondary septum. Before the primary and secondary septa fuse (at birth), the gap between them forms the foramen ovale.

The sinuatrial node (SA node, not illustrated) is embedded in the anterior wall of the atrium at the upper end of the crista terminalis, just below the opening of the superior vena cava.

The atrioventricular node (AV node, 8) is embedded in the interatrial septum, just above and to the left of the opening of the coronary sinus (6).

D Right ventricle
from the front

1 Anterior cusp of tricuspid valve
2 Anterior papillary muscle
3 Ascending aorta
4 Auricle of right atrium
5 Chordae tendineae
6 Inferior vena cava
7 Infundibulum of right ventricle
8 Posterior papillary muscle
9 Pulmonary trunk
10 Right atrium
11 Septomarginal trabecula
12 Superior vena cava
13 Trabeculae on interventricular septum

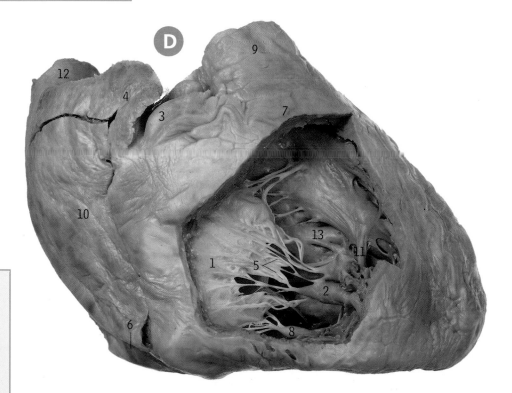

The septomarginal trabecula (11), which conducts part of the right limb of the atrioventricular bundle from the interventricular septum (13) to the anterior papillary muscle (2), was formerly known as the moderator band.

The chordae tendineae (5) connect the cusps of the tricuspid valve to the papillary muscles.

 Cardiac pacemaker, valvular disease, ventricular hypertrophy, see pp 218, 219.

Left ventricle
from the left and below

A

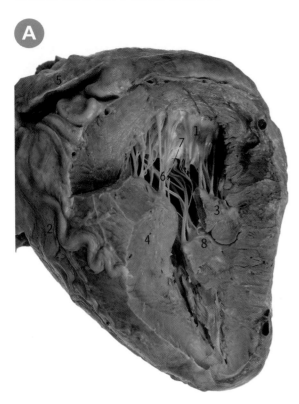

Heart *coronal section of the ventricles*

B

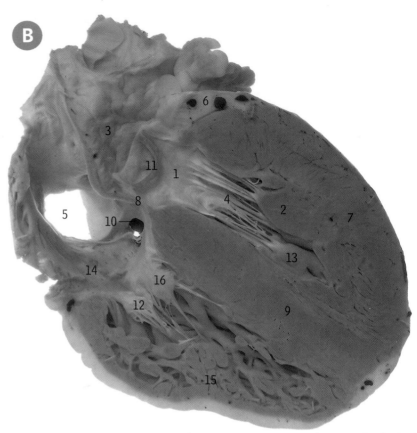

The ventricle has been opened by removing much of the left, anterior and posterior walls, and is viewed from below, looking upwards to the under-surface of the cusps of the mitral valve (1 and 7) which are anchored to the anterior and posterior papillary muscles (3 and 8) by chordae tendineae (6). The posterior cusp (7) is largely hidden by the anterior cusp (1) in this view.

1 Anterior cusp of mitral valve
2 Anterior interventricular branch of left coronary artery
3 Anterior papillary muscle
4 Anterior ventricular wall
5 Auricle of left atrium
6 Chordae tendineae
7 Posterior cusp of mitral valve
8 Posterior papillary muscle

The heart has been cut in two in the coronal plane, and this is the posterior section seen from the front, looking towards the back of both ventricles. The section has passed immediately in front of the anterior cusp of the mitral valve (1) and the posterior cusp of the aortic valve (11).

The cusps of the aortic and pulmonary valves are here given their official names but some English texts use slightly different alternatives, as follows:

		Official	English
Aortic		Right	Anterior
		Left	Left posterior
		Posterior	Right posterior
Pulmonary		Left	Posterior
		Anterior	Left anterior
		Right	Right anterior

1 Anterior cusp of mitral valve
2 Anterior papillary muscle
3 Ascending aorta
4 Chordae tendineae
5 Inferior vena cava
6 Left coronary artery branches and great cardiac vein
7 Left ventricular wall
8 Membranous part of interventricular septum
9 Muscular part of interventricular septum
10 Opening of coronary sinus
11 Posterior cusp of aortic valve
12 Posterior cusp of tricuspid valve
13 Posterior papillary muscle
14 Right atrium
15 Right ventricular wall
16 Septal cusp of tricuspid valve

Intracardiac injections, see p. 219.

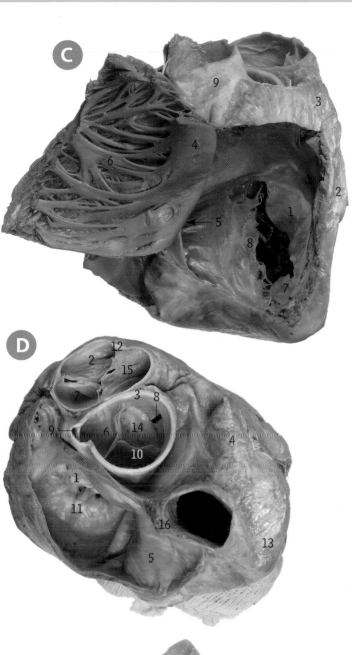

ⓒ Tricuspid valve
from the right atrium

The atrium has been opened by incising the anterior wall (2) and turning the flap outwards so that the atrial surface of the atrioventricular orifice is seen, guarded by the three cusps of the tricuspid valve – anterior (1), posterior (7) and septal (8).

1	Anterior cusp of tricuspid valve	**6**	Pectinate muscles
2	Anterior wall of right atrium	**7**	Posterior cusp of tricuspid valve
3	Auricle of right atrium		
4	Crista terminalis	**8**	Septal cusp of tricuspid valve
5	Interatrial septum	**9**	Superior vena cava

The posterior cusp (7) of the tricuspid valve is the smallest.

ⓓ Pulmonary, aortic and mitral valves *from above*

The pulmonary trunk (12) and ascending aorta (3) have been cut off immediately above the three cusps of the pulmonary and aortic valves (7, 2 and 15, and 14, 10 and 6). The upper part of the left atrium (5) has been removed to show the upper surface of the mitral valve cusps (11 and 1).

1	Anterior cusp of mitral valve	**9**	Ostium of left coronary artery
2	Anterior cusp of pulmonary valve	**10**	Posterior cusp of aortic valve
3	Ascending aorta	**11**	Posterior cusp of mitral valve
4	Auricle of right atrium	**12**	Pulmonary trunk
5	Left atrium	**13**	Right atrium
6	Left cusp of aortic valve	**14**	Right cusp of aortic valve
7	Left cusp of pulmonary valve	**15**	Right cusp of pulmonary valve
8	Marker in ostium of right coronary artery	**16**	Superior vena cava

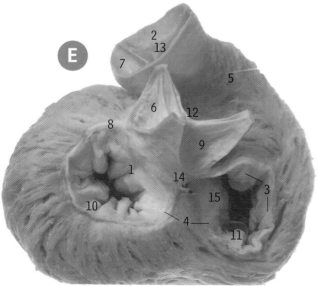

ⓔ Heart *fibrous framework*

The heart is seen from the right and behind after removing both atria, looking down on to the fibrous rings (4) that surround the mitral and tricuspid orifices and form the attachments for the bases of the valve cusps. The cusps of the pulmonary valve (7, 2 and 13) are seen at the top of the infundibulum of the right ventricle (5), and the aortic valve cusps (12, 9 and 6) have been dissected out from the beginning of the ascending aorta.

1	Anterior cusp of mitral valve	**8**	Left fibrous trigone
2	Anterior cusp of pulmonary valve	**9**	Posterior cusp of aortic valve
3	Anterior cusp of tricuspid valve	**10**	Posterior cusp of mitral valve
4	Fibrous ring	**11**	Posterior cusp of tricuspid valve
5	Infundibulum of right ventricle	**12**	Right cusp of aortic valve
6	Left cusp of aortic valve	**13**	Right cusp of pulmonary valve
7	Left cusp of pulmonary valve	**14**	Right fibrous trigone
		15	Septal cusp of tricuspid valve

Coronary arteries

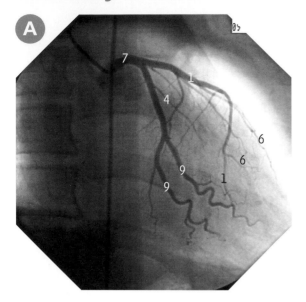

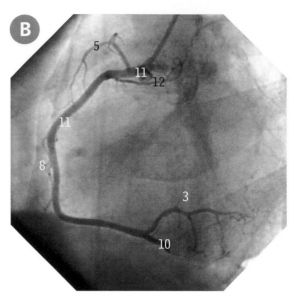

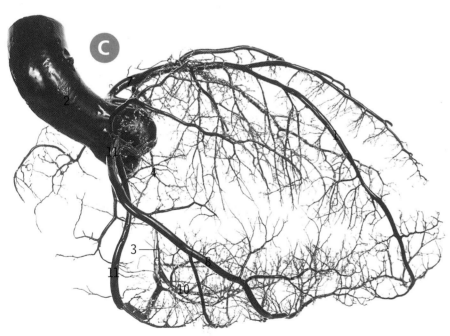

A left coronary arteriogram, right anterior oblique projection

B right coronary arteriogram, left anterior oblique projection

C cast of the coronary arteries, from the front

The interventricular branches are often called by clinicians the descending branches (anterior interventricular = left anterior descending; posterior interventricular = posterior descending).

1 Anterior interventricular branch of left coronary artery
2 Ascending aorta
3 Atrioventricular nodal artery
4 Circumflex branch of left coronary artery
5 Conus artery
6 Diagonal artery
7 Left coronary artery
8 Marginal branch of right coronary artery
9 Obtuse marginal artery
10 Posterior interventricular branch of right coronary artery
11 Right coronary artery
12 Sinuatrial nodal artery

 Angina pectoris, balloon angioplasty, cardiac angiography, see p. 218.

Colour Doppler echocardiographs

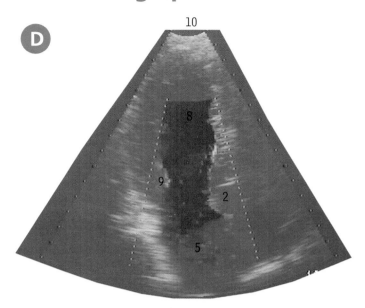

D

E

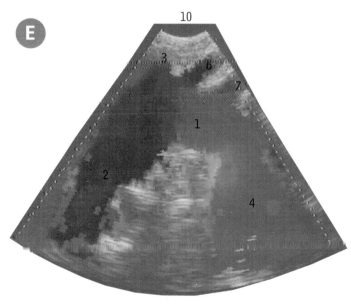

F Cast of the heart and great vessels *from below and behind*

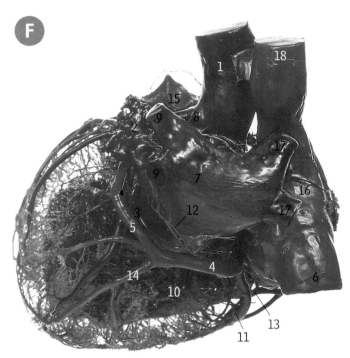

This specimen shows the coronary sinus (4) in the atrioventricular groove, and various tributaries (see notes).

1	Ascending aorta	**11**	Middle cardiac vein
2	Auricle of left atrium	**12**	Oblique vein of left atrium
3	Circumflex branch of left coronary artery	**13**	Posterior interventricular branch of right coronary artery
4	Coronary sinus	**14**	Posterior vein of left ventricle
5	Great cardiac vein	**15**	Pulmonary trunk
6	Inferior vena cava	**16**	Right atrium
7	Left atrium	**17**	Right pulmonary veins
8	Left coronary artery	**18**	Superior vena cava
9	Left pulmonary veins		
10	Left ventricle		

D apical long axis – left ventricle

E suprasternal notch view of aortic arch

1	Aortic arch	**6**	Left common carotid artery
2	Ascending aorta	**7**	Left subclavian artery
3	Brachiocephalic artery	**8**	Left ventricle
4	Descending aorta	**9**	Mitral valve
5	Left atrium	**10**	Site of transducer

Colour code: red = blood coming towards transducer; blue = away from the transducer

This technique enables both anatomy and pathology of blood vessels to be visualized in the living subject without exposure to radiation.

The base of the heart (like the base of the prostate) is its posterior surface, formed largely by the left atrium (F7). Note that the base is not the part of the heart which joins the superior vena cava, aorta and pulmonary trunk; this part has no special name.

The very small oblique vein of the left atrium (F12) marks the point where the great cardiac vein (F5) becomes the coronary sinus (F4), but in F the junction is unusually far to the right so that the posterior vein of the left ventricle (F14) joins the great cardiac vein (F5) instead of the coronary sinus itself.

The coronary sinus (F4), which receives most of the venous blood from the heart, lies in the posterior part of the atrioventricular groove between the left atrium and left ventricle (page 190, B2), and opens into the right atrium (page 191, C6).

The coronary sinus normally receives as tributaries the great cardiac vein (F5), middle cardiac vein (F11), and the small cardiac vein, the posterior vein of the left ventricle (F14) and the oblique vein of the left atrium (F12).

Right lung root and mediastinal pleura

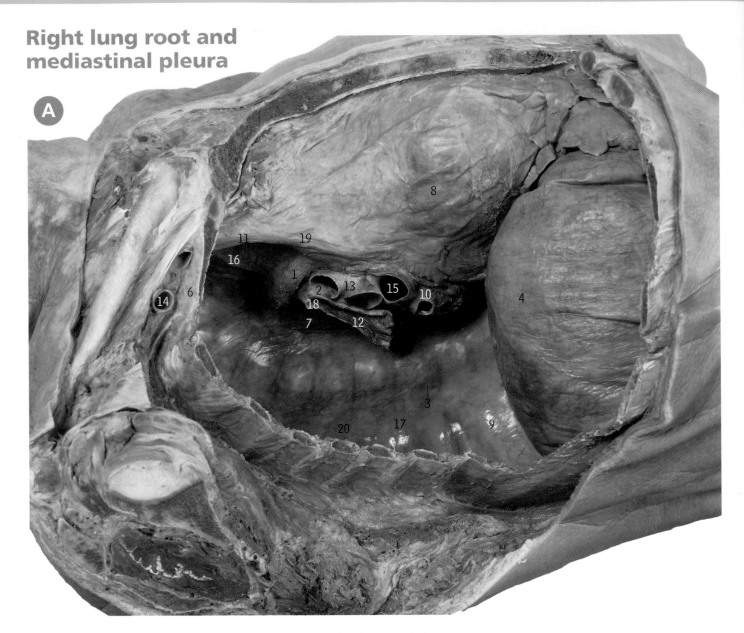

This is the view of the right side of the mediastinum after removing the lung but with the parietal pleura still intact (with the body lying on its back, head towards the left).

1   Azygos vein
2   Branch of right pulmonary artery to superior lobe
3   Branches of sympathetic trunk to greater splanchnic nerve
4   Diaphragm
5   Inferior vena cava
6   Neck of first rib
7   Oesophagus
8   Pericardium over right atrium
9   Pleura, costal
10 Right inferior pulmonary vein
11 Right phrenic nerve
12 Right principal bronchus
13 Right pulmonary artery
14 Right subclavian artery
15 Right superior pulmonary vein
16 Right vagus nerve
17 Sixth right posterior intercostal vessels under parietal pleura
18 Superior lobe bronchus
19 Superior vena cava
20 Sympathetic trunk and ganglion

ⓑ Right lung root and mediastinum

In a similar specimen to A, most of the pleura has been removed to display the underlying structures. The azygos vein (1) arches over the structures forming the lung root to enter the superior vena cava (23). The highest structures in the lung root are the artery (2) and bronchus (22) to the superior lobe of the lung. The right superior pulmonary vein (16) is in front of the right pulmonary artery, with the right inferior pulmonary vein (10) the lowest structure in the root. Above the arch of the azygos vein the trachea (26), with the right vagus nerve (17) in contact with it, lies in front of the oesophagus (7). Part of the first rib has been cut away to show the structures lying in front of its neck (6) – the sympathetic trunk (25), supreme intercostal vein (24), superior intercostal artery (20) and the ventral ramus of the first thoracic nerve (27). The right recurrent laryngeal nerve (14) hooks underneath the right subclavian artery (15). The right phrenic nerve (11) runs down over the superior vena cava (23) and the pericardium overlying the right atrium (8), and pierces the diaphragm (4) beside the inferior vena cava (5). Contributions from the sympathetic trunk (3) pass over the sides of vertebral bodies superficial to posterior intercostal arteries and veins (as at 19 and 18) to form the greater splanchnic nerve. The lower part of the oesophagus (7) behind the lung root and heart has the azygos vein (1) on its right side.

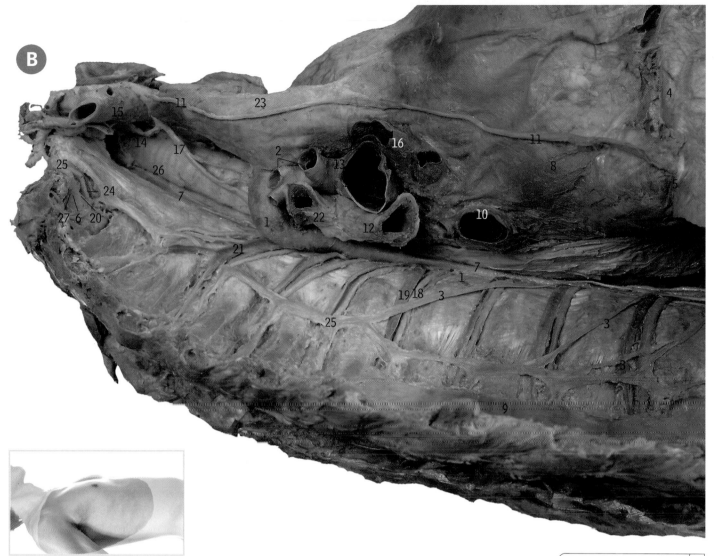

1   Azygos vein
2   Branch of right pulmonary artery to superior lobe
3   Branches of sympathetic trunk to greater splanchnic nerve
4   Diaphragm
5   Inferior vena cava
6   Neck of first rib
7   Oesophagus
8   Pericardium over right atrium
9   Pleura (cut edge)
10 Right inferior pulmonary vein
11 Right phrenic nerve
12 Right principal bronchus
13 Right pulmonary artery
14 Right recurrent laryngeal nerve
15 Right subclavian artery
16 Right superior pulmonary vein
17 Right vagus nerve
18 Sixth right posterior intercostal artery
19 Sixth right posterior intercostal vein
20 Superior intercostal artery
21 Superior intercostal vein
22 Superior lobe bronchus
23 Superior vena cava
24 Supreme intercostal vein
25 Sympathetic trunk and ganglion
26 Trachea
27 Ventral ramus of first thoracic nerve

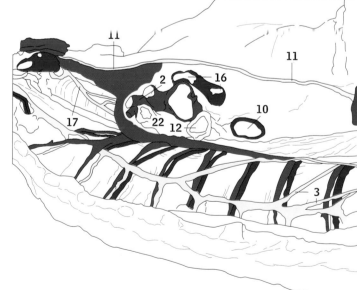

Pleural effusion, see p. 219.

Left lung root and mediastinal pleura

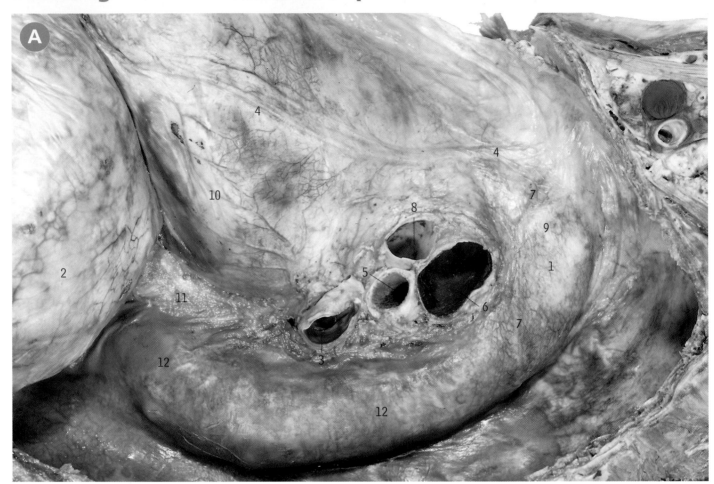

This is the view of the left side of the mediastinum after removing the lung but with the parietal pleura still intact (with the body lying on its back, head towards the right). Compare the features seen here with those in the dissection opposite (a different specimen), from which the pleura has been removed.

On the left side above the diaphragm, the lower end of the oesophagus lies in a triangle bounded by the diaphragm below (A2), the heart in front (A10 and B24) and the descending aorta behind (A12 and B27).

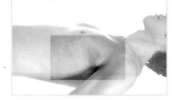

1 Arch of aorta
2 Diaphragm
3 Left inferior pulmonary vein
4 Left phrenic nerve and pericardiacophrenic vessels
5 Left principal bronchus
6 Left pulmonary artery
7 Left superior intercostal vein
8 Left superior pulmonary vein
9 Left vagus nerve
10 Mediastinal pleura and pericardium overlying left ventricle
11 Oesophagus
12 Thoracic aorta

Aortic aneurysm, pleurisy, pneumothorax, see pp 218, 219.

Left lung root and mediastinum

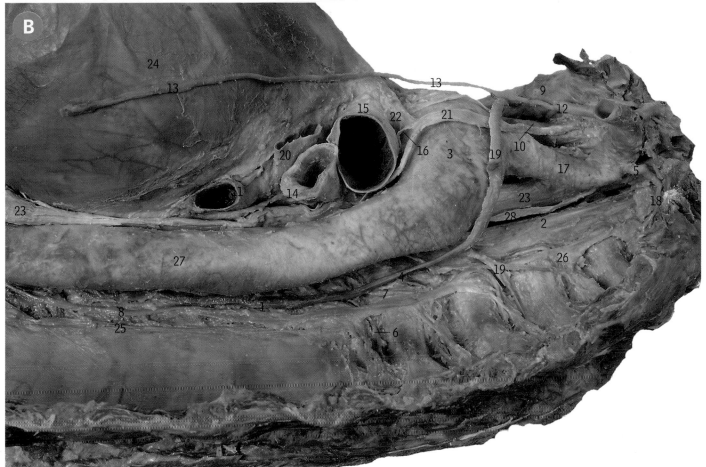

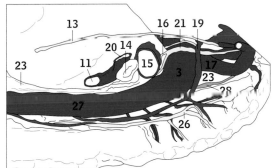

In a similar specimen to that on the opposite page, most of the pleura has been removed to show the underlying structures seen in A. The left vagus nerve (21) crosses the arch of the aorta (3) with the left phrenic nerve (13) anterior to it; the superior intercostal vein (19) runs over the vagus and under the phrenic. The left recurrent laryngeal nerve (16) hooks round the ligamentum arteriosum (22) while the vagus nerve continues behind the structures forming the lung root. The left pulmonary artery (15) is the highest structure in the root, and the inferior pulmonary vein (11) the lowest. The left superior pulmonary vein (20) is in front of the principal bronchus. The thoracic duct (28) is seen behind the left edge of the oesophagus (23), and the origin of the left superior intercostal artery (18) from the costocervical trunk (5) of the subclavian artery (17) is shown. In this specimen there is an uncommon communication (4) between the left superior intercostal vein (19) and the accessory hemi-azygos vein (1). Above the diaphragm (not shown, having been pushed beyond the edge of the picture with the lower end of the phrenic nerve, 13) the oesophagus (23) bulges towards the left between the heart and pericardium (24) in front and the descending aorta (27) behind.

1 Accessory hemi-azygos vein
2 Anterior longitudinal ligament
3 Arch of aorta
4 Communication between 19 and 1
5 Costocervical trunk
6 Fifth left posterior intercostal vein
7 Fourth left posterior intercostal artery
8 Hemi-azygos vein
9 Left brachiocephalic vein
10 Left common carotid artery
11 Left inferior pulmonary vein
12 Left internal thoracic artery
13 Left phrenic nerve
14 Left principal bronchus
15 Left pulmonary artery
16 Left recurrent laryngeal nerve
17 Left subclavian artery
18 Left superior intercostal artery
19 Left superior intercostal vein
20 Left superior pulmonary vein
21 Left vagus nerve
22 Ligamentum arteriosum
23 Oesophagus
24 Pericardium overlying left ventricle
25 Pleura (cut edge)
26 Sympathetic trunk and ganglion
27 Thoracic aorta
28 Thoracic duct

 Coarctation of the aorta, see p. 218.

Axial CT images *with contrast*

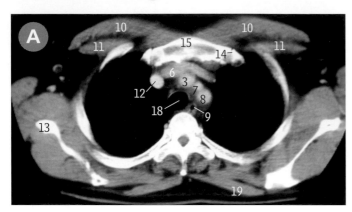

Level of T2

1	Arch aorta	**6**	Left brachiocephalic vein
2	Azygos vein	**7**	Left common carotid artery
3	Brachiocephalic trunk (artery)	**8**	Left subclavian artery
4	Descending aorta	**9**	Oesophagus
5	Hemi-azygos vein	**10**	Pectoralis major

Level of T4

11	Pectoralis minor	**16**	Superior vena cava
12	Right brachiocephalic vein	**17**	Thoracic duct
13	Scapula	**18**	Trachea
14	Sternoclavicular joint	**19**	Trapezius
15	Sternum		

Chest radiograph

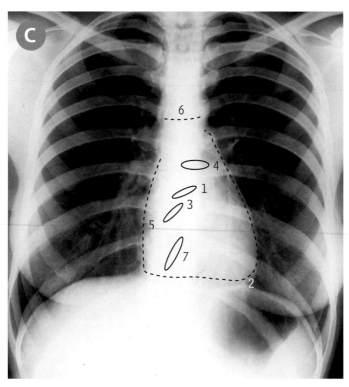

The surface markings of the heart valves are outlined by the ellipses.

1	Aortic valve	**5**	Right atrium
2	Apex of heart	**6**	Site of manubriosternal joint
3	Mitral valve	**7**	Tricuspid valve
4	Pulmonary valve		

Thorax *coronal MR image*

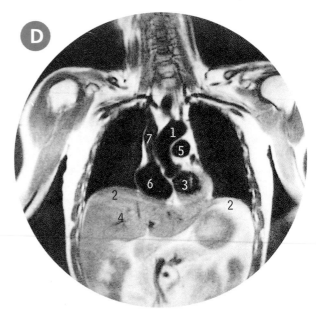

The section shows the heart and great vessels in the mediastinum, above the domes of the diaphragm (2) and liver (4). The plane of the image is through the left ventricle (3) and right atrium (6).

1	Arch of aorta	**5**	Pulmonary trunk
2	Dome of diaphragm	**6**	Right atrium
3	Left ventricle	**7**	Superior vena cava
4	Liver		

 Phrenic nerve palsy, see p. 219.

Cast of the lower trachea and bronchi

Ⓐ *vertical from the front* **Ⓑ** *oblique from the left*

The main bronchi and lobar bronchi are labelled with letters; the segmental bronchi are labelled with their conventional numbers. In the side view in B the cast has been tilted to avoid overlap, and the right side is more anterior than the left.

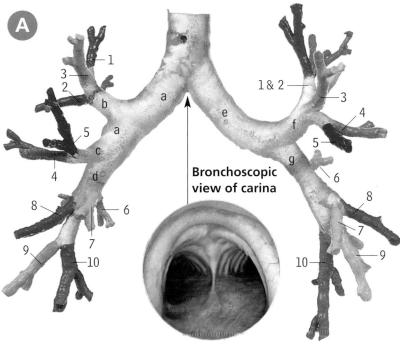

Bronchoscopic view of carina

Image courtesy of Prof. J. F. Dumon, France.

RIGHT LUNG	LEFT LUNG

Lobar bronchi

a	Principal		**e**	Principal
b	Superior lobe		**f**	Superior lobe
c	Middle lobe		**g**	Inferior lobe
d	Inferior lobe			

Segmental bronchi

Superior lobe	Superior lobe
1 Apical	**1 & 2** Apicoposterior
2 Posterior	**3** Anterior
3 Anterior	**4** Superior lingular
	5 Inferior lingular

Middle lobe	
4 Lateral	
5 Medial	

Inferior lobe	Inferior lobe
6 Apical (superior)	**6** Apical (superior)
7 Medial basal	**7** Medial basal
8 Anterior basal	**8** Anterior basal
9 Lateral basal	**9** Lateral basal
10 Posterior basal	**10** Posterior basal

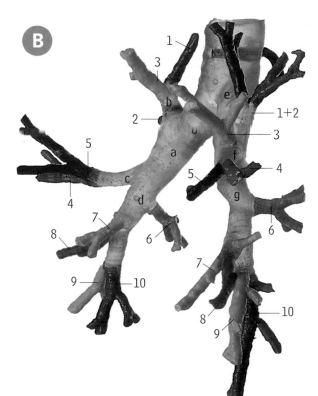

The trachea divides into right and left principal bronchi (a and e).

The right principal bronchus (a) is shorter, wider and more vertical than the left (e).

The left principal bronchus (e) is longer and narrower and lies more transversely than the right. Foreign bodies are therefore more likely to enter the right principal bronchus than the left.

The right principal bronchus (a) gives off a superior lobe bronchus (b) and then enters the hilum of the right lung before dividing into middle and inferior lobe bronchi (c and d).

The left principal bronchus (e) enters the hilum of the lung before dividing into superior and inferior lobe bronchi (f and g).

The branches of the lobar bronchi are called segmental bronchi and each supplies a segment of lung tissue – bronchopulmonary segment. The segmental bronchi and the bronchopulmonary segments have similar names, and the ten segments of each lung are officially numbered (as here and page 202) as well as being named.

The segmental bronchi of the left and right lungs are essentially similar except that the apical and posterior bronchi of the superior lobe of the left lung arise from a common stem, thus called the apicoposterior bronchus and labelled here as 1 and 2; also there is no middle lobe of the left lung, and so the corresponding segments bear similar numbers; and the medial basal bronchus (7) of the left lung usually arises in common with the anterior basal (8).

The apical (superior) bronchus of the inferior lobe (6) of both lungs is the first or highest bronchus to arise from the posterior surface of the bronchial tree, as illustrated in B. When lying on the back fluid may therefore gravitate into this bronchus.

Cast of the bronchial tree

The bronchus and bronchopulmonary segments have been coloured and labelled with their conventional numbers.

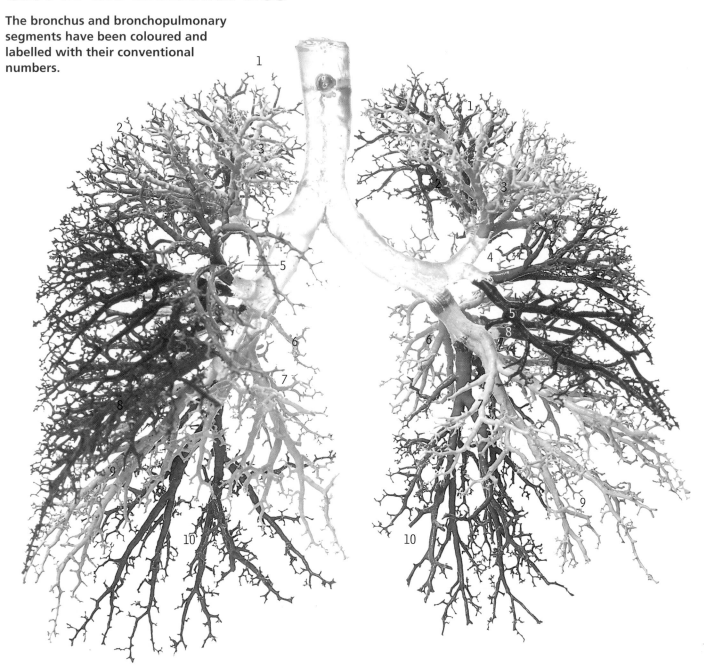

RIGHT LUNG

Superior lobe
1 Apical
2 Posterior
3 Anterior

Middle lobe
4 Lateral
5 Medial

Inferior lobe
6 Apical (superior)
7 Medial basal
8 Anterior basal
9 Lateral basal
10 Posterior basal

LEFT LUNG

Superior lobe
1 Apical
2 Posterior
3 Anterior
4 Superior lingular
5 Inferior lingular

Inferior lobe
6 Apical (superior)
7 Medial basal (cardiac)
8 Anterior basal
9 Lateral basal
10 Posterior basal

Bronchoscopy, see p. 218.

Bronchopulmonary segments of the right lung

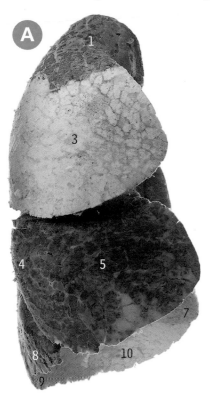

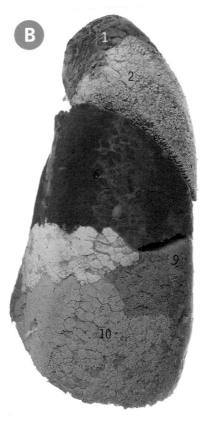

A from the front

B from behind

Superior lobe
1 Apical
2 Posterior
3 Anterior

Middle lobe
4 Lateral
5 Medial

Inferior lobe
6 Apical (superior)
7 Medial basal
8 Anterior basal
9 Lateral basal
10 Posterior basal

A subapical (subsuperior) segmental bronchus and bronchopulmonary segment are present in over 50 per cent of lungs; in this specimen this additional segment is shown in white.

The posterior basal segment (10) is coloured with two different shades of yellow ochre.

Bronchopulmonary segments of the left lung

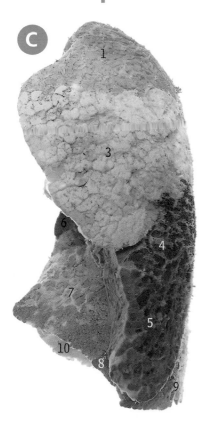

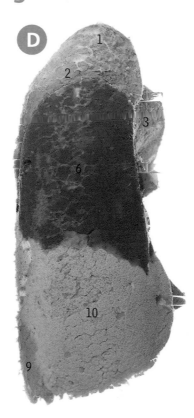

C from the front

D from behind

Superior lobe
1 Apical
2 Posterior
3 Anterior
4 Superior lingular
5 Inferior lingular

Inferior lobe
6 Apical (superior)
7 Medial basal (cardiac)
8 Anterior basal
9 Lateral basal
10 Posterior basal

The apical and posterior segments (1 and 2) are both coloured green, having been filled from the common apicoposterior bronchus (see page 201).

Bronchopulmonary segments of the right lung *from the lateral side*

Right bronchogram

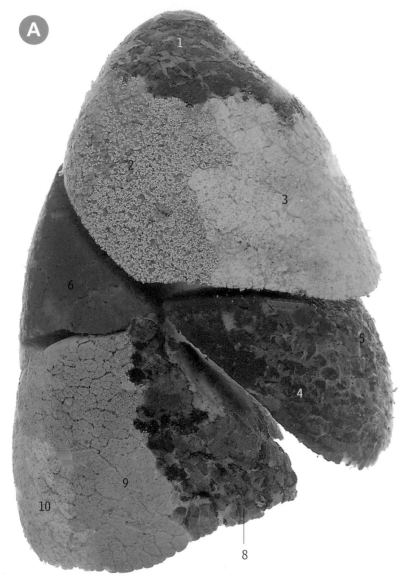

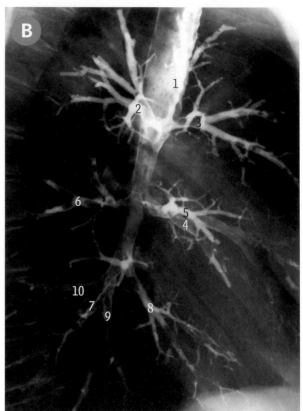

Superior lobe
1 Apical
2 Posterior
3 Anterior

Middle lobe
4 Lateral
5 Medial

Inferior lobe
6 Apical (superior)
7 Medial basal
8 Anterior basal
9 Lateral basal
10 Posterior basal

The medial basal segment (7) is not seen in the view in A.

The posterior basal segment in A (10) is coloured with two different shades of green.

Pneumonia, see p. 219.

Bronchopulmonary segments of the left lung *from the lateral side*

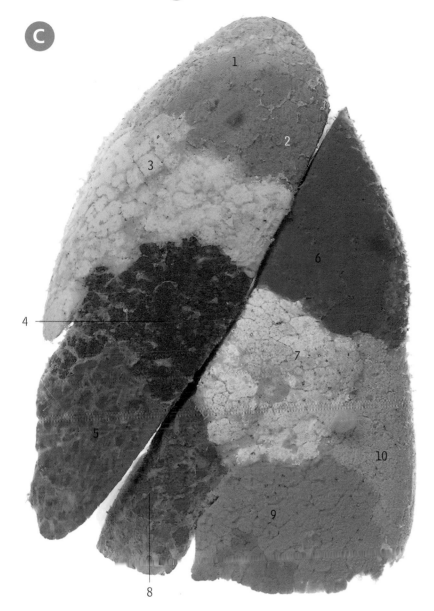

Left bronchogram

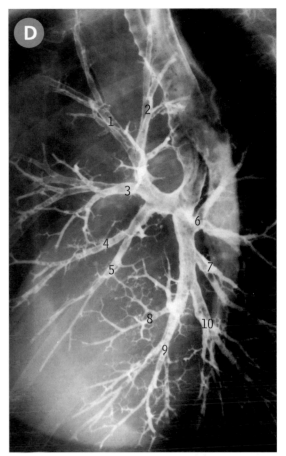

Superior lobe
1 Apical
2 Posterior
3 Anterior
4 Superior lingular
5 Inferior lingular

Inferior lobe
6 Apical (superior)
7 Medial basal (cardiac)
8 Anterior basal
9 Lateral basal
10 Posterior basal

The apical and posterior segments (1 and 2) are both coloured green, having been filled from the common apicoposterior bronchus (see page 201).

Cast of the bronchial tree and pulmonary vessels *from the front*

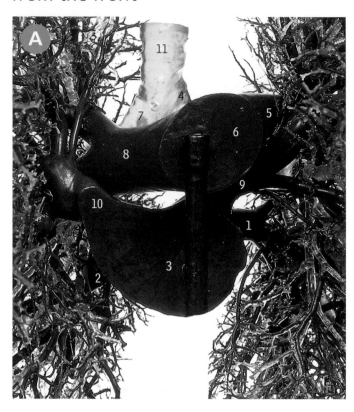

The pulmonary trunk (6) divides into the left and right pulmonary arteries (5 and 8), and these vessels have been injected with red resin. The four pulmonary veins (9, 1, 2 and 10) which drain into the left atrium (3) have been filled with blue resin. Note that in the living body the pulmonary veins are filled with oxygenated blood from the lungs and would normally be represented by a red colour; similarly the pulmonary arteries contain deoxygenated blood and should be represented by a blue colour.

1 Inferior left pulmonary vein	6 Pulmonary trunk
2 Inferior right pulmonary vein	7 Right principal bronchus
3 Left atrium	8 Right pulmonary artery
4 Left principal bronchus	9 Superior left pulmonary vein
5 Left pulmonary artery	10 Superior right pulmonary vein
	11 Trachea

Lung roots and bronchial arteries *right side from above*

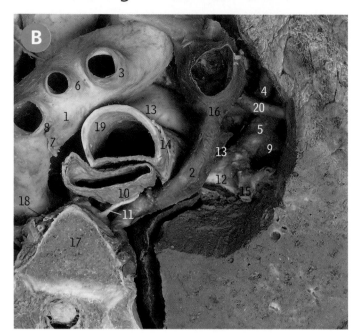

The thorax has been sectioned transversely at the level of the third thoracic vertebra (17), just above the arch of the aorta (1) whose three larger branches have been removed (8, 6 and 3), and lung tissue at the hilum has been dissected away from above. The oesophagus (10) and trachea (19) have been tilted forwards to show one of the bronchial arteries (11).

1 Arch of aorta	12 Right principal bronchus
2 Azygos vein	13 Right pulmonary artery
3 Brachiocephalic trunk	14 Right vagus nerve
4 Inferior lobe artery	15 Superior lobe bronchus
5 Inferior lobe bronchus	16 Superior vena cava
6 Left common carotid artery	17 Third thoracic vertebra
7 Left recurrent laryngeal nerve	18 Thoracic duct
8 Left subclavian artery	19 Trachea
9 Middle lobe bronchus	20 Tributary of inferior
10 Oesophagus	pulmonary vein
11 Right bronchial artery	

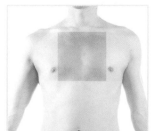

C Azygos vein *endoscopic view*

1 Azygos vein
2 Right lung
3 Superior vena cava
4 Visceral pleura

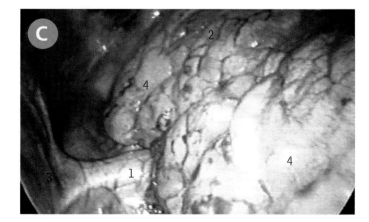

Pulmonary embolism, see p. 219.

D Cast of the pulmonary arteries and bronchi *from the front*
E Pulmonary arteriogram

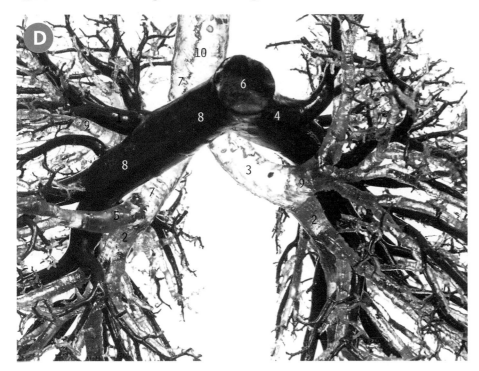

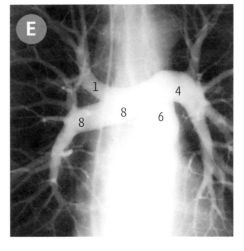

The upper part of the pulmonary trunk (6) is seen end-on after cutting off the lower part, and the bifurcation of the trunk into the left (4) and right (8) pulmonary arteries is in front of the beginning of the left main bronchus (3). In the living body these pulmonary vessels contain deoxygenated blood and would normally be represented by a blue colour, but here they have been filled with red resin. Compare the vessels in the cast with those in the arteriogram E.

1 Branch of right pulmonary artery to superior lobe
2 Inferior lobe bronchus
3 Left principal bronchus
4 Left pulmonary artery
5 Middle lobe bronchus
6 Pulmonary trunk
7 Right principal bronchus
8 Right pulmonary artery
9 Superior lobe bronchus
10 Trachea

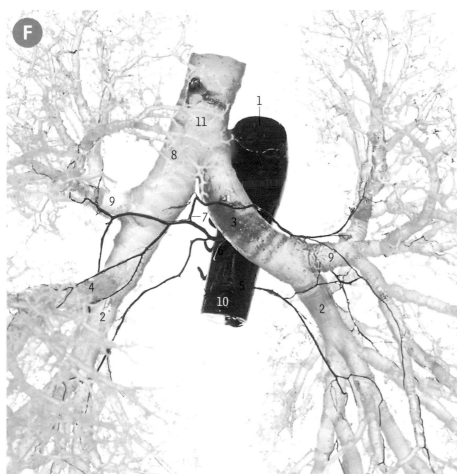

F Cast of the bronchi and bronchial arteries
from the front

Part of the aorta (1 and 10) has been injected with red resin to fill the bronchial arteries. These vessels normally run behind the bronchi and their branches but in this specimen they are in front.

1 Arch of aorta
2 Inferior lobe bronchus
3 Left principal bronchus
4 Middle lobe bronchus
5 Origin of lower left bronchial artery
6 Origin of right bronchial artery
7 Origin of upper left bronchial artery
8 Right principal bronchus
9 Superior lobe bronchus
10 Thoracic aorta
11 Trachea

Right lung *medial surface*

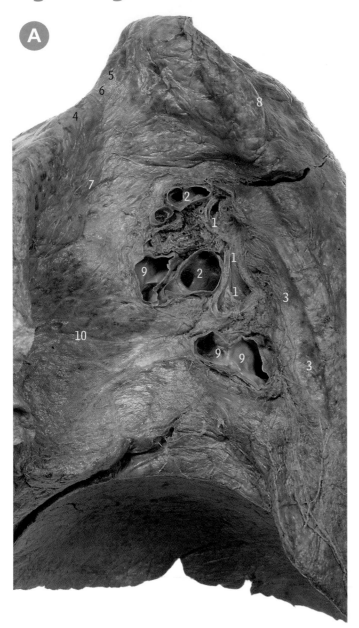

Left lung *medial surface*

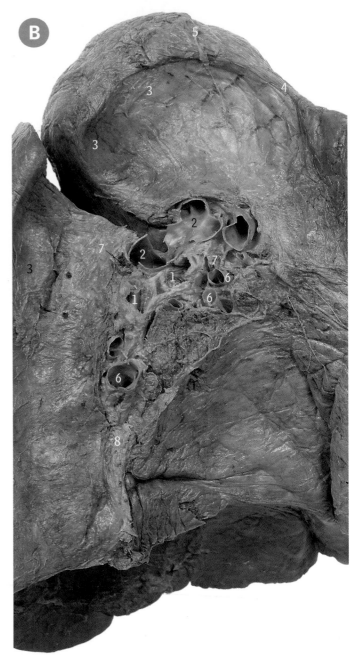

In the hardened dissecting room specimen, adjacent structures make impressions on the medial surface of the lung. The most prominent feature on the right side is the groove for the azygos vein (3), above and behind the structures of the lung root (9, 2 and 1).

Compare with the right lung in A, and note the large size of the impression made by the aorta on the left lung (B3), in contrast to the smaller azygos groove on the right (A3).

1 Branches of right principal bronchus
2 Branches of right pulmonary artery
3 Groove for azygos vein
4 Groove for first rib
5 Groove for subclavian artery
6 Groove for subclavian vein
7 Groove for superior vena cava
8 Oesophageal and tracheal area
9 Right pulmonary veins
10 Transverse fissure

The upper end of the medial surface of the right lung lies against the oesophagus and trachea (A8) with only the pleura intervening, but on the left the subclavian artery (B5) (and the left common carotid in front of it) keep the lung further away from these structures.

1 Branches of left principal bronchus
2 Branches of left pulmonary artery
3 Groove for aorta
4 Groove for first rib
5 Groove for left subclavian artery
6 Left pulmonary veins
7 Lymph node, containing carbon
8 Pulmonary ligament

Lower neck and upper thorax *surface markings*

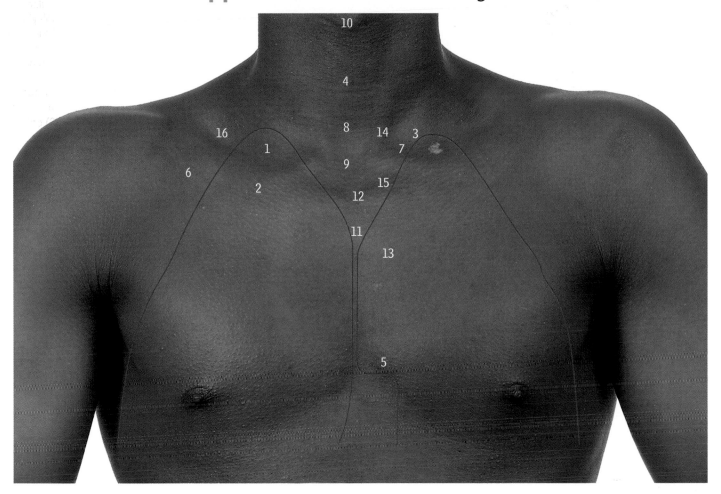

The magenta line indicates the extent of the pleura and lung on each side; the apices of the pleura and lung (1) rise into the neck for about 3 cm above the medial third of the clavicle. The lower end of the internal jugular vein (7) lies behind the interval between the sternal (14) and clavicular (3) heads of sternocleidomastoid. Behind the sternoclavicular joint (15) the internal jugular and subclavian veins unite to form the brachiocephalic vein. The trachea (8) is felt in the midline above the jugular notch (9), and the arch of the cricoid cartilage (4) is 4 to 5 cm above the notch. The manubriosternal joint is at the level of the second costal cartilage (13) and opposite the lower border of the body of the fourth thoracic vertebra, and the horizontal plane through these points indicates the junction between the superior and inferior parts of the mediastinum. The left brachiocephalic vein passes behind the upper half of the manubrium to unite with the right brachiocephalic at the lower border of the right first costal cartilage (to form the superior vena cava). The midpoint of the manubrium (12) marks the highest level of the arch of the aorta and the origin of the brachiocephalic trunk. Compare many of the features mentioned here with the structures in the dissection on page 210.

1 Apex of pleura and lung
2 Clavicle
3 Clavicular head of sternocleidomastoid
4 Cricoid cartilage
5 Fourth costal cartilage
6 Infraclavicular fossa
7 Internal jugular vein
8 Isthmus of thyroid gland overlying trachea
9 Jugular notch (suprasternal)
10 Laryngeal prominence
11 Manubriosternal joint
12 Midpoint of manubrium of sternum
13 Second costal cartilage
14 Sternal head of sternocleidomastoid
15 Sternoclavicular joint
16 Supraclavicular fossa

Thoracic inlet and mediastinum *from the front*

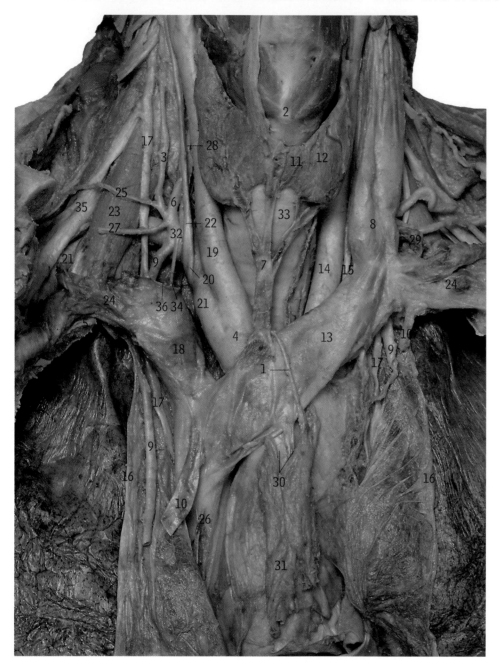

The anterior thoracic wall and the medial ends of the clavicles have been removed, but part of the parietal pleura (16) remains over the medial part of each lung. The right internal jugular vein has also been removed, displaying the thyrocervical trunk (32) and the origin of the internal thoracic artery (9). Inferior thyroid veins (7) run down over the trachea (33) to enter the left brachiocephalic vein (13). The thymus (31) has been dissected out from mediastinal fat; thymic veins (30) enter the left brachiocephalic vein, and an unusual thymic artery (1) arises from the brachiocephalic trunk (4).

The remains of the thymus (31) are in front of the pericardium, but in the child, where the thymus is much larger (see page 188B), it may extend upwards in front of the great vessels as high as the lower part of the thyroid gland (12).

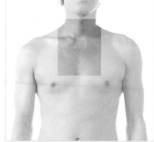

1	A thymic artery	13	Left brachiocephalic vein	25	Superficial cervical artery
2	Arch of cricoid cartilage	14	Left common carotid artery	26	Superior vena cava
3	Ascending cervical artery	15	Left vagus nerve	27	Suprascapular artery
4	Brachiocephalic trunk	16	Parietal pleura (cut edge) over lung	28	Sympathetic trunk
5	First rib	17	Phrenic nerve	29	Thoracic duct
6	Inferior thyroid artery	18	Right brachiocephalic vein	30	Thymic veins
7	Inferior thyroid veins	19	Right common carotid artery	31	Thymus
8	Internal jugular vein	20	Right recurrent laryngeal nerve	32	Thyrocervical trunk
9	Internal thoracic artery	21	Right subclavian artery	33	Trachea
10	Internal thoracic vein	22	Right vagus nerve	34	Unusual cervical tributary of 18
11	Isthmus of thyroid gland	23	Scalenus anterior	35	Upper trunk of brachial plexus
12	Lateral lobe of thyroid gland	24	Subclavian vein	36	Vertebral vein

 Pancoast's tumour, thoracic outlet syndromes, see p. 219.

Thoracic inlet *right upper ribs, from below*

ANTERIOR

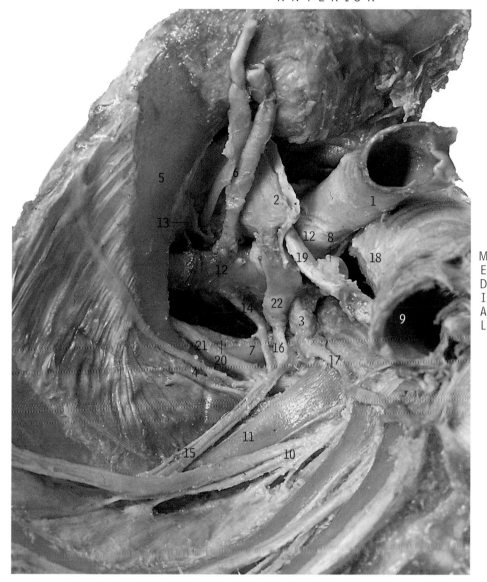

MEDIAL

1 Brachiocephalic trunk
2 Brachiocephalic vein
3 Cervicothoracic (stellate) ganglion
4 First intercostal nerve
5 First rib
6 Internal thoracic vessels
7 Neck of first rib
8 Recurrent laryngeal nerve
9 Right principal bronchus
10 Second intercostal nerve
11 Second rib
12 Subclavian artery
13 Subclavian vein
14 Superior intercostal artery
15 Superior intercostal vein
16 Supreme intercostal vein (unusually large)
17 Sympathetic trunk
18 Trachea
19 Vagus nerve
20 Ventral ramus of eighth cervical nerve
21 Ventral ramus of first thoracic nerve
22 Vertebral vein

> The neck of the first rib (7) is crossed in order from medial to lateral by the sympathetic trunk (17), supreme intercostal vein (16), superior intercostal artery (14) and the ventral ramus of the first thoracic nerve (21).

This is the view looking upwards into the right side of the thoracic inlet – the region occupied by the cervical pleura, here removed. The under-surface of most of the first rib (5) is seen from below, with the subclavian artery (12) passing over the top of it after giving off the internal thoracic branch (6) which runs towards the top of the picture (to the anterior thoracic wall), and the costocervical trunk whose superior intercostal branch (14) runs down over the neck of the first rib (7). The vertebral vein (22) has come down from the neck and is labelled on its posterior surface before entering the brachiocephalic vein (2, labelled at its opened cut edge). The vertebral vein receives an unusually large supreme intercostal vein (16). On its medial side is the sympathetic trunk (17) with the cervicothoracic ganglion (3). The neck of the first rib (7) has the ventral ramus of the first thoracic nerve (21) below it.

 Horner's syndrome, subclavian vein catheterization, see p. 219.

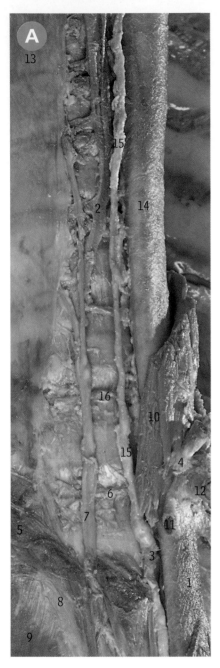

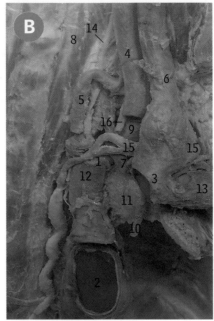

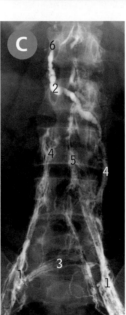

Ⓐ Thoracic duct
thoracic part

All viscera and part of the pleura have been removed to show the aorta (14 and 1) in front of the vertebral column and viewed from the right, with the thoracic duct (15) lying between the aorta (14) and azygos vein (2); the lower part of the vein was overlying the duct and has been removed. The cisterna chyli (3), where the thoracic duct begins, is in the abdomen under cover of the right crus of the diaphragm (10).

1	Abdominal aorta	10	Right crus of
2	Azygos vein		diaphragm
3	Cisterna chyli	11	Right renal artery
4	Coeliac trunk	12	Superior mesenteric
5	Diaphragm		artery
6	First lumbar artery	13	Sympathetic trunk
	and first lumbar		underlying pleura
	vertebra	14	Thoracic aorta
7	Greater splanchnic	15	Thoracic duct
	nerve	16	Twelfth thoracic
8	Medial arcuate		vertebra and
	ligament		subcostal artery
9	Psoas major		

Ⓑ Thoracic duct *cervical part*

In this deep dissection of the left side of the root of the neck and upper thorax, the internal jugular vein (6) joins the subclavian vein (13) to form the left brachiocephalic vein (3). The thoracic duct (15) is double for a short distance just before passing in front of the vertebral artery (9) and behind the common carotid artery (4, whose lower end has been cut away to show the duct). The duct then runs behind the internal jugular vein (6) before draining into the junction of that vein with the subclavian vein (13).

1	Ansa subclavia	9	Origin of vertebral artery
2	Arch of aorta	10	Phrenic nerve
3	Brachiocephalic vein	11	Pleura
4	Common carotid artery	12	Subclavian artery
5	Inferior thyroid artery	13	Subclavian vein
6	Internal jugular vein	14	Sympathetic trunk
7	Internal thoracic artery	15	Thoracic duct
8	Longus colli	16	Vagus nerve

From the cisterna chyli (A3), situated under cover of the left margin of the right crus of the diaphragm (A10) at the level of the first and second lumbar vertebrae, the thoracic duct passes upwards (through the aortic opening in the diaphragm) on the right side of the front of the thoracic vertebral column between the aorta (A14) and azygos vein (A2), crossing to the left at the level of the fifth to sixth thoracic vertebra and ending by opening into the left side of the union of the left internal jugular (B6) and subclavian (B13) veins after passing between the common carotid artery (in front, B4) and the vertebral artery (behind, B9).

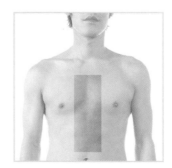

Ⓒ **First day lymphangiogram**

1	Common iliac vessels	4	Para-aortic vessels
2	Cysterna chyli	5	Pre-aortic vessels
3	Lumbar crossover	6	Thoracic duct

Chylothorax, see p. 218.

Ⓐ **Oesophagus** *lower thoracic part, from the front*

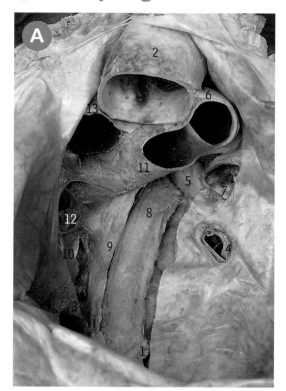

The heart has been removed from the pericardial cavity by transecting the great vessels, the pulmonary trunk being cut at the point where it divides into the two pulmonary arteries (11 and 6). Part of the pericardium (9) at the back has been removed to reveal the oesophagus (8). It is seen below the left principal bronchus (5) and is being crossed by the beginning of the right pulmonary artery (11).

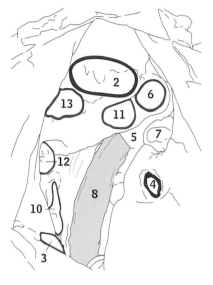

1	Anterior vagal trunk
2	Ascending aorta
3	Inferior vena cava
4	Left inferior pulmonary vein
5	Left principal bronchus
6	Left pulmonary artery
7	Left superior pulmonary vein
8	Oesophagus
9	Pericardium (cut edge)
10	Right inferior pulmonary vein
11	Right pulmonary artery
12	Right superior pulmonary vein
13	Superior vena cava

Ⓑ **Intercostal spaces**
posterior internal view

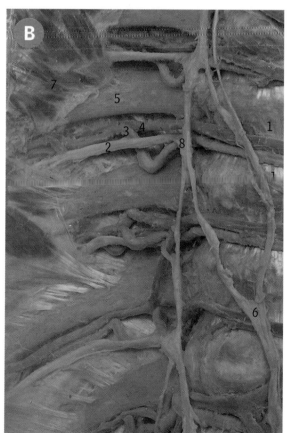

This dissection shows the medial ends of some intercostal spaces of the right side, viewed from the front and slightly from the right. The pleura has been removed, revealing subcostal muscles (7) laterally, the nerves and vessels (4, 3 and 2) in the intercostal spaces, and the sympathetic trunk (8) and greater splanchnic nerve (6) on the sides of the vertebral bodies (as at 1).

1	Body of ninth thoracic vertebra
2	Eighth intercostal nerve
3	Eighth posterior intercostal artery
4	Eighth posterior intercostal vein

5	Eighth rib
6	Greater splanchnic nerve
7	Subcostal muscle
8	Sympathetic trunk and ganglia

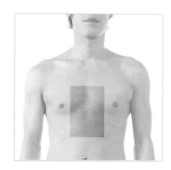

 Intercostal drainage, see p. 219.

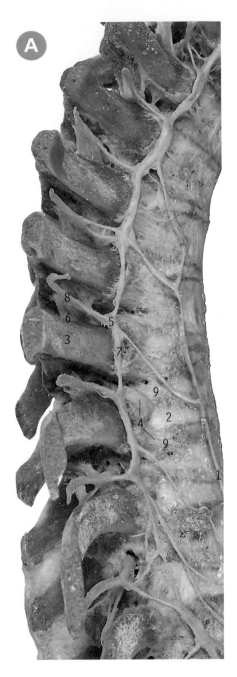

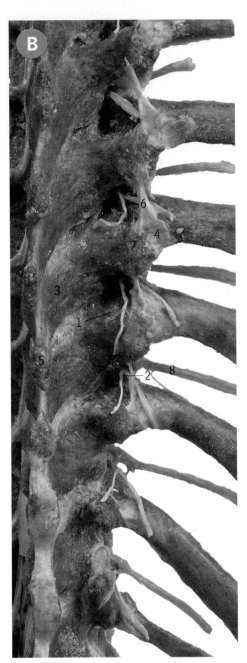

Ⓐ Joints of the heads of the ribs
from the right

In this part of the right mid-thoracic region, the ribs have been cut short beyond their tubercles, and the joints that the two facets of the head of a rib make with the facets on the sides of adjacent vertebral bodies and the intervening disc are shown, as at 4, 9 and 2, where the radiate ligament (4) covers the capsule of these small synovial joints.

1 Greater splanchnic nerve
2 Intervertebral disc
3 Neck of rib
4 Radiate ligament of joint of head of rib
5 Rami communicantes
6 Superior costotransverse ligament
7 Sympathetic trunk
8 Ventral ramus of spinal nerve
9 Vertebral body

Ⓑ Costotransverse joints *from behind*

In this view of the right half of the thoracic vertebral column from behind, costotransverse joints between the transverse processes of vertebrae and the tubercles of ribs are covered by the lateral costotransverse ligaments (as at 4). The dorsal rami of spinal nerves (2) pass medial to the superior costotransverse ligaments (6); ventral rami (8) run in front of these ligaments.

1 Costotransverse ligament
2 Dorsal ramus of spinal nerve
3 Lamina
4 Lateral costotransverse ligament
5 Spinous process
6 Superior costotransverse ligament
7 Transverse process
8 Ventral ramus of spinal nerve

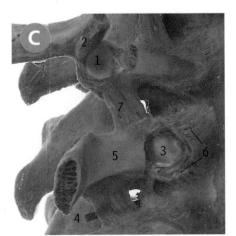

Ⓒ Costovertebral joints
disarticulated, from the right

In the upper part of the figure, the upper rib has been severed through its neck (5) and the part with the tubercle attached has been turned upwards after cutting through the capsule of the costotransverse joint, to show the articular facet of the tubercle (2) and the transverse process (1). The head of the lower rib has been removed after transecting the radiate ligament (6) and underlying capsule of the joint of the head of the rib (3).

1 Articular facet of transverse process
2 Articular facet of tubercle of rib
3 Cavity of joint of head of rib
4 Marker between anterior and posterior
   parts of superior costotransverse ligament
5 Neck of rib
6 Radiate ligament
7 Superior costotransverse ligament

Cast of the aorta and associated vessels

A *from the right* **B** *from the left*

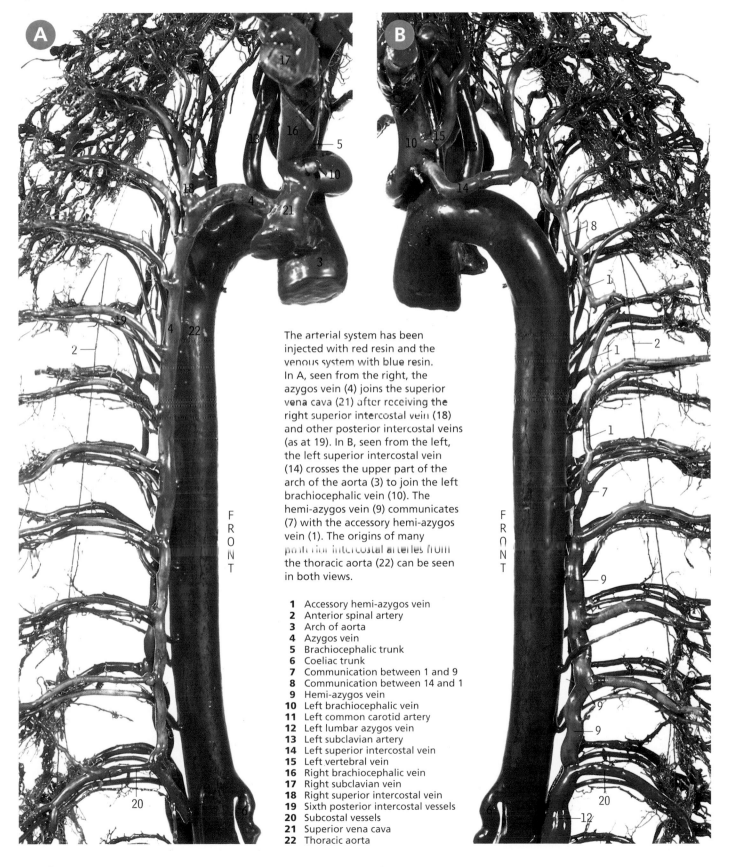

The arterial system has been injected with red resin and the venous system with blue resin. In A, seen from the right, the azygos vein (4) joins the superior vena cava (21) after receiving the right superior intercostal vein (18) and other posterior intercostal veins (as at 19). In B, seen from the left, the left superior intercostal vein (14) crosses the upper part of the arch of the aorta (3) to join the left brachiocephalic vein (10). The hemi-azygos vein (9) communicates (7) with the accessory hemi-azygos vein (1). The origins of many posterior intercostal arteries from the thoracic aorta (22) can be seen in both views.

1	Accessory hemi-azygos vein
2	Anterior spinal artery
3	Arch of aorta
4	Azygos vein
5	Brachiocephalic trunk
6	Coeliac trunk
7	Communication between 1 and 9
8	Communication between 14 and 1
9	Hemi-azygos vein
10	Left brachiocephalic vein
11	Left common carotid artery
12	Left lumbar azygos vein
13	Left subclavian artery
14	Left superior intercostal vein
15	Left vertebral vein
16	Right brachiocephalic vein
17	Right subclavian vein
18	Right superior intercostal vein
19	Sixth posterior intercostal vessels
20	Subcostal vessels
21	Superior vena cava
22	Thoracic aorta

Diaphragm *from above*

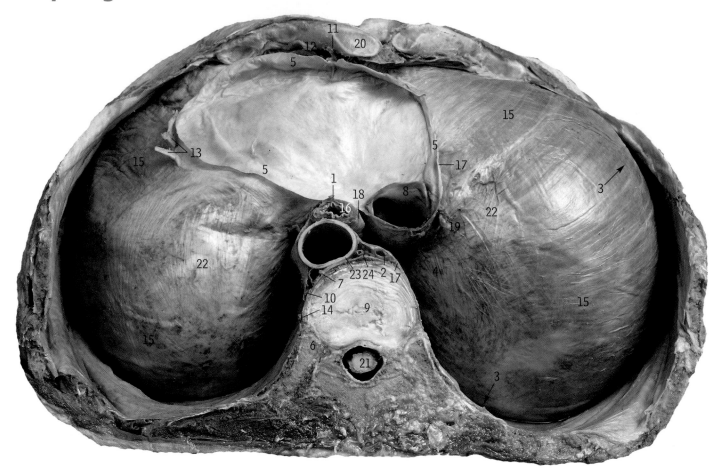

The thorax has been transected at the level of the disc between the ninth and tenth thoracic vertebrae.

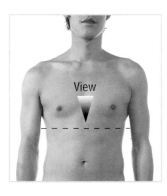

View

1	Anterior vagal trunk
2	Azygos vein
3	Costodiaphragmatic recess
4	Costomediastinal recess
5	Fibrous pericardium (cut edge)
6	Head of left ninth rib
7	Hemi-azygos vein
8	Inferior vena cava
9	Intervertebral disc
10	Left greater splanchnic nerve
11	Left internal thoracic artery
12	Left musculophrenic artery
13	Left phrenic nerve
14	Left sympathetic trunk
15	Muscle of diaphragm
16	Oesophagus
17	Pleura (cut edge)
18	Posterior vagal trunk
19	Right phrenic nerve
20	Seventh left costal cartilage
21	Spinal cord
22	Tendon of diaphragm
23	Thoracic aorta
24	Thoracic duct

According to the standard textbook description, the foramen for the vena cava is at the level of the disc between the eighth and ninth thoracic vertebrae, the oesophageal opening at the level of the tenth thoracic vertebra and the aortic opening opposite the twelfth thoracic vertebra. However, it is common for the oesophageal opening to be nearer the midline, as in this specimen (16), and the vena caval foramen (8) is lower than usual.

The vena caval foramen is in the tendinous part of the diaphragm and the oesophageal opening in the muscular part. The so-called aortic opening is not *in* the diaphragm but behind it (page 261).

The central tendon of the diaphragm has the shape of a trefoil leaf and has no bony attachment.

The right phrenic nerve (19) passes through the vena caval foramen, i.e. through the tendinous part, but the left phrenic nerve (13) pierces the muscular part in front of the central tendon just lateral to the overlying pericardium.

The phrenic nerves are the *only motor* nerves to the diaphragm, including the crura. The supply from lower thoracic (intercostal and subcostal) nerves is purely afferent. Damage to one phrenic nerve completely paralyses its own half of the diaphragm.

Gastro-oesophageal reflux, see p. 218.

Oesophageal radiographs *during a barium swallow*

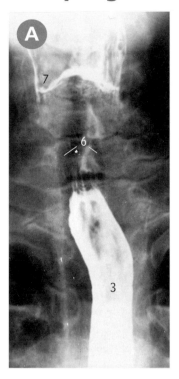

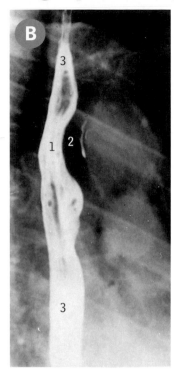

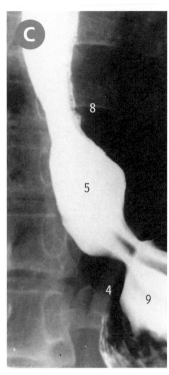

A lower pharynx and upper oesophagus

B middle part

C lower end

1 Aortic impression in oesophagus
2 Arch of aorta with plaque of calcification
3 Barium in oesophagus
4 Diaphragm
5 Lower thoracic oesophagus
6 Margins of trachea (translucent with contained air)
7 Piriform recess in laryngeal part of pharynx
8 Position of left atrium
9 Stomach

In A, viewed from the front, some of the barium paste adheres to the pharyngeal wall, outlining the piriform recesses (7), but most of it has passed into the oesophagus (3). In B, viewed obliquely from the left, the oesophagus is indented by the arch of the aorta (2) which shows some calcification in its wall – a useful aid to its identification. In C there is some dilatation at the lower end of the thoracic oesophagus (5) and it is constricted where it passes through the diaphragm (4) to join the stomach (9). The left atrium of the heart (8) lies in front of the lower thoracic oesophagus (page 213, A8), but only when enlarged does the atrium cause an indentation in the oesophagus.

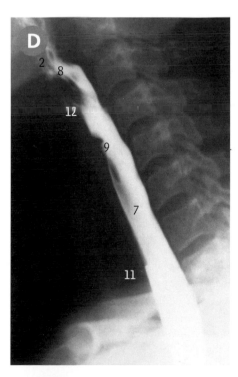

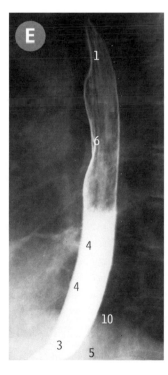

D cervical part

E thoracic part

1 Aortic arch impression
2 Base of tongue
3 Gastro-oesophageal junction
4 Left atrium position
5 Left hemidiaphragm
6 Left principal bronchus impression
7 Oesophagus
8 Oropharynx
9 Postcricoid venous plexus impression
10 Right hemidiaphragm
11 Trachea
12 Vallecula

Dysphagia, see p. 218.

Thorax
Clinical notes

Angina pectoris, an intermittent, relatively transient constricting central chest pain usually brought on by effort or exercise, is commonly due to coronary artery insufficiency secondary to atherosclerosis. (page 194)

Aortic aneurysm is a 'ballooning' of either the thoracic or abdominal aorta, occasionally with dissection or rupture causing sudden death. On a plain X-ray an aneurysm may be seen as an enlargement or unfolding of the aortic shadow. (page 198)

Balloon angioplasty is a procedure, similar to that for cardiac angiography, in which a catheter is inserted, usually via the femoral artery, and the tip of the catheter advanced into the narrowed coronary artery segment. A balloon at the end of the catheter is then blown up to stretch the coronary artery at this site. (page 194)

Bone marrow aspiration. The sternum is a site containing red marrow, even in adulthood, and is a convenient site to obtain a bone marrow biopsy. Another common site is the posterior iliac crest. (page 180)

Breast examination. A retracted nipple or a dimpling of the skin on breast examination are signs that should be taken seriously and may indicate an underlying pathology. Examination of the axillary lymph nodes is an important part of all breast examinations. (page 183)

Bronchoscopy is a technique that uses an instrument inserted in through the mouth to look at the trachea and main bronchi. The 'keel-like' carina is a particularly important region to note. If the tracheobronchial lymph nodes are enlarged the sharp edge of the carina becomes rounded, often an indication of carcinoma of the lung. (page 202)

Carcinoma of the breast is one of the most common causes of death in women. Most commonly found in the upper outer quadrant of the breast, metastases from these cancers often spread to the axillary lymph nodes. Surgeons may remove nodes from the axilla to 'stage' the disease. (page 183)

Cardiac angiography is a radiographic record of the functional cardiac circulation. It is carried out by means of a long catheter passed through the ascending aorta via the femoral or brachial arteries. The tip of the catheter is placed just inside the opening of a coronary artery and a small injection of radio-opaque contrast material will then show a moving coronary angiogram. This technique is used to find sites of coronary occlusion that may present clinically as angina or myocardial infarction. (page 194)

Cardiac pacemaker. This is an electrical impulse-generating device that is inserted under the skin of the anterior chest wall, from which wires pass to the heart tissue to maintain a regular heart beat. The insertion is a relatively minor surgical procedure, with the pacemaker lying on the pectoralis major muscle. (page 191)

Cardiac tamponade occurs when sufficient fluid, usually blood, accumulates within the pericardial cavity to restrict filling of the heart during diastole, leading to reduced blood pressure, tachycardia and eventually cardiac arrest if the tamponade is not relieved by a pericardial puncture. (page 189)

Chylothorax is the accumulation of lymph within the pleural cavity; i.e. between the visceral and parietal pleurae. (page 212)

Clicking-rib syndrome is a form of costochondritis along the costal margin due to subluxation of a rib causing irritation of the intercostal nerves. This may be confused clinically with upper abdominal problems. (page 186)

Coarctation of the aorta is a narrowing of the aorta that is usually congenital, causing reversal of flow through the intercostal arteries. This may present as the radiological sign of 'rib-notching'. (page 199)

Coronary bypass surgery is performed to provide a reliable arterial supply to cardiac muscle distal to stenosis (narrowing) of a coronary artery. Many different techniques have been used over the last thirty years but most commonly the internal thoracic arteries are freed from the anterior thoracic wall and anastomosed to coronary artery segments distal to the obstructions. (page 190)

Costochondritis, sometimes known as Tietze's syndrome, is inflammation of the costochondral and chondrosternal joints. It is commonly misdiagnosed as cardiac disease. (page 181)

Dysphagia. Difficulty in swallowing may be due to intrinsic (peptic stricture) or extrinsic (structures pressing on the oesophagus such as an unfolding aorta, swollen lymph nodes from the trachea or an enlarged left atrium) pathology. (page 217)

Flail chest is the result of multiple rib fractures, most commonly following a motor vehicle accident. The section of the broken ribs moves paradoxically during respiration, making breathing extremely painful and distressing. (page 185)

Gastro-oesophageal reflux, also known as heartburn, is commonly associated with either a hiatus hernia or increased acid production in the stomach and peptic ulceration. (page 216)

Heart sounds (sites of auscultation). The four heart valves are best heard in specific places on the anterior chest wall related to the direction of blood flow through that valve – the aortic over the second right intercostal space just lateral to the sternum; the pulmonary in the second left intercostal space just lateral to the sternum; the tricuspid valve in the midline at the lower end of the sternum; the mitral valve towards the apex at the level of the fourth or fifth left costal cartilage usually just medial to the nipple. (page 182)

Horner's syndrome features ptosis, a constricted pupil (miosis), and a dry and flushed side of the face due to damage or interruption of the sympathetic trunk usually in the upper thoracic or lower cervical region. It is sometimes due to tumours (carcinoma of the lung), but may also be iatrogenic following a stellate ganglion block or cervical sympathectomy. (page 211)

Intercostal drainage, known also as thoracocentesis, is a procedure in which a needle is inserted through the intercostal muscles into the pleural cavity to remove excess fluid. The needle is inserted along the top of the rib to avoid damage to the neurovascular bundle which lies in the subcostal groove of each intercostal space. (page 213)

Intercostal nerve block. Using an anaesthetic agent this may be performed at any point along the course of an intercostal nerve in the subcostal groove, just below each rib. (page 186)

Intracardiac injections. In acute emergencies, when drugs need to be delivered directly into the heart, a long needle may be inserted through the anterior chest wall to the right of the sternum. (page 192)

Mastectomy is the removal of a breast. It is now a less popular operation, the most common procedure being a lumpectomy or removal of the tumour and possibly surrounding lymph nodes in the axilla. This more conservative surgical procedure can be followed by chemotherapy and/or radiotherapy, depending on the underlying pathology. (page 183)

Myocardial infarction, better known as a 'heart attack', is death of a section of heart muscle due to prolonged, progressive ischaemia. Occasionally the dead heart muscle may then thin and expand, causing an aneurysm. (page 190)

Orange-peel texture of the skin, also known as 'peau d'orange', is a pitting oedema of the breast often seen with an underlying malignancy due to blocked lymphatics. Dimpling of the breast, particularly associated with fixation of a lump, may be due to contraction of the suspensory ligaments of the breast caused by an underlying pathology. Retraction of the nipple. Many women have congenitally inverted nipples and this should not be a cause for concern except when preparing to breast feed. As a new occurrence this should have a high index of suspicion for malignancy. (page 183)

Pancoast's tumour is a tumour of the apex of the lung, usually a bronchogenic carcinoma, which compresses the brachial plexus and the sympathetic trunk with a resultant Horner's syndrome. (page 210)

Pericardial effusion is an accumulation of fluid within the pericardial sac; i.e. between the visceral and parietal serous layers of the pericardium. If a large amount of fluid accumulates this can lead to cardiac tamponade. (page 189)

Phrenic nerve palsy will cause paralysis of the ipsilateral dome of the diaphragm. This can be seen radiographically by noticing paradoxical movement; i.e. instead of descending on inspiration, the diaphragm is pushed upwards by pressure from the underlying abdominal viscera. (page 200)

Pleural effusion is the accumulation of fluid within the pleural cavity (between the visceral and parietal layers of pleura). (page 197)

Pleurisy is a painful inflammation of the pleura. The pain is referred from the parietal pleura to the cutaneous distribution of the intercostal nerve. (page 198)

Pneumonia is an infection of the lung by either bacteria, fungi or viruses and will show up on an X-ray as a white shadow in the normally radiolucent lung tissue. (page 204)

Pneumothorax is the introduction of air between the visceral and parietal pleurae. This may result from a stab wound damaging the parietal pleura or, more commonly, from the spontaneous bursting of an air sac tearing the visceral pleura. (page 198)

Pulmonary embolism is a serious or fatal condition caused by blood clots, usually from the deep veins of the leg or pelvis, which dislodge and travel through the venous side of the heart to block the pulmonary trunk or its branches. (page 206)

Rib/sternal fractures are most commonly seen following motor vehicle accidents (where the chest is crushed against the steering wheel) or during contact sports. In both situations a common complication is pneumothorax, the broken rib edge having torn the visceral pleura, allowing air to enter the pleural cavity, collapsing the lung. (page 181)

Subclavian vein catheterization takes advantage of the vascular relations on the superior aspect of the first rib to place a central venous line, normally by an infraclavicular route. The tip of the needle should be pointed as anteriorly as possible towards the jugular notch to avoid injury to posterior structures (apex of the lung, subclavian artery and the brachial plexus). A supraclavicular approach puts the needle into the origin of the brachiocephalic vein. (page 211)

Thoracic outlet syndromes, complex in both terminology and pathogenesis, are neural or vascular complications in the upper extremity caused by compression of subclavian vessels and/or nerve roots of the brachial plexus in the scalene triangle above the first rib. Common causes are cervical ribs or constriction bands from cervical outgrowths. Common signs include cold hands, tingling or paralysis of the fourth and fifth digits or weakness of the intrinsic hand muscles. (page 210)

Valvular disease, a common complication of rheumatic fever, produces valvular incompetence most frequently in the mitral and aortic valves. This can be readily seen on video colour Doppler ultrasonography. (page 191, 195)

Ventricular hypertrophy is the enlargement of the ventricular heart muscle. Ischaemia, cardiomyopathy and valvular disease are common causes. (page 191)

Abdomen and pelvis

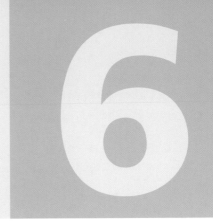

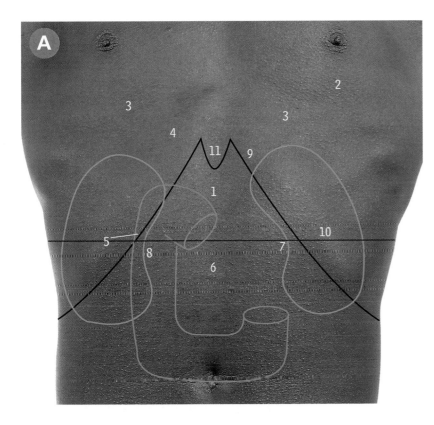

6

Ⓐ Anterior abdominal wall
surface markings, above the umbilicus

The solid black line indicates the costal margin. The magenta line indicates the transpyloric plane. The C-shaped duodenum is outlined in blue, and the kidneys in green.

1 Aortic opening in diaphragm
2 Apex of heart in fifth intercostal space
3 Dome of diaphragm and upper margin of liver
4 Foramen for inferior vena cava in diaphragm
5 Fundus of gall bladder, and junction of ninth costal cartilage and lateral border of rectus sheath
6 Head of pancreas and level of second lumbar vertebra
7 Hilum of left kidney
8 Hilum of right kidney
9 Oesophageal opening in diaphragm
10 Transpyloric plane
11 Xiphisternal joint

> The transpyloric plane (10) lies midway between the jugular notch of the sternum and the upper border of the pubic symphysis, or approximately a hand's breadth below the xiphisternal joint (11), and level with the lower part of the body of the first lumbar vertebra.

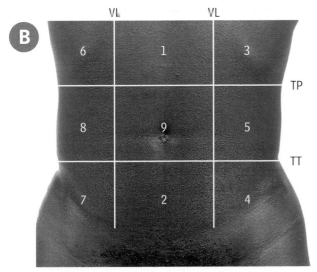

Ⓑ Regions of the abdomen

The abdomen may be divided into regions by two vertical and two horizontal lines. The vertical lines (VL) pass through the midinguinal points: the upper horizontal line corresponds to the transpyloric plane (TP, A10), the lower line is drawn between the tubercles of the iliac crests (transtubercular (or supracristal) plane, TT).

1 Epigastric region
2 Hypogastrium or suprapubic
3 Left hypochondrium
4 Left iliac region or iliac fossa
5 Left lumbar region
6 Right hypochondrium
7 Right iliac region or iliac fossa
8 Right lumbar region
9 Umbilical region

Abdominal paracentesis, see p. 281.

Anterior abdominal wall

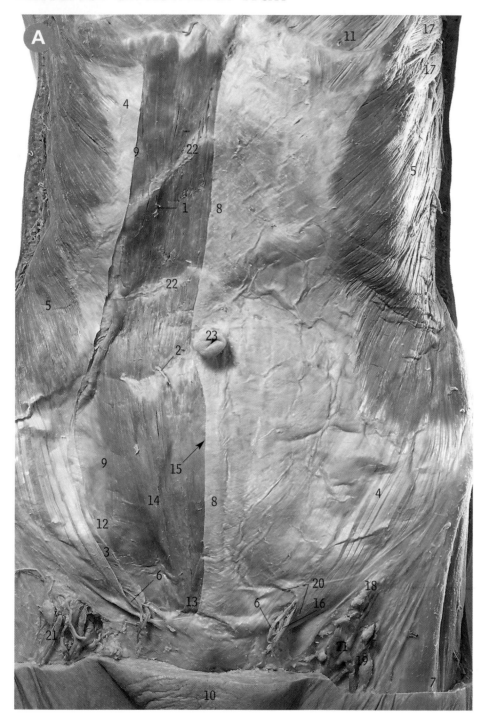

1 Anterior cutaneous nerve
   (eighth intercostal)
2 Anterior cutaneous nerve
   (tenth intercostal)
3 Anterior layer internal oblique
   aponeurosis
4 External oblique aponeurosis
5 External oblique muscle
6 Ilioinguinal nerve
7 Iliotibial tract
8 Linea alba
9 Linea semilunaris
10 Mons pubis
11 Pectoralis major muscle
12 Posterior layer internal oblique
   aponeurosis
13 Pyramidalis muscle
14 Rectus abdominis
15 Rectus sheath, anterior
16 Round ligament of uterus
17 Serratus anterior muscle
18 Superficial inguinal lymph node
   (horizontal group)
19 Superficial inguinal lymph node
   (vertical group)
20 Superficial inguinal ring
21 Superficial inguinal veins
22 Tendinous intersection
23 Umbilicus

The rectus sheath (A15) is formed by
the internal oblique aponeurosis (A3)
which splits at the lateral border of
the rectus muscle (A9) into two layers.
The posterior (A12) passes behind the
muscle to blend with the aponeurosis of
transversus abdominis (B19) to form the
posterior wall of the sheath (B13), and
the anterior layer (A3) passes in front of
the muscle to blend with the external
oblique aponeurosis (A4) as the anterior
wall (A15).

The anterior and posterior walls of the
sheath unite at the medial border of the
rectus muscle to form the midline linea
alba (A8, B11).

Haematoma of the rectus sheath, see p. 282.

Rectus sheath

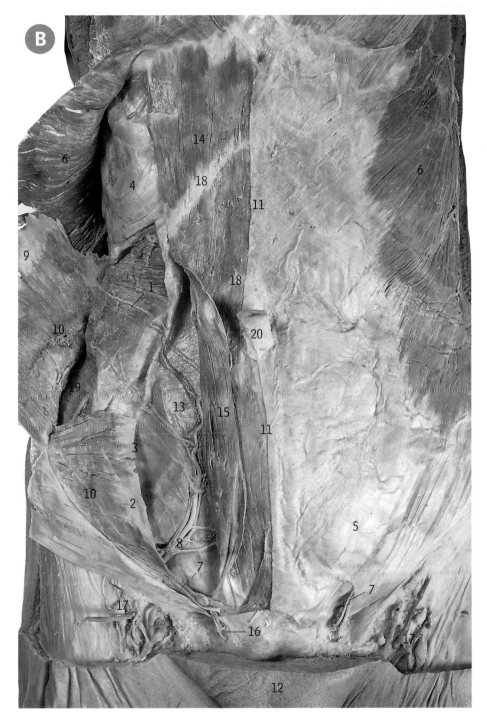

B

1 Anterior cutaneous nerve
  (tenth intercostal)
2 Anterior layer of internal oblique
  aponeurosis
3 Anterior wall of rectus sheath
4 Eighth rib
5 External oblique aponeurosis
6 External oblique muscle
7 Ilioinguinal nerve
8 Inferior epigastric vessels
9 Internal oblique aponeurosis
10 Internal oblique muscle
11 Linea alba
12 Mons pubis
13 Posterior wall of rectus sheath
14 Rectus abdominis
15 Rectus abdominis, reflected
16 Round ligament of uterus
17 Superficial inguinal lymph nodes
18 Tendinous intersection
19 Transversus abdominis
20 Umbilicus

There is no posterior rectus sheath in the
lower third of rectus abdominis, below
the arcuate line (page 227, A1).

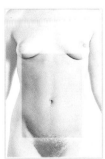

Anterior abdominal wall *abdominal contents*

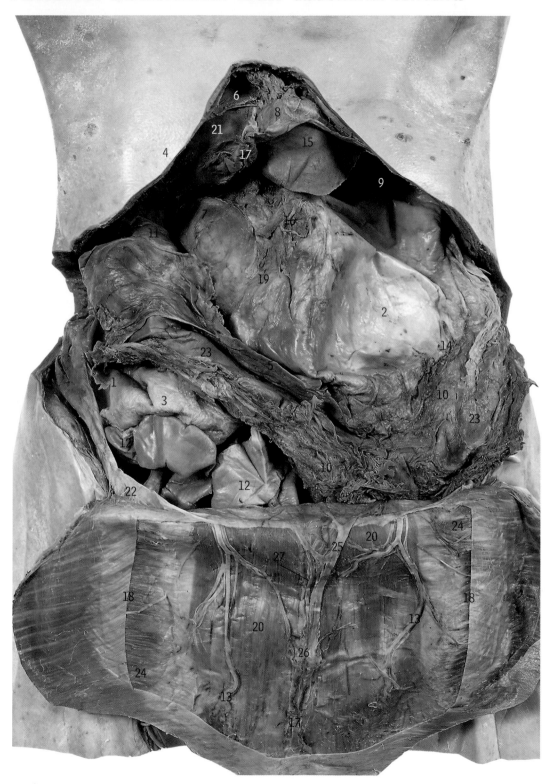

The anterior abdominal wall, cut along the costal margins (4), has been reflected downwards. The posterior wall of rectus sheath, fascia transversalis (22) and parietal peritoneum (18) have been excised and the abdominal contents exposed *in situ*.

1 Ascending colon
2 Body of stomach
3 Caecum
4 Costal margin
5 Cut edge of greater omentum
6 Diaphragm
7 Duodenum
8 Falciform ligament
9 Fundus of stomach
10 Greater omentum
11 Hepatic flexure, colon
12 Ileum
13 Inferior epigastric vessels
14 Left gastro-epiploic vessels
15 Left lobe, liver
16 Lesser omentum
17 Ligamentum teres
18 Parietal peritoneum, cut edge
19 Pyloric sphincter
20 Rectus abdominis muscle
21 Right lobe, liver
22 Transversalis fascia
23 Transverse colon
24 Transversus abdominis muscle
25 Umbilical artery, remnant
26 Umbilicus
27 Urachus

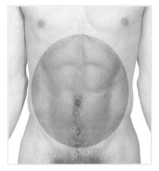

Groin

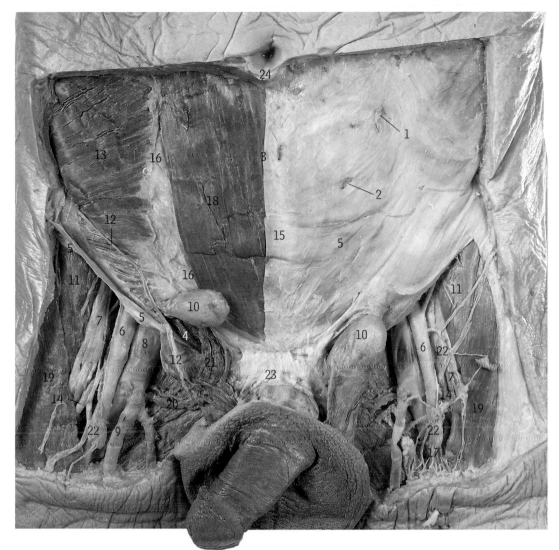

1 Anterior cutaneous nerve (eleventh intercostal)
2 Anterior cutaneous nerve (twelfth intercostal)
3 Anterior rectus sheath (cut edge)
4 Ductus deferens (vas)
5 External oblique aponeurosis
6 Femoral artery
7 Femoral nerve
8 Femoral vein
9 Great saphenous vein
10 Hernial sac (indirect)
11 Iliacus muscle
12 Ilioinguinal nerve
13 Internal oblique muscle
14 Lateral circumflex femoral artery
15 Linea alba
16 Linea semilunaris
17 Lymphatic vessels
18 Rectus abdominis muscle
19 Sartorius muscle
20 Scrotal venous connections
21 Spermatic cord
22 Superficial inguinal lymph node
23 Suspensory ligament of penis
24 Umbilicus

The hernial sac (10), shown here, is not present in normal subjects.

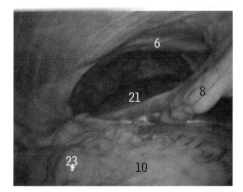

Laparoscopic view of upper abdominal cavity

Labels refer to key on page 224, opposite.

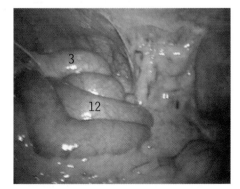

Laparoscopic view of abdominal cavity

Labels refer to key on page 224, opposite.

Laparoscopic images on this page and pages 230, 231, 232, 233, 245, 250, 253 and 276, all appear courtesy of Mr Simon Dexter DM FRCS, LIMIT Unit, Leeds University.

 Hernia repair, see p. 282.

Anterior abdominal wall *surface markings, right iliac fossa*

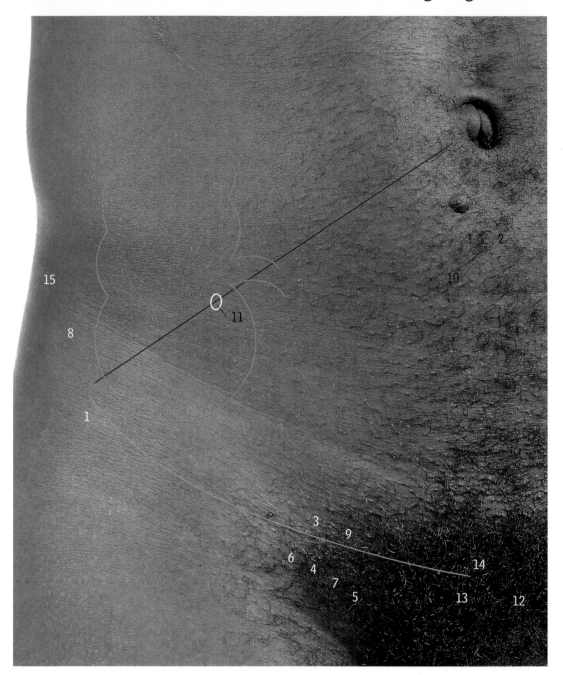

1 Anterior superior iliac spine
2 Bifurcation of aorta (fourth lumbar vertebra)
3 Deep inguinal ring
4 Femoral artery
5 Femoral canal
6 Femoral nerve
7 Femoral vein
8 Iliac crest
9 Inferior epigastric vessels
10 Lower end of inferior vena cava (fifth lumbar vertebra)
11 McBurney's point
12 Pubic symphysis
13 Pubic tubercle
14 Superficial inguinal ring
15 Tubercle of iliac crest

The femoral artery (4, whose pulsation should normally be palpable) enters the thigh midway between the pubic symphysis (12) and the anterior superior iliac spine (1). This is often referred to as the midinguinal point.

The caecum with the ileum opening into it from the left and the ascending colon continuing upwards from it are indicated by the blue line. The inguinal ligament, between the anterior superior iliac spine (1) and the pubic tubercle (13), is indicated by the green line. The femoral artery (4) has the femoral vein (7) on its medial side and the femoral nerve (6) on its lateral side. The femoral canal (5) is on the medial side of the vein. The deep inguinal ring (3) and inferior epigastric vessels (9) are above the femoral artery, while the superficial inguinal ring (14) is above and lateral to the pubic tubercle (13). McBurney's point (11) is a site on the surface of the anterior abdominal wall indicating the usual location of the base of the appendix internally. It lies one-third of the way along a line from the right anterior superior iliac spine to the umbilicus (red line).

McBurney's point, see p. 282.

Anterior abdominal wall *umbilical folds, from behind*

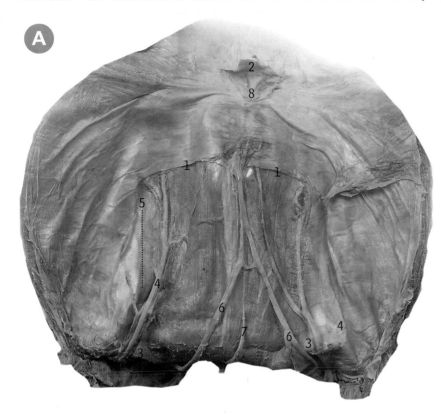

This view of the peritoneal surface of the central region of the anterior abdominal wall shows the peritoneal folds raised by underlying structures. There is one fold above the umbilicus – the falciform ligament – and there are five below it: the median umbilical fold (7) in the midline, and a pair of medial and lateral umbilical folds on each side (6 and 4).

1 Arcuate line
2 Falciform ligament
3 Inguinal triangle (Hesselbach)
4 Lateral umbilical fold
5 Linea semilunaris
6 Medial umbilical fold
7 Median umbilical fold
8 Umbilicus

The inguinal triangle of Hesselbach is a naturally weak region between rectus abdominis and the inferior epigastric vessels. Direct inguinal hernia appear through this region.

Fetal anterior abdominal wall *from behind*

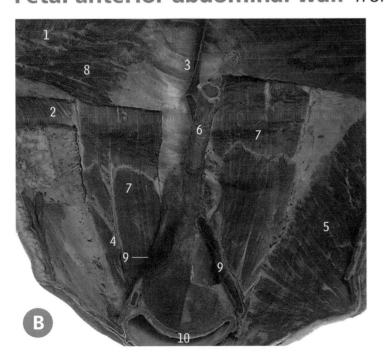

In this at term fetus the peritoneum and extraperitoneal tissues have been removed from the anterior abdominal wall to show the umbilical arteries (9) and left umbilical vein (6) converging at the back of the (unlabelled) umbilicus.

1 Diaphragm
2 External oblique
3 Falciform ligament
4 Inferior epigastric vessels
5 Internal oblique
6 Left umbilical vein
7 Rectus abdominis
8 Transversus abdominis
9 Umbilical artery
10 Urinary bladder

Caput medusae, peritoneal pain, umbilical hernia, see pp 281, 283.

Direct inguinal hernia *laparoscopic view, right side*

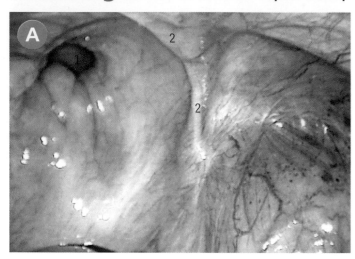

1 Direct inguinal hernia
2 Inferior epigastric vessels

Anterior abdominal wall *abdominal view*

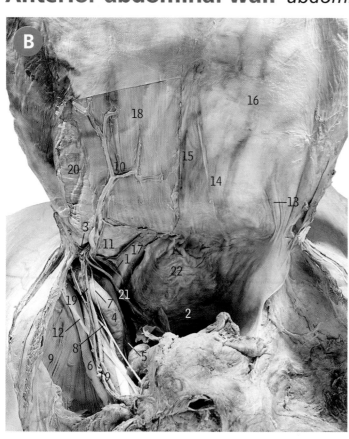

Abdominal viscera have been removed and the anterior abdominal wall detached laterally and reflected anteriorly and inferiorly to reveal the internal surface of the abdominal wall. The parietal peritoneum has been removed from the left side to show deeper structures in the pelvic and abdominal walls.

1 Accessory obturator artery
2 Bladder
3 Deep inguinal ring
4 External iliac artery
5 External iliac vein
6 Femoral nerve
7 Genitofemoral nerve, femoral branch
8 Genitofemoral nerve, genital branch
9 Iliacus
10 Inferior epigastric vessels
11 Inguinal triangle (Hesselbach)
12 Lateral cutaneous nerve of the thigh
13 Lateral umbilical fold (inferior epigastric vessels)
14 Medial umbilical fold (umbilical artery)
15 Median umbilical fold (urachus)
16 Parietal peritoneum
17 Pelvic brim
18 Posterior rectus sheath
19 Testicular vessels
20 Transversus abdominis
21 Vas deferens
22 Visceral peritoneum

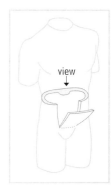

view

Direct inguinal hernia, indirect inguinal hernia, see p. 282.

Upper abdominal viscera *in transverse section*

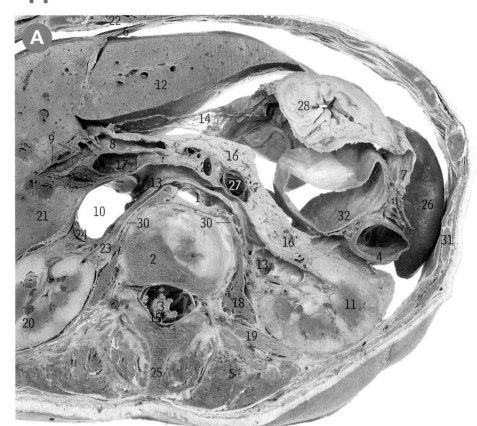

1 Abdominal aorta
2 Body of first lumbar vertebra
3 Conus medullaris of spinal cord
4 Descending colon
5 Erector spinae
6 Falciform ligament
7 Greater omentum
  (gastrosplenic ligament)
8 Hepatic artery
9 Hepatic ducts
10 Inferior vena cava
11 Left kidney
12 Left lobe of liver
13 Left renal vein
14 Lesser omentum
15 Nerve roots of cauda equina
16 Pancreas
17 Portal vein
18 Psoas major
19 Quadratus lumborum
20 Right kidney
21 Right lobe of liver
22 Right rectus abdominis
23 Right renal artery
24 Right renal vein
25 Spine of first lumbar vertebra
26 Spleen
27 Splenic vein
28 Stomach
29 Superior mesenteric artery
30 Sympathetic trunk
31 Tenth rib
32 Transverse colon

This section through the upper abdomen at the level of the first lumbar vertebra, seen from below looking towards the thorax, shows the general disposition of some of the viscera. The vertebral column (2) bulges forwards into the abdominal cavity, with the kidneys (11 and 20) lying in the trough on either side. The bulk of the liver (21) is on the right side, extending towards the left (12) to overlap part of the stomach (28), and the pancreas (16) lies centrally, also extending towards the left (but on a deeper plane) to overlap part of the left kidney (11). Parts of the colon (32 and 4) are adjacent to the spleen (26), which lies against the part of the diaphragm attached to the thoracic wall in the region of the tenth rib (31).

CT scan of the upper abdomen *at the level of the coeliac trunk*

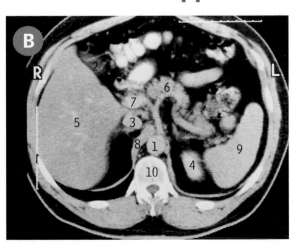

All CT (computerized tomography) scans of the trunk are, by convention, viewed from below (as with the body lying on the back and the viewer looking towards the head). In B both oral and intravenous contrast media have been used (to emphasize the outlines of the gut and vascular system). To avoid too many labels, only some key features have been numbered, and the various parts of the alimentary tract are unlabelled. The coeliac trunk arising from the aorta (1) is seen to divide as a Y into the splenic artery running towards the left behind the pancreas (6) and the common hepatic artery passing to the right near the portal vein (7). On the left side the spleen (9) and the upper pole of the kidney (4) are shown, but on the right the plane of the scan is too high to show the right kidney.

1 Abdominal aorta
2 Gall bladder
3 Inferior vena cava
4 Left kidney
5 Liver
6 Pancreas
7 Portal vein
8 Right crus of diaphragm
9 Spleen
10 Twelfth thoracic vertebra

Upper abdominal viscera *from the front*

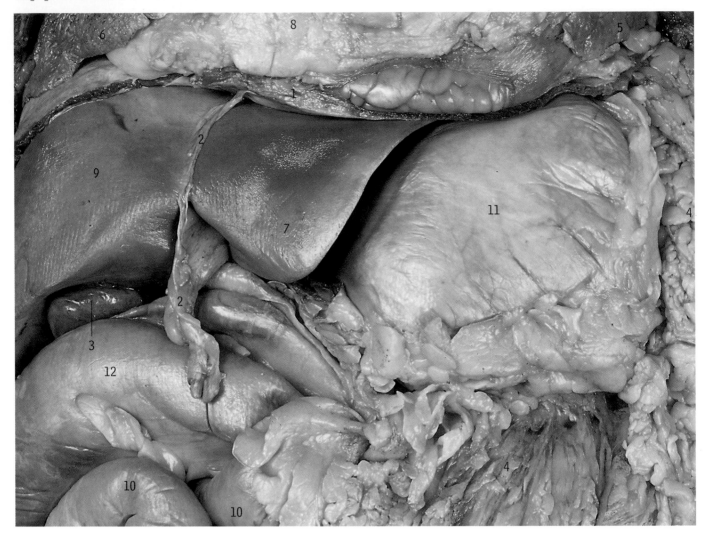

The thoracic and abdominal walls and the anterior part of the diaphragm have been removed to show the undisturbed viscera. The liver (9 and 7) and stomach (11) are immediately below the diaphragm (1). The greater omentum (4) hangs down from the greater curvature (lower margin) of the stomach (11), overlying much of the small and large intestine but leaving some of the transverse colon (12) and small intestine (10) uncovered. The fundus (tip) of the gall bladder (3) is seen between the right lobe of the liver (9) and transverse colon (12).

1	Diaphragm	**7**	Left lobe of liver
2	Falciform ligament	**8**	Pericardial fat
3	Gall bladder	**9**	Right lobe of liver
4	Greater omentum	**10**	Small intestine
5	Inferior lobe of left lung	**11**	Stomach
6	Inferior lobe of right lung	**12**	Transverse colon

For an explanation of peritoneal structures see the diagrams on page 236.

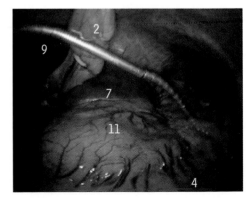

Laparoscopic view of upper abdominal viscera

 Liver biopsy, see p. 282.

Upper abdominal viscera *from the front*

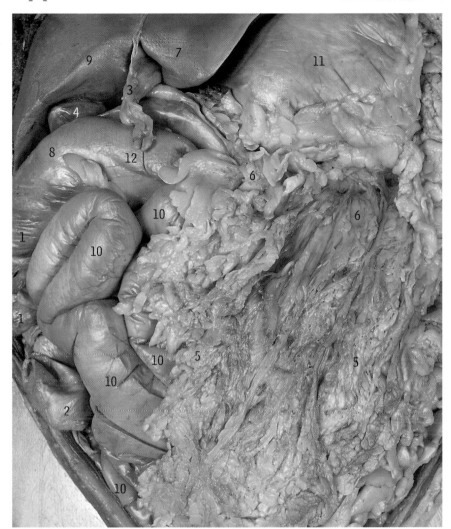

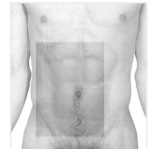

In this view of the undisturbed abdomen the upper part of the greater omentum (as at 6) overlies much of the transverse colon and mesocolon (with the right part of the transverse colon seen at 12). The lower part of the omentum (5) covers coils of small intestine, some of which (10) are visible beyond the right margin of the omentum. The caecum (2) is at the proximal end of the ascending colon (1) which continues upwards into the right colic flexure (hepatic flexure, 8) and then becomes the transverse colon (12).

1 Ascending colon
2 Caecum
3 Falciform ligament
4 Fundus of gall bladder
5 Greater omentum overlying coils of small intestine
6 Greater omentum overlying transverse colon and mesocolon
7 Left lobe of liver
8 Right colic flexure
9 Right lobe of liver
10 Small intestine
11 Stomach
12 Transverse colon

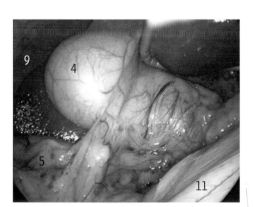

Laparoscopic view of gall bladder

 Cholecystectomy, laparoscopy, see pp 281, 282.

Upper abdominal viscera *from the front*

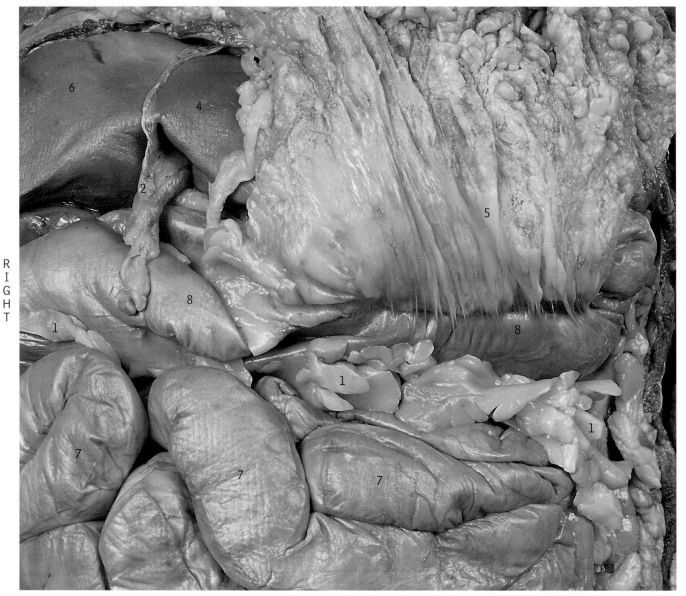

In this view of the same specimen as on page 230, the greater omentum (5) has been lifted upwards to show its adherence to the transverse colon (8) (see page 236, C).

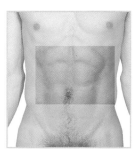

1 Appendices epiploicae
2 Falciform ligament
3 Gall bladder (fundus)
4 Left lobe of liver
5 Posterior surface of greater omentum
6 Right lobe of liver
7 Small intestine
8 Transverse colon

The appendices epiploicae (1) are fat-filled appendages of peritoneum on the various parts of the colon (ascending, transverse, descending and sigmoid). They are not present on the small intestine or the rectum, and may be rudimentary on the caecum and appendix. In abdominal operations they are one feature that helps to distinguish colon from other parts of the intestine.

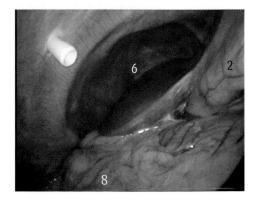

Laparoscopic view of abdominal viscera

 Peritoneal lavage, peritoneal dialysis, see p. 283.

Lesser omentum and epiploic foramen
Ⓐ *from the front*   Ⓑ *from the front and the right*

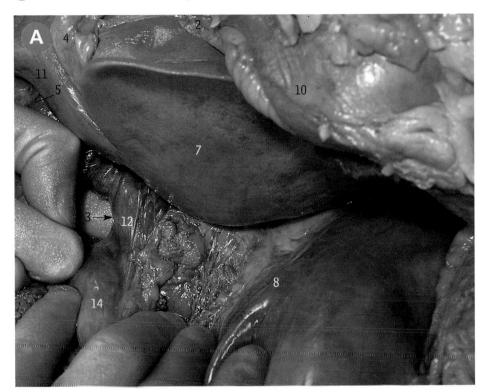

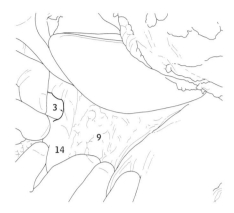

1   Descending (second) part of duodenum
2   Diaphragm
3   Epiploic foramen
4   Falciform ligament
5   Gall bladder
6   Inferior vena cava
7   Left lobe of liver
8   Lesser curvature of stomach
9   Lesser omentum
10 Pericardium
11 Quadrate lobe of liver
12 Right free margin of lesser omentum
13 Right lobe of liver
14 Superior (first) part of duodenum
15 Upper pole of right kidney

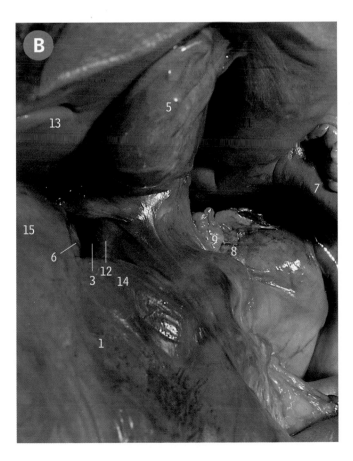

In A a finger has been placed in the epiploic foramen (3) behind the right free margin of the lesser omentum (12), and the tip can be seen in the lesser sac, through the transparent lesser omentum (9) which stretches between the liver (7) and the lesser curvature of the stomach (8). In the more lateral view in B, looking into the foramen from the right, the foramen (3) is identified between the right free margin of the lesser omentum (12) in front and the inferior vena cava (6) behind, above the first part of the duodenum (14).

> The epiploic foramen (of Winslow, A3 and B3) is the communication between the general peritoneal cavity (sometimes called the greater sac) and the lesser sac (omental bursa), a space lined by peritoneum behind the stomach (A8 and B8) and lesser omentum (A9 and A12) and in front of parts of the pancreas and left kidney.

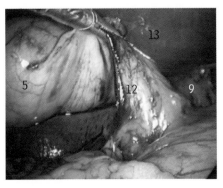

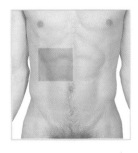

Laparoscopic view of lesser omentum (free margin)

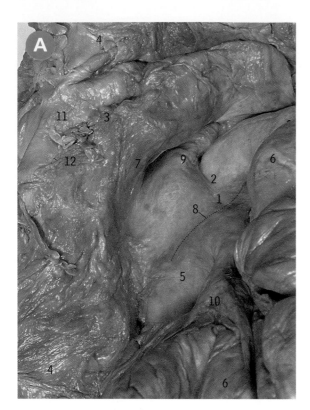

Ⓐ Upper abdominal viscera
from the front

In this view the stomach (3 and 7), transverse colon (11) and greater omentum (4) have been lifted up to show the region of the duodenojejunal flexure (2). The left end of the horizontal (third) part of the duodenum (5) turns upwards as the ascending (fourth) part (1) which is continuous with the jejunum at the duodenojejunal flexure (2) below the lower border of the pancreas (9).

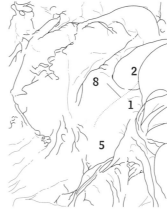

1   Ascending (fourth) part of duodenum
2   Duodenojejunal flexure
3   Greater curvature of stomach
4   Greater omentum (posterior surface)
5   Horizontal (third) part of duodenum
6   Jejunum
7   Lesser curvature of stomach
8   Line of attachment of root of mesentery
9   Lower border of pancreas
10   Mesentery
11   Transverse colon (posterior surface)
12   Transverse mesocolon (posterior surface)

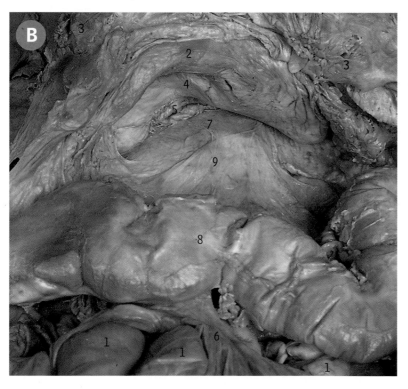

Ⓑ Lesser sac and transverse mesocolon
from the front

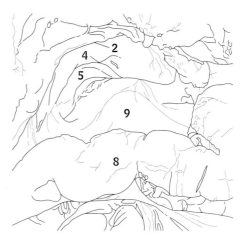

The greater omentum (3) hanging down from the greater curvature of the stomach (2) has been separated from the underlying transverse colon (8) and mesocolon (9) and lifted upwards, and an opening made into the lesser sac (as in D on page 236). This view therefore shows the posterior surface of the greater omentum (3), stomach and lesser omentum (5), and the anterior surface of the transverse mesocolon (9).

1   Coils of jejunum and ileum
2   Greater curvature of stomach
3   Greater omentum (posterior surface)
4   Lesser curvature of stomach
5   Lesser omentum (posterior surface)
6   Mesentery
7   Peritoneum of lesser sac overlying pancreas
8   Transverse colon
9   Transverse mesocolon overlying horizontal (third) part of duodenum

Ascites, see p. 281.

Mesentery and descending colon *from the front*

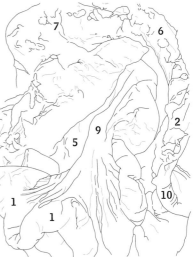

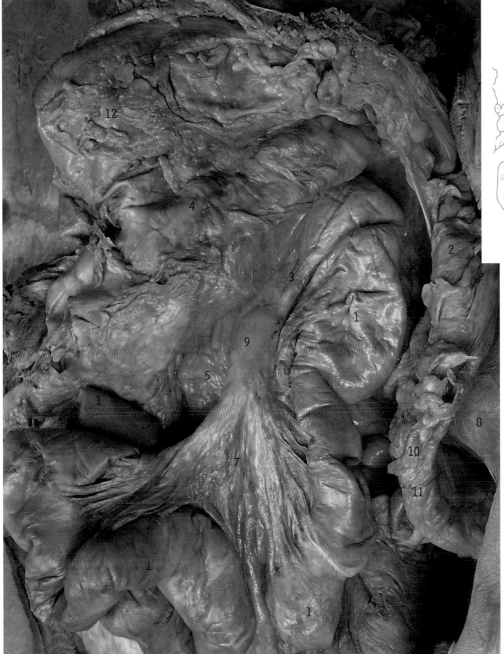

1 Coils of jejunum and ileum
2 Descending colon
3 Duodenojejunal flexure
4 Greater curvature of stomach
5 Horizontal (third) part of
   duodenum
6 Left colic (splenic) flexure
7 Mesentery
8 Peritoneum overlying external
   iliac vessels
9 Root of mesentery
10 Sigmoid colon
11 Sigmoid mesocolon
12 Transverse colon

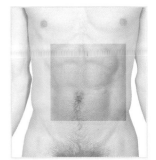

The stomach (4) and transverse colon (12) have been displaced upwards to show the left end of the root of the mesentery (9) at the duodenojejunal flexure (3). The descending colon (2), which is retroperitoneal, becomes the sigmoid colon (10) when it ceases to be retroperitoneal and acquires a mesentry (11).

 Drainage of peritoneal abscesses, volvulus, see pp 282, 284.

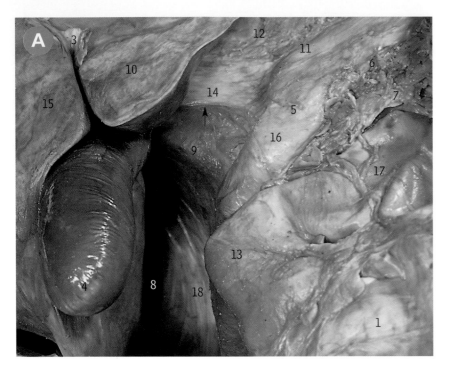
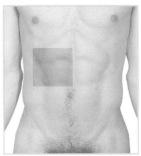

Ⓐ Hepatorenal pouch of peritoneum
from the right and below

With the body lying on its back and seen from the right (with the head towards the left), the liver (15) has been turned upwards (towards the left) to open up the gap between the liver and upper pole of the right kidney (18) – the hepatorenal pouch of peritoneum (8, Morison's pouch or the right subhepatic compartment of the peritoneal cavity).

1 Ascending colon	**7** Greater omentum	**13** Right colic (hepatic) flexure
2 Epiploic foramen	**8** Hepatorenal (Morison's) pouch	**14** Right free margin of lesser omentum
3 Falciform ligament	**9** Inferior vena cava	**15** Right lobe of liver
4 Gall bladder	**10** Left lobe of liver	**16** Superior (first) part of duodenum
5 Gastroduodenal junction	**11** Lesser curvature of stomach	**17** Transverse colon
6 Greater curvature of stomach	**12** Lesser omentum overlying pancreas	**18** Upper pole of right kidney

Diagrams of peritoneum

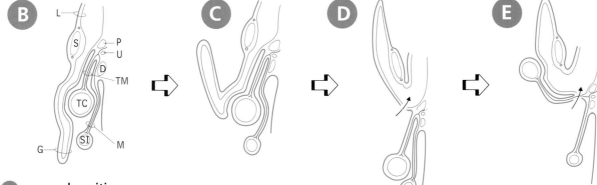

Ⓑ **normal position**

Ⓒ **with the lower part of the greater omentum lifted up**

Ⓓ **with the greater omentum lifted up and separated from the transverse mesocolon and colon, with an opening into the lesser sac**

Ⓔ **with the greater omentum and transverse mesocolon and colon lifted up, with an opening into the lesser sac through the mesocolon**

These drawings of a sagittal section through the middle of the abdomen, viewed from the left, illustrate theoretically how the peritoneum forms the lesser omentum (L, passing down to the stomach, S), greater omentum (G), transverse mesocolon (TM) passing to the transverse colon (TC), and the mesentery (M) of the small intestine (SI). The layer in blue represents the peritoneum of the lesser sac. The superior mesenteric artery passes between the head and uncinate process of the pancreas (P and U), and continues across the duodenum (D) into the mesentery (M) to the small intestine (SI), giving off the middle colic artery which runs in the transverse mesocolon (TM) to the transverse colon (TC). The greater omentum (G) is formed by four layers fused together and also fused with the front of the transverse mesocolon (TM, two layers) and transverse colon. On dissection, no separation between any layers is possible except between the greater omentum and the transverse mesocolon. The six layers between the stomach and transverse colon are sometimes collectively known as the gastrocolic omentum. B corresponds to the dissections on pages 230 and 231, C to page 232, D to page 234B, and E to page 239. The small arrows in D and E indicate the layers cut to make artificial openings into the lesser sac.

Coeliac trunk *and surrounding area*

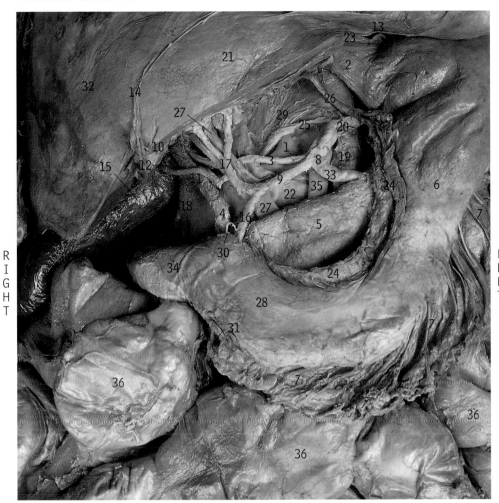

1 Abdominal aorta
2 Abdominal part of oesophagus
3 Accessory hepatic artery
4 Bile duct
5 Body of pancreas
6 Body of stomach
7 Branches of left and right gastroepiploic arteries in greater omentum
8 Coeliac trunk
9 Common hepatic artery
10 Common hepatic duct
11 Cystic artery
12 Cystic duct
13 Diaphragm
14 Falciform ligament
15 Gall bladder
16 Gastroduodenal artery
17 Hepatic artery and right and left branches
18 Inferior vena cava
19 Left crus of diaphragm
20 Left gastric artery
21 Left lobe of liver
22 Left renal vein
23 Left triangular ligament
24 Lesser omentum containing right and left gastric arteries
25 Median arcuate ligament of diaphragm
26 Oesophageal branch of left gastric artery
27 Portal vein
28 Pyloric part of stomach
29 Right crus of diaphragm
30 Right gastric artery
31 Right gastro-epiploic artery
32 Right lobe of liver
33 Splenic artery
34 Superior (first) part of duodenum
35 Superior mesenteric artery
36 Transverse colon

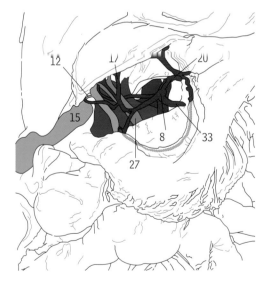

Part of the left lobe of the liver (21), and most of the lesser and greater omenta (24 and 7) have been removed, together with peritoneum of the central part of the posterior abdominal wall (posterior wall of the lesser sac), to show some of the most important structures in the upper abdomen: the coeliac trunk (8) and its branches (20, 33 and 9), the portal vein (27), and the bile duct (4) formed by the union of the cystic duct (12) from the gall bladder (15) with the common hepatic duct (10) from the liver (32 and 21). Note the unusual origin of the right gastric artery (30) from the gastroduodenal artery (16).

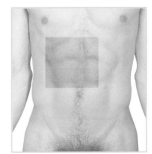

The left gastric artery (20) passes upwards and to the left and then turns down to run along the lesser curvature of the stomach between the two layers of peritoneum that form the lesser omentum (24). It gives off an oesophageal branch which passes up through the oesophageal opening in the diaphragm and supplies the lower part of the oesophagus (2). The accompanying veins (not shown here) drain to the left gastric vein and thence to the portal vein, making the lower end of the oesophagus one of the most important sites of portal–systemic anastomosis.

Carcinoma of the pancreas, portocaval shunt, see pp 281, 283.

Superior mesenteric vessels

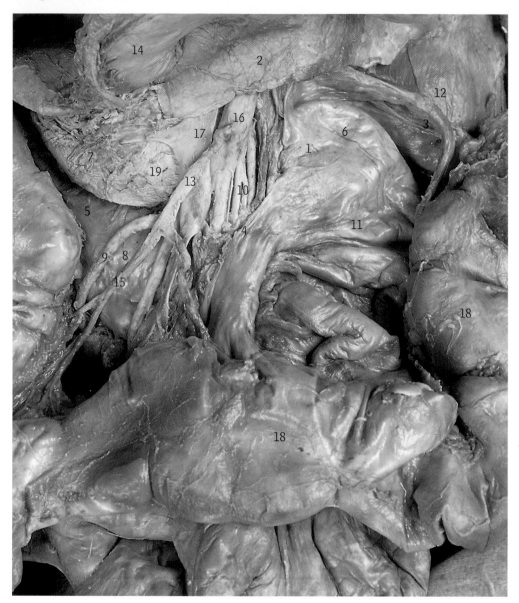

1 Ascending (fourth) part of duodenum
2 Body of pancreas
3 Branches of inferior mesenteric vessels
4 Cut edge of peritoneum at root of mesentery
5 Descending (second) part of duodenum
6 Duodenojejunal flexure
7 Head of pancreas
8 Horizontal (third) part of duodenum
9 Ileocolic artery
10 Jejunal and ileal arteries
11 Jejunum
12 Lower pole of left kidney
13 Middle colic artery
14 Posterior surface of pyloric part of stomach
15 Right colic artery
16 Superior mesenteric artery
17 Superior mesenteric vein
18 Transverse colon
19 Uncinate process of pancreas

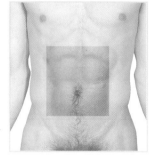

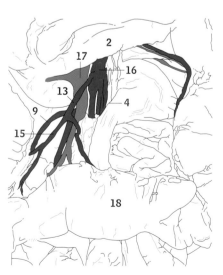

The stomach (14) has been lifted upwards and transverse mesocolon removed, leaving the transverse colon (18) in its normal position. Part of the peritoneum of the mesentery (4) has been dissected away to show branches of the superior mesenteric artery (16).

Superior mesenteric vessels

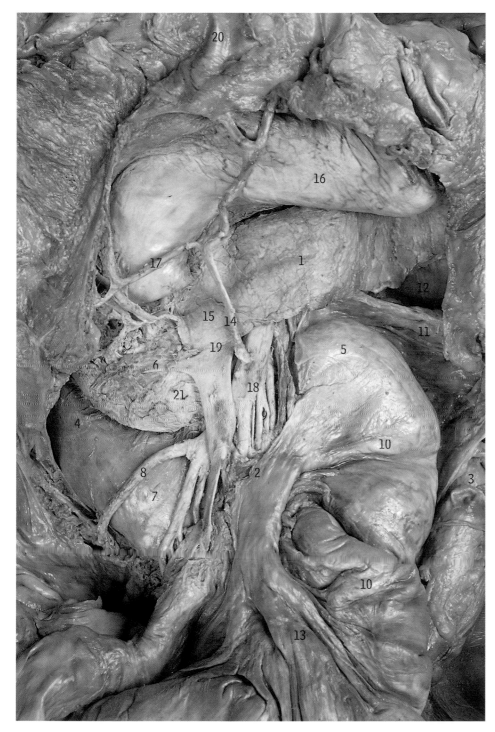

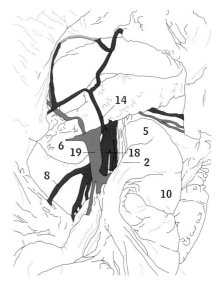

1 Body of pancreas
2 Cut edge of peritoneum at root of mesentery
3 Descending colon
4 Descending (second) part of duodenum
5 Duodenojejunal flexure
6 Head of pancreas
7 Horizontal (third) part of duodenum
8 Ileocolic artery
9 Jejunal and ileal arteries
10 Jejunum
11 Left colic vessels (inferior mesenteric)
12 Left kidney
13 Mesentery
14 Middle colic artery
15 Neck of pancreas
16 Posterior surface of body of stomach
17 Right branch of middle colic artery
18 Superior mesenteric artery
19 Superior mesenteric vein
20 Transverse colon
21 Uncinate process of pancreas

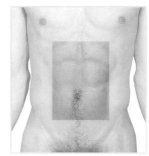

This dissection is similar to that opposite, but here the stomach (16) and transverse colon (20) have both been lifted upwards, so lifting the middle colic artery (14) upwards also. The root of the mesentery (2) begins at the duodenojejunal flexure (5) and passes obliquely downwards to the right over the horizontal (third) part of the duodenum (7), where the superior mesenteric vessels and their branches (19, 18 and 9) become enclosed between the two layers of the peritoneum that form the mesentery (see B on page 236).

Inferior mesenteric vessels *from the front*

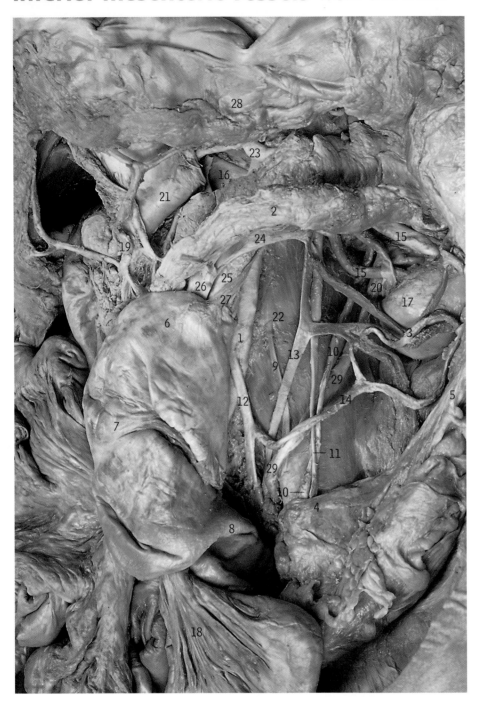

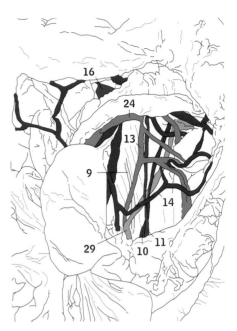

1   Abdominal aorta
2   Body of pancreas
3   Branches of left colic vessels
4   Cut edge of peritoneum
5   Descending colon
6   Duodenojejunal flexure
7   Duodenum: ascending (fourth)
8   Duodenum: horizontal (third)
9   Genitofemoral nerve
10 Gonadal artery
11 Gonadal vein
12 Inferior mesenteric artery
13 Inferior mesenteric vein
14 Left colic artery
15 Left renal artery
16 Left renal vein
17 Lower pole of left kidney
18 Mesentery
19 Middle colic artery
20 Pelvis of kidney
21 Posterior surface of pyloric
    part of stomach
22 Psoas major
23 Splenic artery
24 Splenic vein
25 Superior mesenteric artery
26 Superior mesenteric vein
27 Suspensory muscle of duodenum
    (muscle of Treitz)
28 Transverse colon
29 Ureter

The stomach (21) and transverse colon (28) are lifted
upwards. The peritoneum of the posterior abdominal wall
has been removed and the left-sided parts of the duodenum
(7 and 6) reflected towards the right, to show the origin
of the inferior mesenteric artery (12) from the aorta (1).
The lower border of the pancreas (2) has been lifted up,
revealing the splenic vein (24) with the inferior mesenteric
(13) running into it. The ureter (29) has the gonadal vessels
(10 and 11) in front of it and the genitofemoral nerve (9)
behind it, lying on psoas major (22).

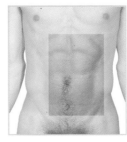

  Bowel ischaemia, see p. 281.

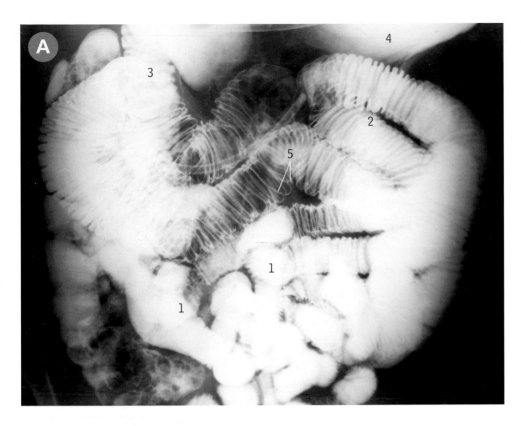

A Small bowel radiograph

enema via a tube in the duodenum

1 Coils of ileum
2 Coils of jejunum
3 Descending (second) part of duodenum
4 Stomach
5 Valvulae conniventes

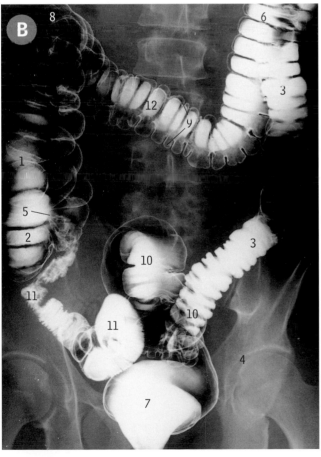

B Large intestine *radiograph*

In this double-contrast barium enema (barium and air), the sacculations (haustrations, 9) of the various parts of the colon allow it to be distinguished from the narrower terminal ileum (11), which has become partly filled by barium flowing into it through the ileocaecal junction (5).

1 Ascending colon
2 Caecum
3 Descending colon
4 Hip joint
5 Ileocaecal junction
6 Left colic (splenic) flexure
7 Rectum
8 Right colic (hepatic) flexure
9 Sacculations
10 Sigmoid colon
11 Terminal ileum
12 Transverse colon

Colostomy, see p. 281.

Stomach *with vessels and vagus nerves, from the front*

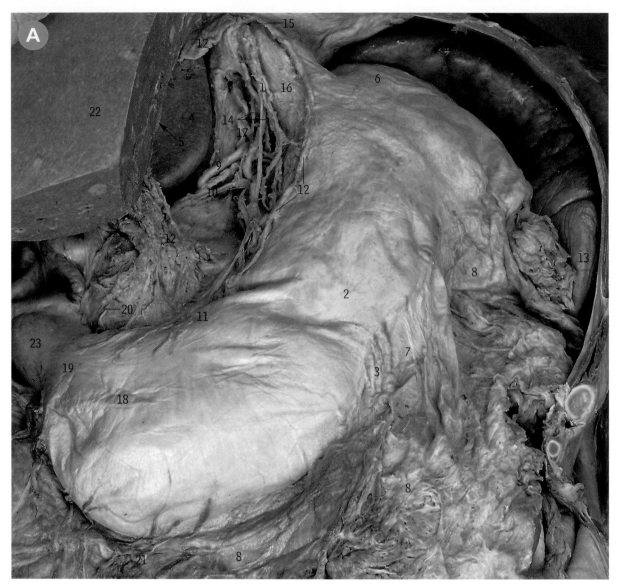

The anterior thoracic and abdominal walls and the left lobe of the liver have been removed, with part of the lesser omentum (12), to show the stomach (6, 2, 18 and 19) in its undisturbed position.

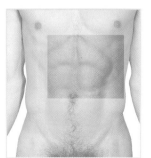

1 Anterior (left) vagal trunk	**13** Lower end of spleen
2 Body of stomach	**14** Oesophageal branches of left gastric vessels
3 Branches of left gastro-epiploic vessels	**15** Oesophageal opening in diaphragm
4 Caudate lobe of liver	**16** Oesophagus
5 Fissure for ligamentum venosum	**17** Posterior vagal trunk
6 Fundus of stomach	**18** Pyloric antrum
7 Greater curvature of stomach	**19** Pyloric canal
8 Greater omentum	**20** Right gastric artery
9 Left gastric artery	**21** Right gastro-epiploic vessels and branches
10 Left gastric vein	**22** Right lobe of liver
11 Lesser curvature of stomach	**23** Superior (first) part of duodenum
12 Lesser omentum (cut edge)	

Oesophageal varices, vagotomy, see pp 282, 284.

Stomach Ⓑ *radiograph after barium meal*

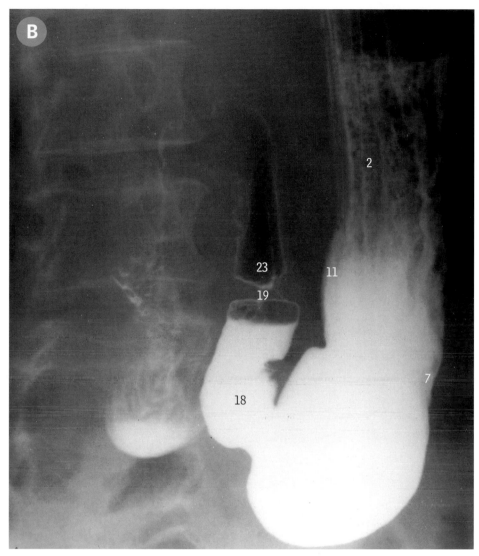

Labels key is shown on opposite page (242).

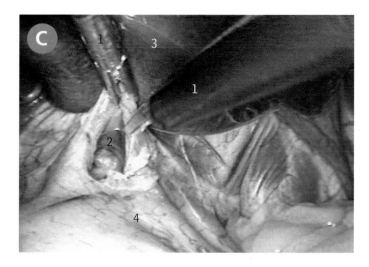

Ⓒ **Hiatus hernia**
laparoscopic view

1 Forceps
2 Hiatus hernia
3 Left lobe of liver
4 Stomach

Hiatus hernia, see p. 282.

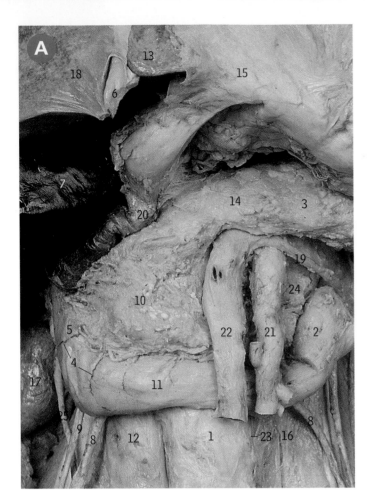

A Duodenum and pancreas

The stomach (15) has been lifted up, the colon and the peritoneum of the posterior abdominal wall removed and branches of the superior mesenteric vessels (21 and 22) cut off. The C-shaped duodenum (20, 5, 11 and 2) is seen embracing the head of the pancreas (10); the neck (14) and body (3) of the pancreas have been displaced slightly upwards to show the splenic vein (19) joining the superior mesenteric vein (22) (to form the portal vein behind the neck of the pancreas). The descending (second) part of the duodenum (5) overlaps the hilum of the right kidney (17). The superior mesenteric artery (21) and vein (22) cross anterior to the uncinate process (24) of the pancreas and then the horizontal (third) part of the duodenum (11).

1	Abdominal aorta	19	Splenic vein
2	Ascending (fourth) part of duodenum	20	Superior (first) part of duodenum
3	Body of pancreas	21	Superior mesenteric artery
4	Branches of pancreaticoduodenal vessels	22	Superior mesenteric vein
5	Descending (second) part of duodenum	23	Sympathetic trunk
6	Falciform ligament	24	Uncinate process of pancreas
7	Gall bladder	25	Ureter
8	Gonadal artery		
9	Gonadal vein		
10	Head of pancreas		
11	Horizontal (third) part of duodenum		
12	Inferior vena cava		
13	Left lobe of liver		
14	Neck of pancreas		
15	Posterior surface of greater omentum overlying stomach		
16	Psoas major muscle		
17	Right kidney		
18	Right lobe of liver		

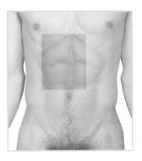

Duodenal papillae

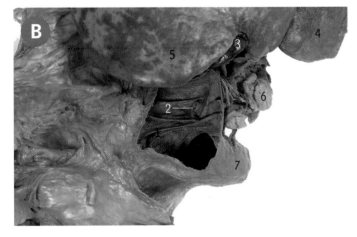

The anterior wall of the descending (second) part of the duodenum has been removed.

1	Circular folds of mucous membrane	4	Liver, left lobe
2	Duodenal papilla	5	Liver, right lobe
3	Gall bladder	6	Pancreas
		7	Third part of duodenum

Endoscopic retrograde cholangiopancreatogram *(ERCP)*

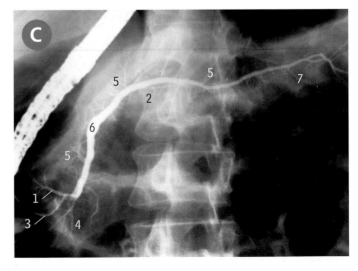

See page 248 for explanation.

1	Accessory pancreatic duct (Santorini)	4	Head of pancreas
2	Body of pancreas	5	Intralobular ducts
3	Cannula in ampulla	6	Pancreatic duct (Wirsung)
		7	Tail of pancreas

Upper abdominal viscera *from the front*

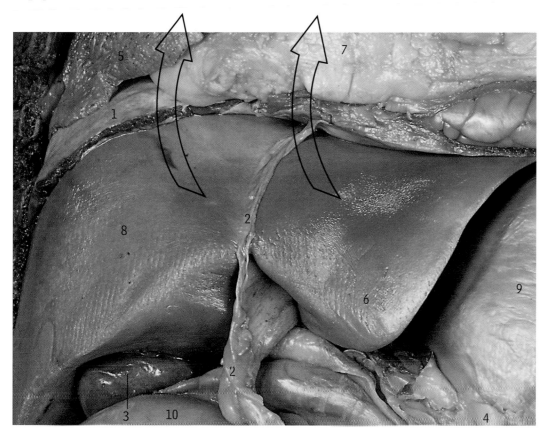

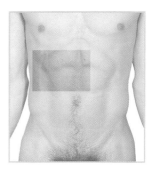

1 Diaphragm
2 Falciform ligament
3 Gall bladder
4 Greater omentum
5 Inferior lobe of right lung
6 Left lobe of liver
7 Pericardial fat
8 Right lobe of liver
9 Stomach
10 Transverse colon

For an explanation of
peritoneal structures see
the diagrams on page 236.

The thoracic and abdominal walls and the anterior part of the diaphragm have been removed to show
the undisturbed viscera. The liver (6 and 8) and stomach (9) are immediately below the diaphragm (1).
The greater omentum (4) hangs down from the greater curvature (lower margin) of the stomach (9),
overlying much of the small and large intestine but leaving some of the transverse colon (10) uncovered.
The fundus (tip) of the gall bladder (3) is seen between the right lobe of the liver (8) and transverse
colon (10). Arrows indicate the direction of liver reflection for view on following page (page 246).

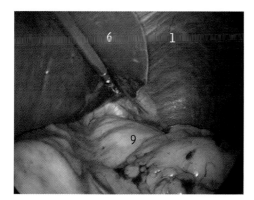

**Laparoscopic view of upper abdominal
viscera**

 Rupture of the liver, see p. 283.

Liver *from below and behind*

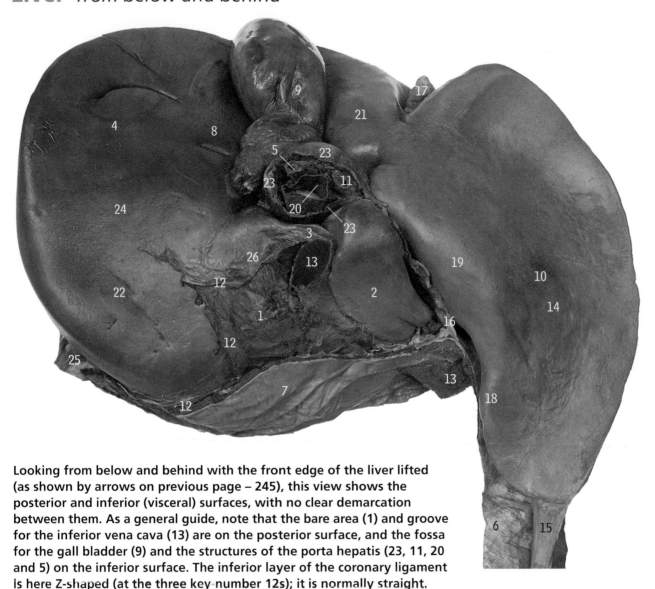

Looking from below and behind with the front edge of the liver lifted (as shown by arrows on previous page – 245), this view shows the posterior and inferior (visceral) surfaces, with no clear demarcation between them. As a general guide, note that the bare area (1) and groove for the inferior vena cava (13) are on the posterior surface, and the fossa for the gall bladder (9) and the structures of the porta hepatis (23, 11, 20 and 5) on the inferior surface. The inferior layer of the coronary ligament is here Z-shaped (at the three key-number 12s); it is normally straight.

1 Bare area	**15** Left triangular ligament
2 Caudate lobe	**16** Lesser omentum in fissure for
3 Caudate process	ligamentum venosum
4 Colic impression	**17** Ligamentum teres and
5 Common hepatic duct	falciform ligament in fissure
6 Diaphragm	for ligamentum teres
7 Diaphragm on part of bare area	**18** Oesophageal groove
(obstructing view of superior layer	**19** Omental tuberosity
of coronary ligament)	**20** Portal vein
8 Duodenal impression	**21** Quadrate lobe
9 Gall bladder	**22** Renal impression
10 Gastric impression	**23** Right free margin of lesser
11 Hepatic artery	omentum in porta hepatis
12 Inferior layer of coronary ligament	**24** Right lobe
13 Inferior vena cava	**25** Right triangular ligament
14 Left lobe	**26** Suprarenal impression

The caudate (2) and quadrate (21) lobes are classified anatomically as part of the right lobe (24), but functionally they belong to the left lobe (14), since they receive blood from the left branches of the hepatic artery and portal vein, and drain bile to the left hepatic duct.

 Liver abscess, portosystemic anastamoses, see pp 282, 283.

Cast of the liver, extrahepatic biliary tract and associated vessels *from below and behind*

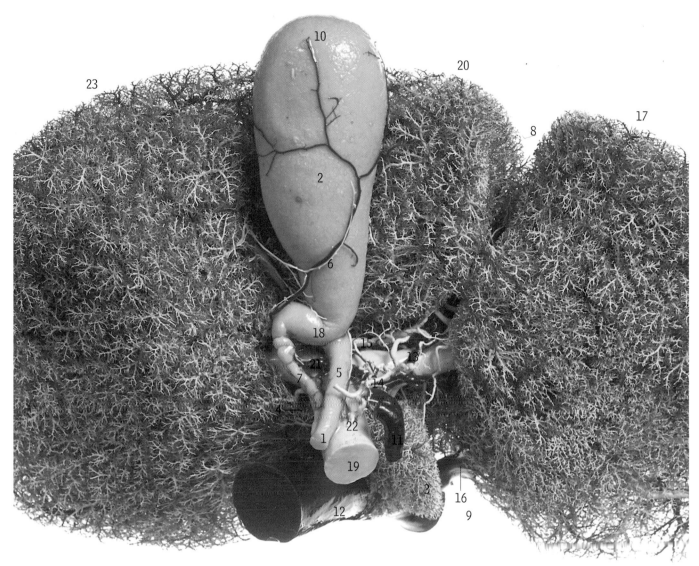

Yellow = gall bladder and biliary tract
Red = hepatic artery and branches
Light blue = portal vein and tributaries
Dark blue = inferior vena cava, hepatic veins and tributaries

This view, like the one opposite, shows the inferior and posterior surfaces, as when looking into the abdomen from below with the lower border of the liver pushed up towards the thorax.

1 Bile duct
2 Body of gall bladder
3 Caudate lobe
4 Caudate process
5 Common hepatic duct
6 Cystic artery and veins
7 Cystic duct
8 Fissure for ligamentum teres
9 Fissure for ligamentum venosum
10 Fundus of gall bladder
11 Hepatic artery
12 Inferior vena cava
13 Left branch of hepatic artery overlying left branch of portal vein

14 Left gastric vein
15 Left hepatic duct
16 Left hepatic vein
17 Left lobe
18 Neck of gall bladder
19 Portal vein
20 Quadrate lobe
21 Right branch of hepatic artery overlying right branch of portal vein
22 Right gastric vein
23 Right lobe

Endoscopic retrograde cholangiopancreatogram *(ERCP)*

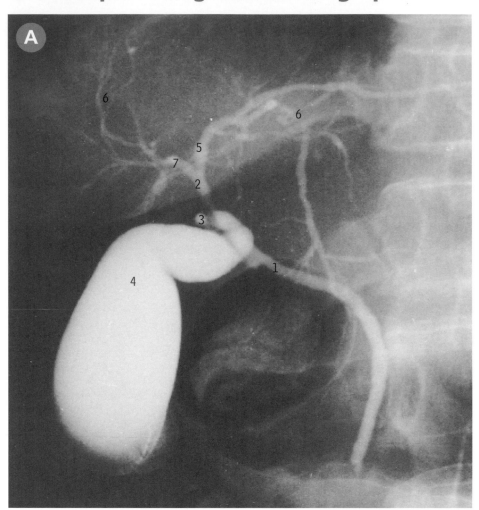

During an ERCP an endoscope is passed through the mouth, pharynx, oesophagus and stomach into the duodenum, and through it a cannula is introduced into the major duodenal papilla (page 244B) and bile duct so that contrast medium can be injected up the biliary tract. (The pancreatic duct can also be cannulated in this way – see C on page 244).

1 Common bile duct
2 Common hepatic duct
3 Cystic duct
4 Gall bladder
5 Left hepatic duct
6 Liver shadow and tributaries of hepatic ducts
7 Right hepatic duct

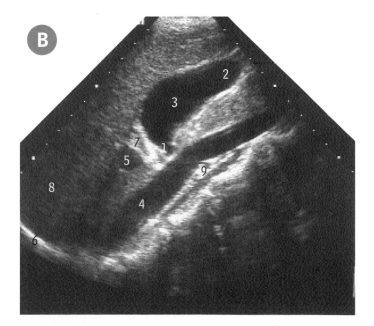

Ⓑ Gall bladder *ultrasound scan*

To an untrained observer, ultrasound scans are difficult to interpret, but here the gall bladder can be distinguished as a sausage-shaped cavity (3).

1 Cystic duct
2 Fundus of gall bladder
3 Gall bladder
4 Inferior vena cava
5 Portal vein
6 Right dome of diaphragm
7 Right hepatic artery
8 Right lobe of liver
9 Right renal artery

> Ultrasound scans are best interpreted by the operator on a screen and not by viewing a hard copy.

Cholecystitis, see p. 281.

Cast of the portal vein and tributaries, and the mesenteric vessels *from behind*

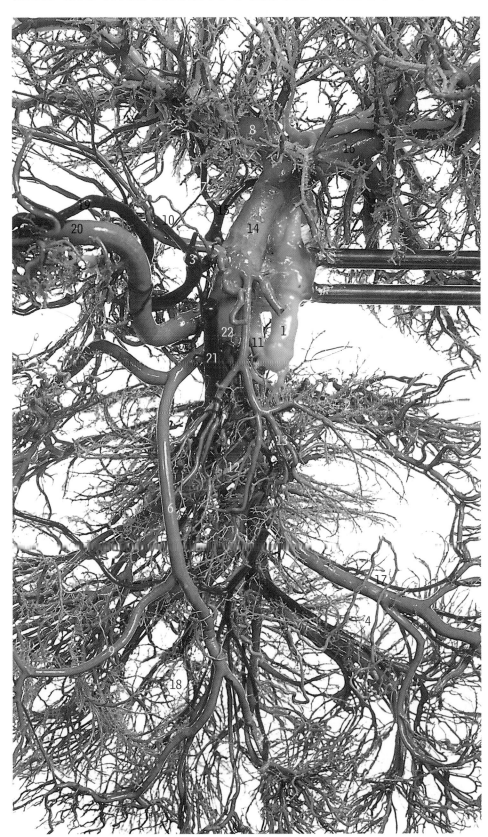

Yellow = biliary tract and pancreatic ducts
Red = arteries
Blue = portal venous system

In this posterior view (chosen in preference to the anterior view, where the many very small vessels to the intestines would have obscured the larger branches), the superior mesenteric vein (22) is seen continuing upwards to become the portal vein (14) after it has been joined by the splenic vein (20). In the porta hepatis the portal vein divides into the left and right branches (8 and 16). Owing to removal of the aorta, the upper part of the inferior mesenteric artery (5) has become displaced slightly to the right and appears to have given origin to the ileocolic artery (4), but this is simply an overlap of the vessels; the origin of the ileocolic from the superior mesenteric is not seen in this view.

 1 Bile duct
 2 Branches of middle colic vessels
 3 Coeliac trunk
 4 Ileocolic vessels
 5 Inferior mesenteric artery
 6 Inferior mesenteric vein
 7 Left branch of hepatic artery
 8 Left branch of portal vein
 9 Left colic vessels
10 Left gastric artery and vein
11 Pancreatic duct
12 Pancreatic ducts in head of pancreas
13 Pancreaticoduodenal vessels
14 Portal vein
15 Right branch of hepatic artery
16 Right branch of portal vein
17 Right colic vessels
18 Sigmoid vessels
19 Splenic artery
20 Splenic vein
21 Superior mesenteric artery
22 Superior mesenteric vein

Spleen *from the front*

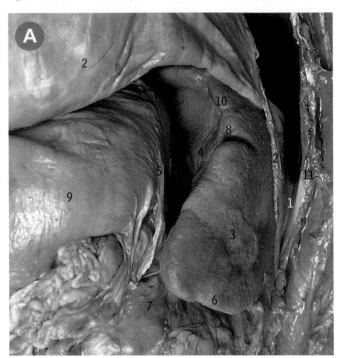

The left upper anterior abdominal and lower anterior thoracic walls have been removed and part of the diaphragm (2) turned upwards to show the spleen in its normal position, lying adjacent to the stomach (9) and colon (7), with the lower part against the kidney (D16 and 9, opposite).

The gastrosplenic ligament contains the short gastric and left gastro-epiploic branches of the splenic vessels.

The lienorenal ligament contains the tail of the pancreas and the splenic vessels.

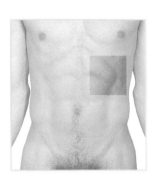

1 Costodiaphragmatic recess
2 Diaphragm
3 Diaphragmatic surface
4 Gastric impression
5 Gastrosplenic ligament
6 Inferior border
7 Left colic flexure
8 Notch
9 Stomach
10 Superior border
11 Thoracic wall

Spleen *visceral surface*

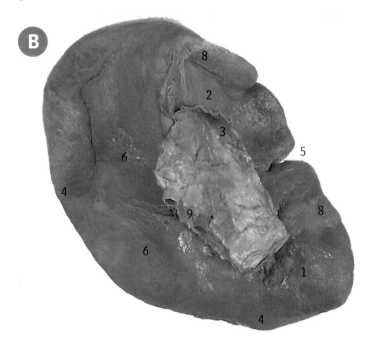

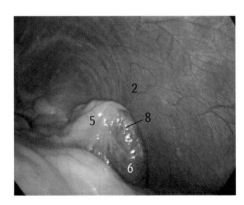

Laparoscopic view of spleen

Labels refer to key above.

1 Colic impression
2 Gastric impression
3 Gastrosplenic ligament containing short gastric and left gastro-epiploic vessels
4 Inferior border
5 Notch
6 Renal impression
7 Spleen
8 Superior border
9 Tail of pancreas and splenic vessels in lienorenal ligament

In B the spleen has been removed and its visceral or medial surface is shown, with a small part of the gastrosplenic (3) and lienorenal (9) ligaments remaining attached.

Splenomegaly, splenectomy, see p. 283.

Spleen *in a transverse section of the left upper abdomen*

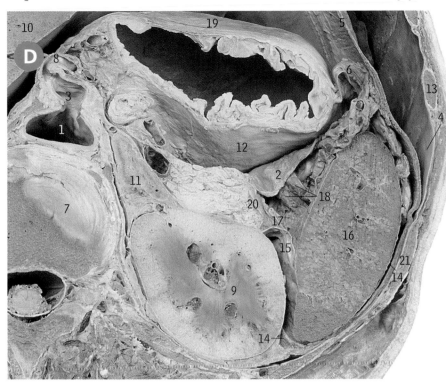

The section is at the level of the disc (7) between the twelfth thoracic and first lumbar vertebrae, and is viewed from below looking towards the thorax.

1 Abdominal aorta
2 Anterior layer of lienorenal ligament
3 Coeliac trunk
4 Costodiaphragmatic recess of pleura
5 Diaphragm
6 Gastrosplenic ligament
7 Intervertebral disc
8 Left gastric artery
9 Left kidney
10 Left lobe of liver
11 Left suprarenal gland
12 Lesser sac
13 Ninth rib
14 Peritoneum of greater sac
15 Posterior layer of lienorenal ligament
16 Spleen
17 Splenic artery
18 Splenic vein
19 Stomach
20 Tail of pancreas
21 Tenth rib

Caecum *in sagittal section, interior view*

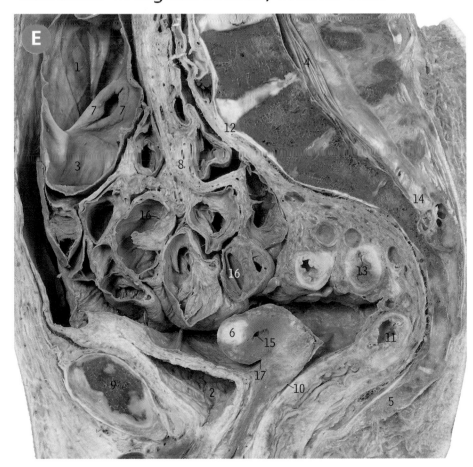

This is a median sagittal section of the pelvis, right side viewed from the left. The anterior wall has been cut open and reflected to show the lips of the ileocaecal valve (7).

1 Ascending colon
2 Bladder
3 Caecum
4 Cauda equina
5 Coccyx
6 Fibroid in uterine fundus
7 Lips of ileocaecal valve
8 Mesentery of small intestine
9 Pubic symphysis
10 Recto-uterine pouch (of Douglas)
11 Rectum
12 Sacral promontory
13 Sigmoid colon
14 Thecal sac termination
15 Uterine cavity
16 Valvulae conniventes
17 Vesico-uterine pouch

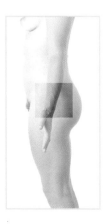

Appendix, ileocolic artery and related structures *from the front*

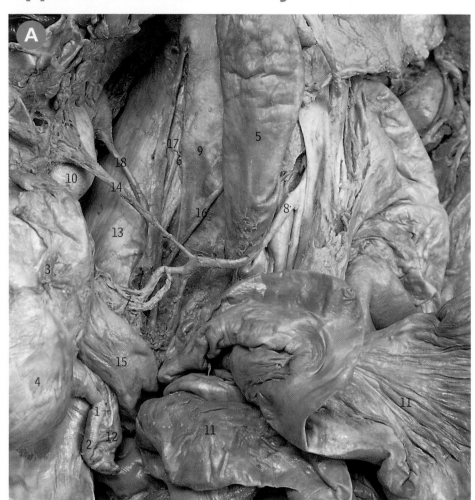

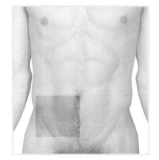

Most of the peritoneum of the mesentery and posterior abdominal wall have been removed, and coils of small intestine (11) have been displaced to the right of the picture, to show the ileocolic artery (8), terminal ileum (15) and appendix (2) with its appendicular artery (1).

1 Appendicular artery in mesoappendix
2 Appendix
3 Ascending colon
4 Caecum
5 Descending (second) part of duodenum
6 Genitofemoral nerve
7 Ileal and caecal vessels
8 Ileocolic artery
9 Inferior vena cava
10 Lower pole of kidney
11 Mesentery and coils of jejunum and ileum
12 Mesoappendix
13 Psoas major
14 Right colic artery
15 Terminal part of ileum
16 Testicular artery
17 Testicular vein
18 Ureter

Caecum and appendix *from the front*

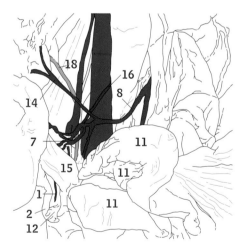

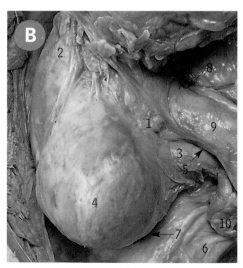

The terminal ileum (9) is seen joining the large intestine at the junction of the caecum (4) and ascending colon (2), and the appendix (3) joins the caecum just below the ileocaecal junction.

1 Anterior taenia coli
2 Ascending colon
3 Base of appendix
4 Caecum
5 Inferior ileocaecal recess
6 Peritoneum overlying external iliac vessels
7 Retrocaecal recess
8 Superior ileocaecal recess
9 Terminal ileum
10 Tip of appendix

Appendicitis, see p. 281.

Small intestine

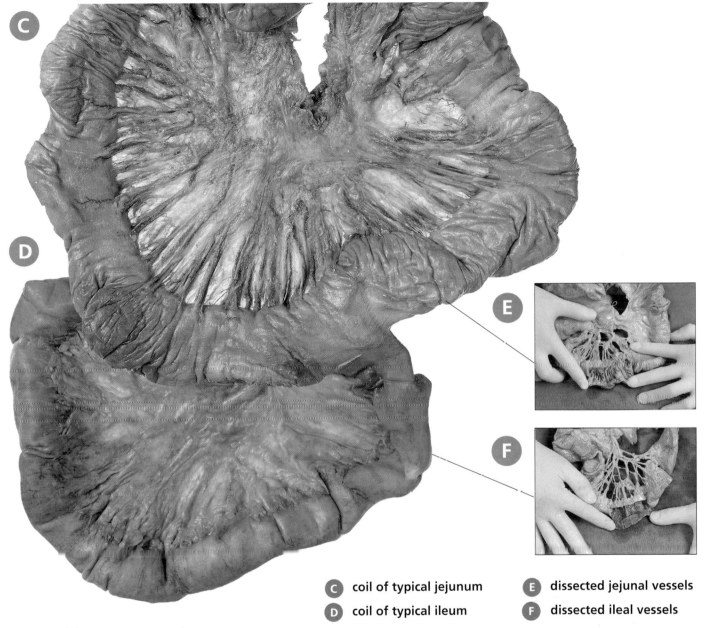

C coil of typical jejunum   E dissected jejunal vessels

D coil of typical ileum   F dissected ileal vessels

In the part of the mesentery supporting the jejunum in C, the vessels anastomose to form one or perhaps two vascular arcades (E) which give off long straight branches that run to the intestinal wall. The fat in the mesentery tends to be concentrated near the root, leaving areas or 'windows' near the gut wall that are devoid of fat. In the mesentery supporting the ileum in D, the vessels form several arcades with shorter branches (F), and there are no fat-free areas. The jejunal wall (C) is thicker than that of the ileum (D) and has a larger lumen. The jejunum also feels thicker, because the folds of its mucous membrane are more numerous than in the ileum.

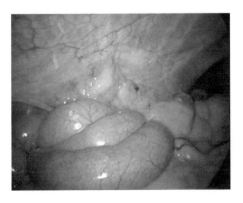

Laparoscopic view of small intestine

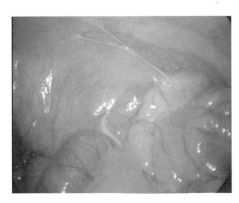

Laparoscopic view of appendix

Kidneys and suprarenal glands

Ⓐ *dissection* Ⓑ *coronal MR image, abdomen*

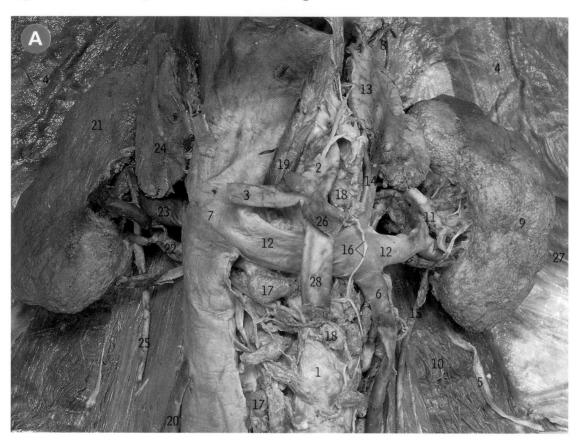

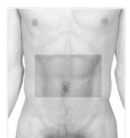

The kidneys (9 and 21) and suprarenal glands (13 and 24) are displayed on the posterior abdominal wall after the removal of all other viscera. The left renal vein (12) receives the left suprarenal (14) and gonadal (6) vein and then passes over the aorta (1) and deep to the superior mesenteric artery (28) to reach the inferior vena cava (7). In the hilum of the right kidney (21) a large branch of the renal artery (22) passes in front of the renal vein (23). The origins of the renal arteries from the aorta are not seen because they underlie the left renal vein (12) and inferior vena cava (7). The MR image in B passes through the kidneys and left suprarenal gland (13).

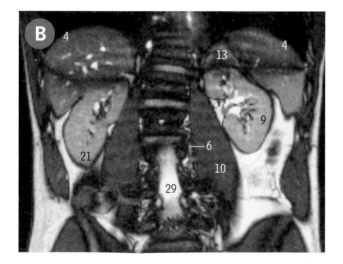

1	Abdominal aorta and aortic plexus	
2	Coeliac trunk	
3	Common hepatic artery	
4	Diaphragm	
5	First lumbar spinal nerve	
6	Gonadal vein, left	
7	Inferior vena cava	
8	Left inferior phrenic vessels	
9	Left kidney	
10	Left psoas major	
11	Left renal artery	
12	Left renal vein	
13	Left suprarenal gland	
14	Left suprarenal vein	
15	Left ureter
16	Lymphatic vessels
17	Para-aortic lymph nodes
18	Pre-aortic lymph nodes
19	Right crus of diaphragm
20	Right gonadal vein
21	Right kidney
22	Right renal artery
23	Right renal vein
24	Right suprarenal gland
25	Right ureter
26	Splenic artery
27	Subcostal nerve, left
28	Superior mesenteric artery
29	Thecal sac

Aortic bruits, see p. 281.

Left kidney, suprarenal gland and related vessels
from the front

Right kidney, suprarenal gland and related vessels
from behind

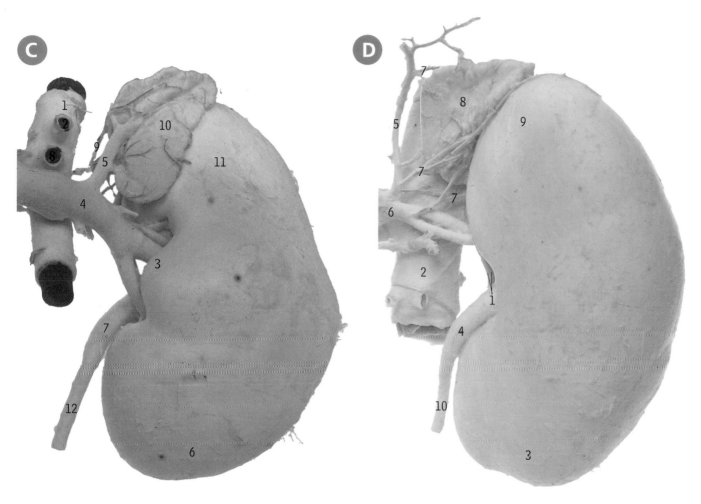

The vessels have been distended by injection of resin, and all fascia has been removed, but the suprarenal gland (10) has been retained in its normal position, lying against the medial side of the upper pole of the kidney (11).

1	Abdominal aorta	**7**	Pelvis of kidney
2	Coeliac trunk	**8**	Superior mesenteric artery
3	Hilum of kidney	**9**	Suprarenal arteries
4	Left renal vein overlying renal artery	**10**	Suprarenal gland
		11	Upper pole of kidney
5	Left suprarenal vein	**12**	Ureter
6	Lower pole of kidney		

Similar to B, but note that this is the right kidney from behind, not the left; the hilum of each kidney faces medially.

1	Hilum of kidney	**6**	Right renal artery
2	Inferior vena cava	**7**	Suprarenal arteries
3	Lower pole of kidney	**8**	Suprarenal gland
4	Pelvis of kidney	**9**	Upper pole of kidney
5	Right inferior phrenic artery	**10**	Ureter

A

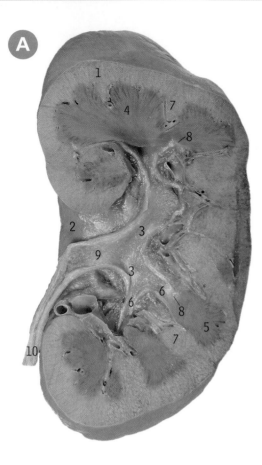

Ⓐ Kidney
internal structure in longitudinal section

The section is through the centre of the kidney and has included the renal pelvis (9) and beginning of the ureter (10). The major vessels in the hilum (2) have been removed.

1	Cortex	**6**	Minor calix
2	Hilum	**7**	Renal column
3	Major calix	**8**	Renal papilla
4	Medulla	**9**	Renal pelvis
5	Medullary pyramid	**10**	Ureter

The two or three major calices (3) unite to form the renal pelvis (9) which passes out through the hilum (2) to become the ureter (10), often with a slight narrowing at the junction. This is known as the pelvi-ureteric junction (PUJ) and is a site of renal stone obstruction.

B

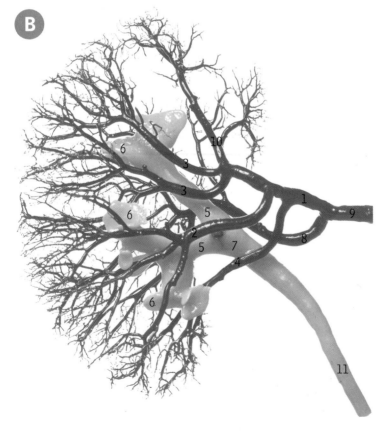

Ⓑ Cast of the right kidney
from the front

Red = renal artery
Yellow = urinary tract

The posterior division (8) of the renal artery (9) here passes behind the pelvis (7) and upper calix (upper 5), but all other vessels are in front of the urinary tract; hence this is a right kidney seen from the front (vein, artery, ureter from front to back, and the hilum on the medial side – see page 255), not a left kidney from behind.

1 Anterior division
2 Anterior inferior segment artery
3 Anterior superior segment artery (double)
4 Inferior segment artery
5 Major calix
6 Minor calix
7 Pelvis of kidney
8 Posterior division (forming posterior segment artery)
9 Renal artery
10 Superior segment artery
11 Ureter

Cast of the aorta and kidneys *from the front*

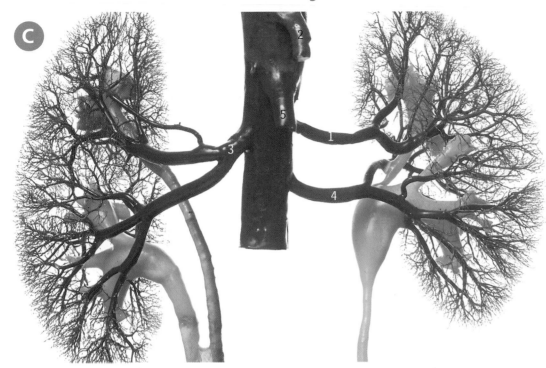

Red = arteries
Yellow = urinary tracts

1 Accessory left renal artery
2 Coeliac trunk
3 Early branching of right renal artery
4 Left renal artery
5 Superior mesenteric artery

Accessory renal arteries represent segmental vessels that arise directly from the aorta. In this specimen, the left accessory vessel (C1) supplies the superior and anterior superior segments, leaving the 'normal' vessel to supply the posterior, anterior inferior and inferior segments.

On the right side the ureters (unlabelled) are double, each arising from a separate set of calices. On the left the arteries are double (1 and 4).

Cast of the kidneys and great vessels *from the front*

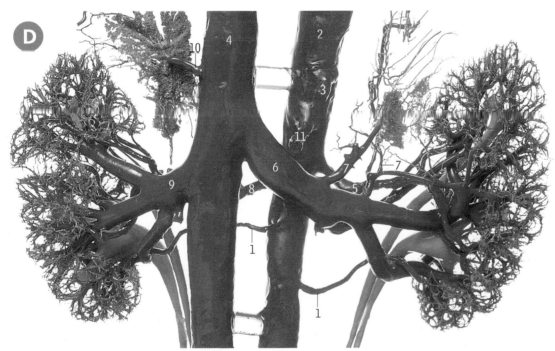

Red = arteries
Blue = veins
Yellow = urinary tracts

1 Accessory renal arteries
2 Aorta
3 Coeliac trunk
4 Inferior vena cava
5 Left renal artery
6 Left renal vein
7 Left suprarenal veins
8 Right renal artery
9 Right renal vein
10 Right suprarenal vein
11 Superior mesenteric artery

Here both kidneys show double ureters (unlabelled), and there are accessory renal arteries (1) to the lower poles of both kidneys. The suprarenal glands (also unlabelled) are outlined by their venous patterns, and the short right suprarenal vein (10) is shown draining directly to the inferior vena cava (4). On the left there are two suprarenal veins (7), both draining to the left renal vein (6). See also page 258, A14, A9, A12.

Left kidney and suprarenal gland *from the front*

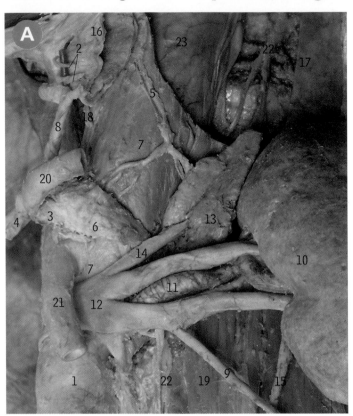

The left kidney (10) and suprarenal gland (13) are seen on the posterior abdominal wall. Much of the diaphragm has been removed but the oesophageal opening remains, with the end of the oesophagus (16) opening out into the cardiac part of the stomach and a (double) anterior vagal trunk (2) overlying the red marker. The posterior vagal trunk (18) is behind and to the right of the oesophagus. Part of the pleura has been cut away (17) to show the sympathetic trunk (22) on the side of the lower thoracic vertebrae. The left coeliac ganglion and the coeliac plexus (6) are at the root of the coeliac trunk (3).

1 Abdominal aorta
2 Anterior vagal trunk (double, over marker)
3 Coeliac trunk
4 Common hepatic artery
5 Inferior phrenic vessels
6 Left coeliac ganglion and coeliac plexus
7 Left crus of diaphragm
8 Left gastric artery
9 Left gonadal vein
10 Left kidney
11 Left renal artery
12 Left renal vein
13 Left suprarenal gland
14 Left suprarenal vein
15 Left ureter
16 Lower end of oesophagus
17 Pleura (cut edge)
18 Posterior vagal trunk
19 Psoas major
20 Splenic artery
21 Superior mesenteric artery
22 Sympathetic trunk
23 Thoracic aorta

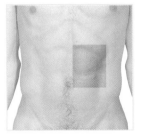

Right kidney and renal fascia *in transverse section from below*

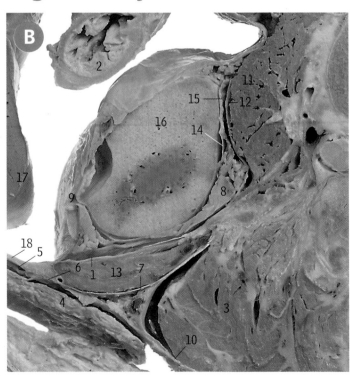

In the transverse section of the lower part of the right kidney (16), seen from below looking towards the thorax, the renal fascia (15) has been dissected out from the perirenal fat (8) and the kidney's own capsule (14). (There was a small cyst on the surface of this kidney.) The section also displays the three layers (10, 7 and 1) of the lumbar fascia (6).

1 Anterior layer of lumbar fascia
2 Coil of small intestine
3 Erector spinae
4 External oblique
5 Internal oblique
6 Lumbar fascia
7 Middle layer of lumbar fascia
8 Perirenal fat
9 Peritoneum
10 Posterior layer of lumbar fascia
11 Psoas major
12 Psoas sheath
13 Quadratus lumborum
14 Renal capsule
15 Renal fascia
16 Right kidney
17 Right lobe of liver
18 Transversus abdominis

Outside the kidney's own capsule (renal capsule, 14), there is variable amount of fat (perirenal fat, 8) and outside this is a condensation of connective tissue forming the renal fascia (15).

 Nephrectomy, superior mesenteric artery syndrome, see p. 283.

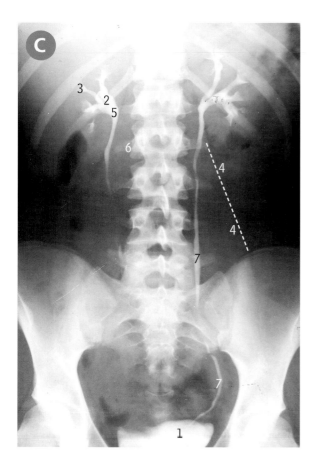

C Intravenous urogram *(IVU)*

Contrast medium injected intravenously is excreted by the kidneys to outline the calices (3 and 2), renal pelvis (5) and the ureters (7) which enter the bladder (1) in the pelvis.

1 Bladder
2 Major calix
3 Minor calix
4 Psoas shadow
5 Renal pelvis
6 Transverse processes of lumbar vertebrae
7 Ureter

> The ureters normally lie near the tips of the transverse processes of the lumbar vertebrae and may kink over the psoas when the muscle is over developed e.g. in rowers.

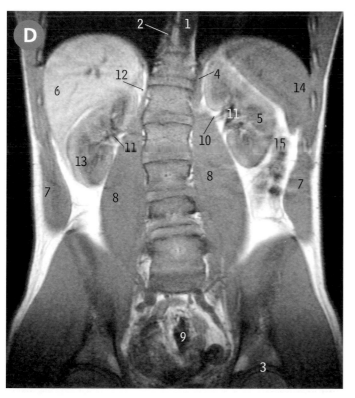

D Abdomen

coronal MR image

1 Aorta
2 Azygos vein
3 Hip joint
4 Left crus of diaphragm
5 Left kidney
6 Liver
7 Oblique muscles of abdomen
8 Psoas major muscle
9 Rectum
10 Renal artery
11 Renal pelvis
12 Right crus of diaphragm
13 Right kidney
14 Spleen
15 Splenic flexure of colon

 Abdominal aortic aneurysm, ureteric calculi, see pp 281, 283.

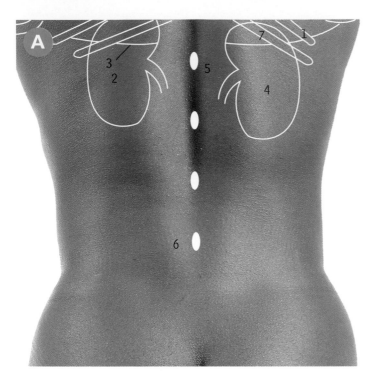

Ⓐ Kidneys
surface markings, from behind

The upper pole of the left kidney rises to the level of the eleventh rib, but the right kidney is slightly lower (due to the bulk of the liver on the right). The hilum of each kidney is 5 cm (2 in) from the midline. The lower edge of the costodiaphragmatic recess of the pleura crosses the twelfth rib; compare with the dissection below (B6).

1 Eleventh rib
2 Left kidney
3 Lower edge of pleura
4 Right kidney
5 Spinous process of first lumbar vertebra
6 Spinous process of fourth lumbar vertebra
7 Twelfth rib

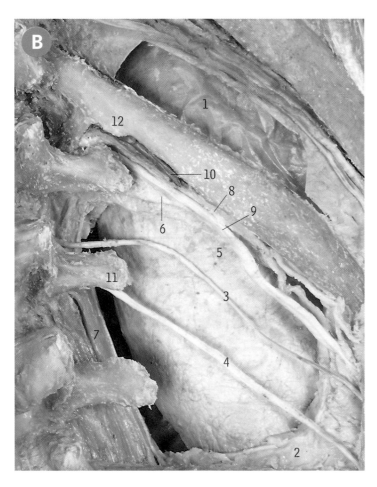

Ⓑ Right kidney *from behind*

Most thoracic and abdominal muscles have been removed to show the three nerves (9, 3 and 4) that lie behind the kidney (5). Much more important is the relationship of the upper part of the kidney to the pleura. A window has been cut in the parietal pleura above the twelfth rib (12) to open into the costodiaphragmatic recess (1), whose lower limit (6) runs transversely behind the kidney and in front of the obliquely placed twelfth rib.

1 Costodiaphragmatic recess of pleura
2 Extraperitoneal tissue
3 Iliohypogastric nerve
4 Ilio-inguinal nerve
5 Kidney
6 Lower edge of pleura
7 Psoas major
8 Subcostal artery
9 Subcostal nerve
10 Subcostal vein
11 Transverse process of second lumbar vertebra
12 Twelfth rib

Renal biopsy, see p. 283.

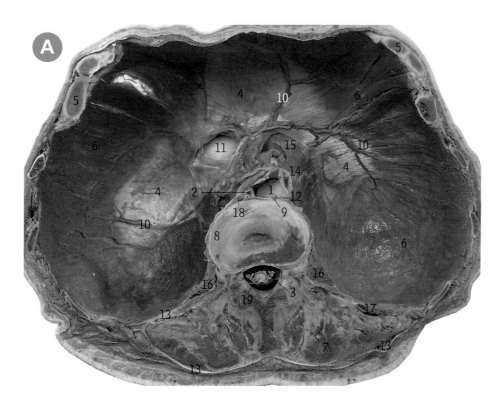

A Diaphragm
from below

1 Aorta
2 Azygos vein
3 Cauda equina
4 Central tendon of diaphragm
5 Costal margin
6 Diaphragm
7 Erector spinae muscles
8 First lumbar intervertebral disc
9 Hemi-azygos vein
10 Inferior phrenic vessels
11 Inferior vena caval opening
12 Left crus
13 Lumbar fascia
14 Median arcuate ligament
15 Oesophageal opening (hiatus)
16 Psoas major
17 Quadratus lumborum
18 Right crus
19 Spinal cord

Fibres of the right crus (A18) form the right and left boundaries of the oesophageal opening or hiatus (A15).

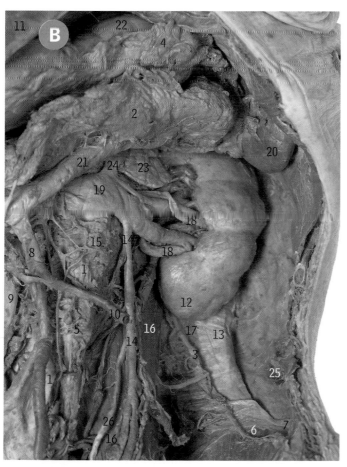

B Posterior abdominal wall
left side

The structures on the posterior abdominal wall are viewed from the front. The body of the pancreas (2) has been turned upwards to expose the splenic vein (21). The suprarenal gland (23) appears detached from the superior pole of the kidney (compared with A13 and 10, page 258).

1 Aorta and aortic plexus
2 Body of pancreas
3 First lumbar spinal nerve
4 Greater omentum
5 Hypogastric plexus
6 Ilio-inguinal nerve
7 Iliohypogastric nerve
8 Inferior mesenteric vein
9 Inferior vena cava
10 Left colic vein
11 Liver
12 Lower pole of kidney
13 Lumbar part of thoracolumbar fascia
14 Ovarian vein
15 Para-aortic lymph node
16 Psoas major
17 Quadratus lumborum
18 Renal artery
19 Renal vein
20 Spleen
21 Splenic vein
22 Stomach
23 Suprarenal gland
24 Suprarenal vein
25 Transversus abdominis
26 Ureter

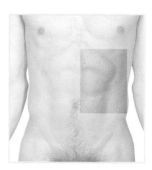

Hiatus hernia, see p. 282.

Posterior abdominal and pelvic walls

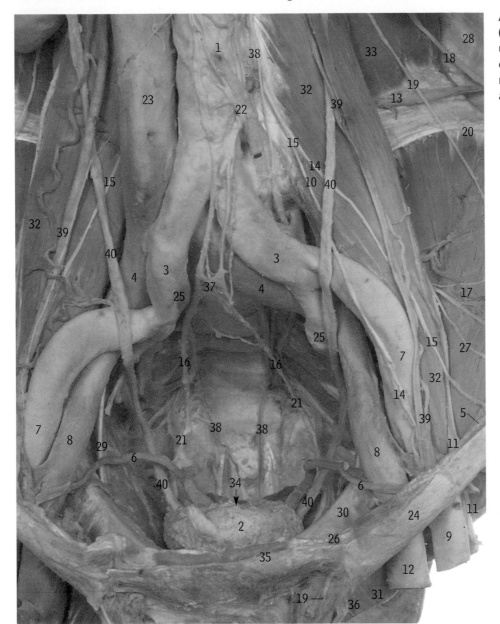

All peritoneum and viscera
(except for the bladder, 2,
ureter, 40, and ductus deferens
or vas deferens, 6) have been
removed, to display vessels
and nerves.

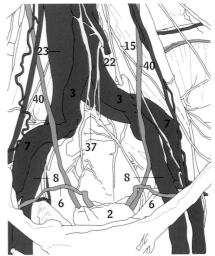

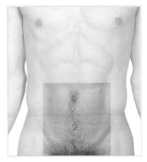

1 Aorta and aortic plexus	**16** Hypogastric nerve	**28** Lumbar part of thoracolumbar fascia
2 Bladder	**17** Iliacus and branches from femoral nerve	**29** Obturator nerve and vessels
3 Common iliac artery	and iliolumbar artery	**30** Pectineal ligament
4 Common iliac vein	**18** Iliohypogastric nerve	**31** Position of femoral canal
5 Deep circumflex iliac artery	**19** Ilio-inguinal nerve	**32** Psoas major
6 Ductus deferens	**20** Iliolumbar ligament	**33** Quadratus lumborum
7 External iliac artery	**21** Inferior hypogastric (pelvic) plexus and	**34** Rectum (cut edge)
8 External iliac vein	pelvic splanchnic nerves	**35** Rectus abdominis
9 Femoral artery	**22** Inferior mesenteric artery and plexus	**36** Spermatic cord
10 Femoral branch of genitofemoral nerve	**23** Inferior vena cava	**37** Superior hypogastric plexus
11 Femoral nerve	**24** Inguinal ligament	**38** Sympathetic trunk and ganglia
12 Femoral vein	**25** Internal iliac artery	**39** Testicular vessels
13 Fourth lumbar artery	**26** Lacunar ligament	**40** Ureter
14 Genital branch of genitofemoral nerve	**27** Lateral femoral cutaneous nerve arising	
15 Genitofemoral nerve	from femoral nerve	

 Psoas sign, see p. 283.

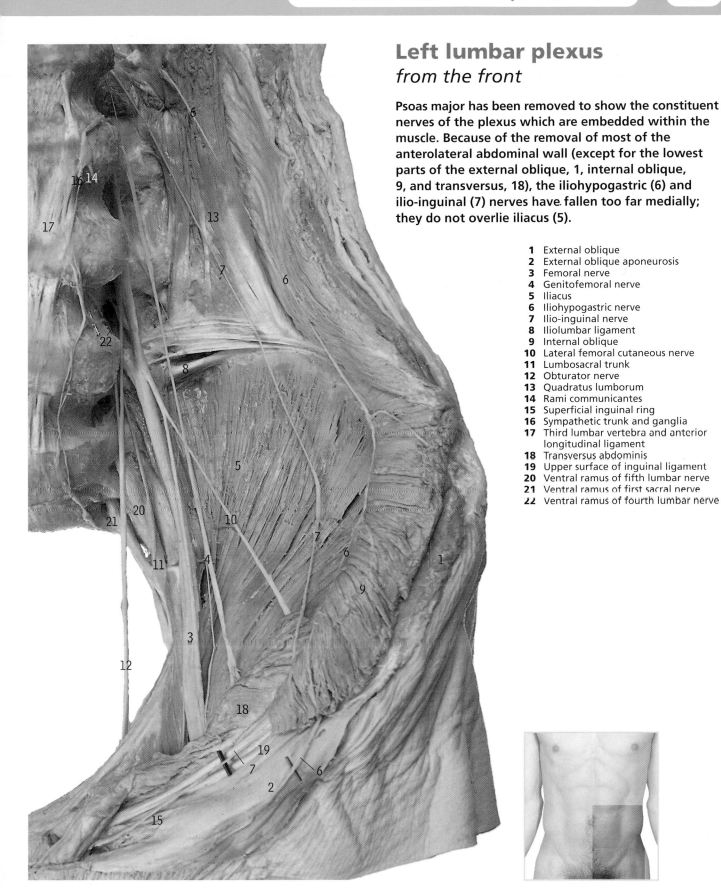

Left lumbar plexus
from the front

Psoas major has been removed to show the constituent nerves of the plexus which are embedded within the muscle. Because of the removal of most of the anterolateral abdominal wall (except for the lowest parts of the external oblique, 1, internal oblique, 9, and transversus, 18), the iliohypogastric (6) and ilio-inguinal (7) nerves have fallen too far medially; they do not overlie iliacus (5).

 1 External oblique
 2 External oblique aponeurosis
 3 Femoral nerve
 4 Genitofemoral nerve
 5 Iliacus
 6 Iliohypogastric nerve
 7 Ilio-inguinal nerve
 8 Iliolumbar ligament
 9 Internal oblique
10 Lateral femoral cutaneous nerve
11 Lumbosacral trunk
12 Obturator nerve
13 Quadratus lumborum
14 Rami communicantes
15 Superficial inguinal ring
16 Sympathetic trunk and ganglia
17 Third lumbar vertebra and anterior
    longitudinal ligament
18 Transversus abdominis
19 Upper surface of inguinal ligament
20 Ventral ramus of fifth lumbar nerve
21 Ventral ramus of first sacral nerve
22 Ventral ramus of fourth lumbar nerve

Lumbar sympathectomy, see p. 282.

Muscles of the left pelvis and proximal thigh
slightly oblique anterior view

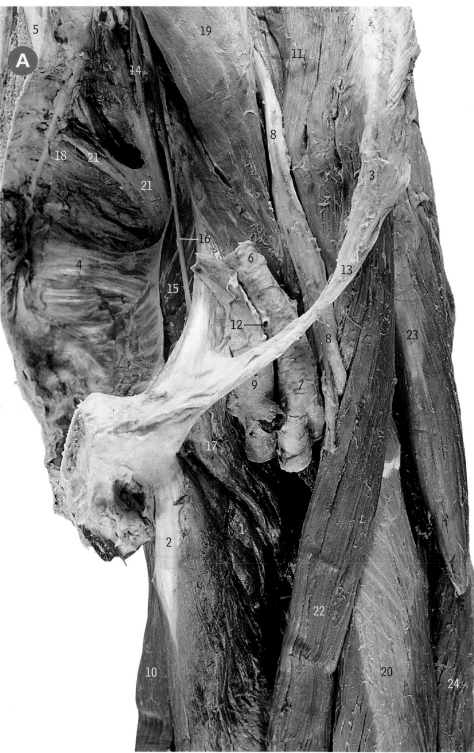

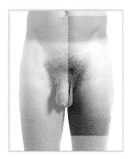

1   Adductor brevis
2   Adductor longus
3   Anterior superior iliac spine
4   Coccygeus
5   Disc, 5th lumbar
6   External iliac artery
7   Femoral artery
8   Femoral nerve
9   Femoral vein
10   Gracilis
11   Iliacus
12   Inferior epigastric artery, origin
13   Inguinal ligament
14   Lumbosacral trunk
15   Obturator internus
16   Obturator nerve
17   Pectineus
18   Piriformis
19   Psoas major
20   Rectus femoris
21   Sacral plexus
22   Sartorius
23   Tensor fasciae latae
24   Vastus lateralis

The anterior superior iliac spine (3) and the pubic tubercle, which give attachment to the ends of the inguinal ligament (13), are important palpable landmarks in the inguinal region (see page 236).

The part of obturator internus (15) *above* the attachment of levator ani is part of the lateral wall of the pelvic cavity, while the part *below* the attachment is in the perineum and forms part of the lateral wall of the ischio-anal (ischiorectal) fossa (pages 279 and 280).

Piriformis (18) passes out of the pelvis into the gluteal region through the *greater* sciatic foramen *above* the ischial spine, while obturator internus (15) passes out through the *lesser* sciatic foramen *below* the ischial spine.

The anterior abdominal wall, most viscera and fasciae have been removed. Segments of the external iliac/femoral vessels and the inferior margin of the external oblique aponeurosis (inguinal ligament) have been retained to assist orientation.

Muscles of the left half of the pelvis

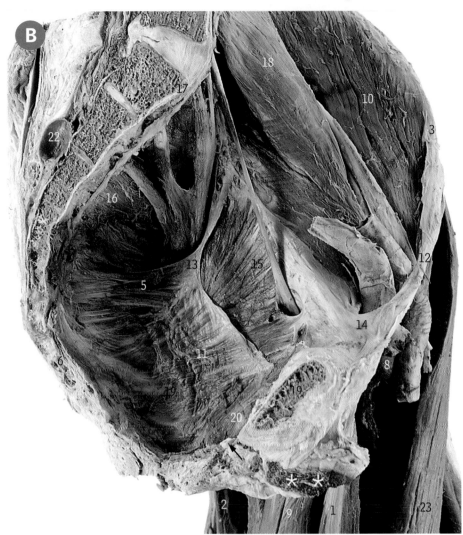

B Male pelvis

The fascia overlying the obturator internus (15) has been removed down to the tendinous origin of the levator ani (11 and 20), a urethral catheter (arrow) indicates the position of the sphincter urethrae, and the plane of section passes through the bulbocavernosus (asterisk).

B and C label key

1 Adductor longus
2 Adductor magnus
3 Anterior superior iliac spine
4 Branch of 4th sacral nerve
5 Coccygeus
6 Coccyx
7 Fascia over obturator internus
8 Femoral vein
9 Gracilis
10 Iliacus
11 Iliococcygeus part of levator ani
12 Inguinal ligament
13 Ischial spine
14 Lacunar ligament
15 Obturator internus, pierced by obturator nerve
16 Piriformis
17 Promontory of sacrum
18 Psoas major
19 Pubic symphysis
20 Pubococcygeus part of levator ani
21 Rectum
22 Sacral canal with cyst
23 Sartorius
24 Urethra
25 Vagina

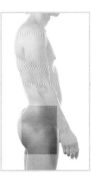

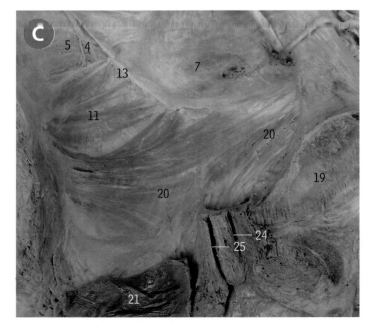

C Female pelvis

The distal ends of the urethra (24), vagina (25) and rectum (21) have been preserved.

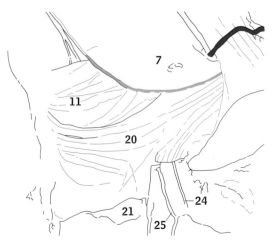

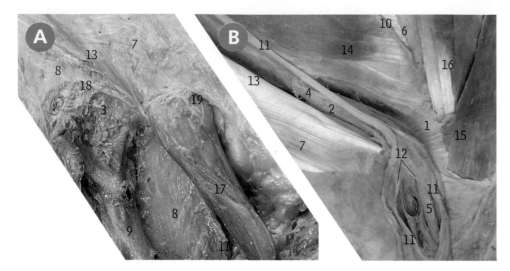

Right inguinal region *in the male*

A superficial dissection

B with the external oblique aponeurosis and spermatic cord incised

In A the spermatic cord (17) is seen emerging from the superficial inguinal ring (19) and covered by the external spermatic fascia. In B, with the external oblique aponeurosis reflected and the anterior wall of the rectus sheath removed, the cord is emerging from the deep inguinal ring (4) with the cremasteric fascia (2) now the most superficial covering. All three coverings of the cord have been incised (12) to show the ductus deferens (5).

1 Conjoint tendon
2 Cremasteric fascia and cremaster muscle over spermatic cord
3 Cribriform fascia
4 Deep inguinal ring
5 Ductus deferens
6 Edge of rectus sheath
7 External oblique aponeurosis
8 Fascia lata
9 Great saphenous vein
10 Iliohypogastric nerve
11 Ilio-inguinal nerve
12 Incised margin of coverings of cord
13 Inguinal ligament
14 Internal oblique
15 Pyramidalis
16 Rectus abdominis
17 Spermatic cord
18 Upper margin of saphenous opening
19 Upper margin of superficial inguinal ring

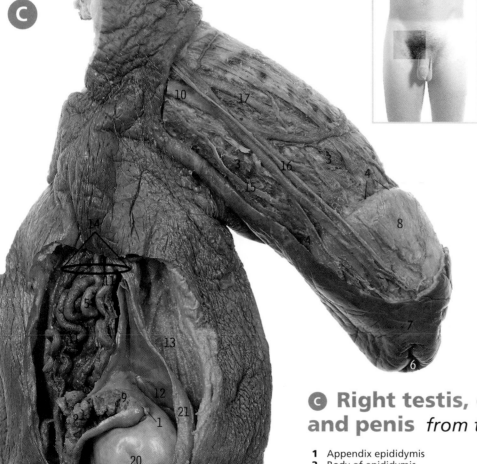

C Right testis, epididymis and penis *from the right*

1 Appendix epididymis
2 Body of epididymis
3 Body of penis
4 Corona of glans
5 Ductus deferens
6 External urethral orifice
7 Foreskin
8 Glans penis
9 Head of epididymis
10 Lateral superficial vein
11 Pampiniform venous plexus
12 Sac of tunica vaginalis

13 Scrotal sac
14 Spermatic cord
15 Superficial dorsal artery
16 Superficial dorsal nerve
17 Superficial dorsal vein
18 Superficial scrotal (dartos) fascia
19 Tail of epididymis
20 Testis
21 Tunica vaginalis, parietal
22 Tunica vaginalis, visceral, overlying tunica alburginea

 Cremasteric reflex, hydrocele, varioceles, vasectomy, see pp 281, 282, 284.

Right inguinal region *in the female*

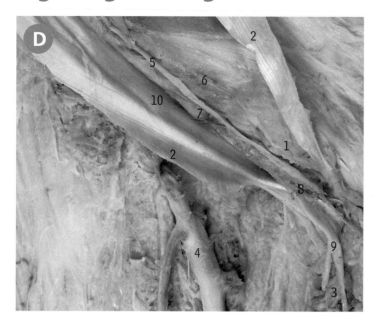

The external oblique aponeurosis (2) has been incised and reflected to show the position of the deep inguinal ring (7) which marks the lateral end of the inguinal canal. The round ligament of the uterus (9) emerges from the superficial inguinal ring (8), which marks the medial end of the canal, and becomes lost in the fat of the labium majus (3). The ilio-inguinal nerve (5) also passes through the canal and out of the superficial ring.

1 Conjoint tendon
2 External oblique aponeurosis
3 Fat of labium majus
4 Great saphenous vein
5 Ilio-inguinal nerve
6 Internal oblique
7 Position of deep inguinal ring
8 Position of superficial inguinal ring
9 Round ligament of uterus
10 Upper surface of inguinal ligament

In the female the inguinal canal contains the round ligament of the uterus and the ilio-inguinal nerve.

The processus vaginalis is normally obliterated, but if it remains patent within the female inguinal canal it is sometimes known as the canal of Nuck.

Right inguinal and femoral regions *in the female*

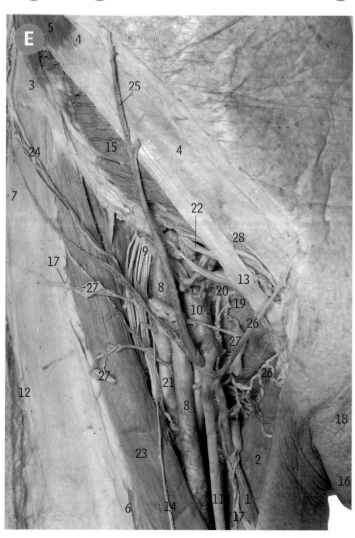

Part of the fascia lata of the thigh has been removed to show the femoral nerve (9), artery (8) and vein (10) beneath the inguinal ligament (13), and also the position of the femoral canal (20), medial to the vein (10). The femoral structures have been included here because of the importance of the femoral canal as a site for hernia in the female (see page 269C).

1 Accessory saphenous vein
2 Adductor longus
3 Anterior superior iliac spine
4 External oblique aponeurosis
5 External oblique muscle
6 Fascia lata, cut edge
7 Fascia lata overlying tensor fasciae latae
8 Femoral artery
9 Femoral nerve
10 Femoral vein
11 Great saphenous vein
12 Iliotibial tract
13 Inguinal ligament
14 Intermediate femoral cutaneous nerve
15 Internal oblique muscle
16 Labium majus
17 Lymph vessels
18 Mons pubis
19 Pectineus
20 Position of femoral canal
21 Profunda femoris artery
22 Round ligament of uterus
23 Sartorius
24 Superficial circumflex iliac vessels
25 Superficial epigastric vein
26 Superficial external pudendal vessels
27 Superficial inguinal lymph nodes
28 Superficial inguinal ring

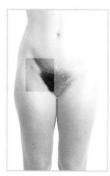

Male pelvis Ⓐ *right half of a midline sagittal section* Ⓑ *sagittal MR image*

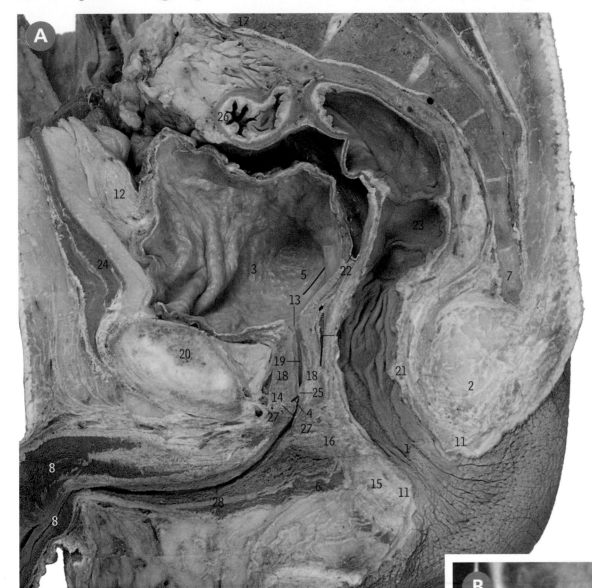

1 Anal canal with anal columns of mucous membrane
2 Anococcygeal body
3 Bladder
4 Bristle in ejaculatory duct
5 Bristle passing up into right ureteral orifice
6 Bulbospongiosus
7 Coccyx
8 Corpus cavernosum
9 Ductus deferens
10 Epididymis
11 External anal sphincter
12 Extraperitoneal fat
13 Internal urethral orifice
14 Membranous part of urethra
15 Perineal body
16 Perineal membrane
17 Promontory of sacrum
18 Prostate
19 Prostatic part of urethra
20 Pubic symphysis
21 Puborectalis fibres of levator ani
22 Rectovesical pouch
23 Rectum
24 Rectus abdominis
25 Seminal colliculus
26 Sigmoid colon
27 Sphincter urethrae
28 Spongy part of urethra and corpus spongiosum
29 Testis

The section (A) has passed exactly through the midline of the anal canal (1) and the prostatic, membranous and spongy parts of the urethra (19, 14 and 28) but has transected the left side of the scrotum and the left testis (29) and epididymis (10). The prostate (18) and bladder (3) are somewhat higher than usual; the empty adult bladder should not extend above the pubic symphysis (20). Compare the features seen in the MR image with the section.

Extravasation of urine, sigmoidoscopy, see pp 282, 283.

Right deep inguinal ring and inguinal triangle *internal view*

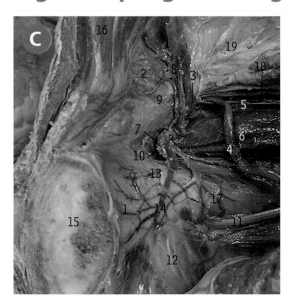

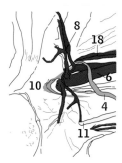

This is the view looking into the right half of the pelvis from the left, showing the posterior surface of the lower part of the anterior abdominal wall, above the pubic symphysis. The femoral ring (7), the entrance to the femoral canal, is below the medial end of the inguinal ligament (9). The inferior epigastric vessels (8) lie medial to the deep inguinal ring (3).

The inguinal triangle (Hesselbach's triangle) is the area bounded laterally by the inferior epigastric vessels (C8), medially by the lateral border of rectus abdominis (C16) and below by the inguinal ligament (C9). A direct inguinal hernia passes forwards through this triangle, medial to the inferior epigastric vessels.

An indirect inguinal hernia passes through the deep inguinal ring (C3) lateral to the inferior epigastric vessels (C8).

1	Body of pubis	**7**	Femoral ring	**12**	Origin of levator ani from fascia overlying obturator internus
2	Conjoint tendon	**8**	Inferior epigastric vessels	**15**	Pubic symphysis
3	Deep inguinal ring			**13**	Pectineal ligament
4	Ductus deferens	**9**	Inguinal ligament	**14**	Pubic branches of inferior epigastric vessels
5	External iliac artery	**10**	Lacunar ligament		
6	External iliac vein	**11**	Obturator nerve		

15	Pubic symphysis
16	Rectus abdominis
17	Superior ramus of pubis
18	Testicular vessels
19	Transversalis fascia overlying transversus abdominis

Right accessory obturator artery *from the left*

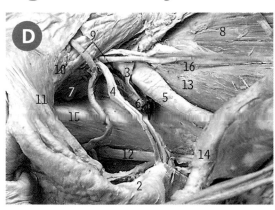

This is a similar view to that in C but showing an accessory obturator artery (1) passing from the inferior epigastric (9) over the superior pubic ramus (15) to enter the obturator foramen with the obturator nerve (12).

1	Accessory obturator artery	**10**	Inguinal ligament
2	Bladder	**11**	Lacunar ligament
3	Deep circumflex iliac vein	**12**	Obturator nerve
4	Ductus deferens	**13**	Psoas major
5	External iliac artery	**14**	Right common iliac artery and vein
6	External iliac vein (cut end)	**15**	Superior ramus of pubis and pectineal ligament
7	Femoral ring	**16**	Testicular vessels
8	Iliacus		
9	Inferior epigastric artery		

The anastomosis between the pubic branches of the inferior epigastric and obturator arteries may be unusually large, forming the vessel known as the accessory or abnormal obturator artery (D1), in which case the normal obturator branch from the internal iliac must be absent.

Pelvis, right inguinal region and penis *from above*

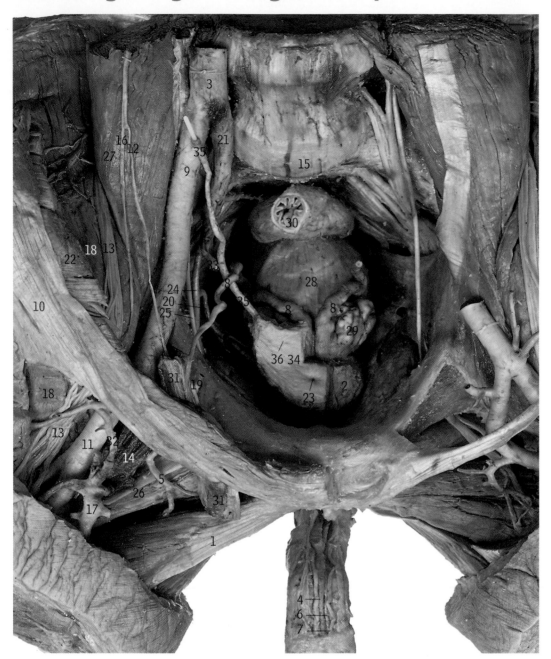

In the pelvis, most of the bladder (34) has been removed to show part of the basal surface of the prostate (2), and the left seminal vesicle (29) lying lateral to the ductus deferens (8). The ductus in the pelvis crosses superficial to the ureter (35). The external iliac artery (9) passes under the inguinal ligament (10) to become the femoral artery (11). On the dorsum of the penis the fascia has been removed, showing the single midline deep dorsal vein (4) with a dorsal artery (6) and dorsal nerve (7) on each side.

The trigone of the bladder (34), at the lower part of the base or posterior surface, is the relatively fixed area with smooth mucous membrane between the internal urethral orifice (23, B16) and the two ureteral openings (36 on the right side, B38 on the left).

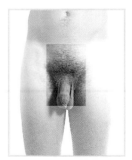

1 Adductor longus	**13** Femoral nerve	**26** Pectineus
2 Base of prostate	**14** Femoral vein	**27** Psoas major
3 Common iliac artery	**15** Fifth lumbar intervertebral disc	**28** Rectum
4 Deep dorsal vein of penis	**16** Genital branch of	**29** Seminal vesicle
5 Deep external pudendal artery	genitofemoral nerve	**30** Sigmoid colon (cut lower end)
6 Dorsal artery of penis	**17** Great saphenous vein	**31** Spermatic cord
7 Dorsal nerve of penis	**18** Iliacus	**32** Superficial circumflex iliac vein
8 Ductus deferens	**19** Inferior epigastric artery	**33** Superior vesical artery
9 External iliac artery	**20** Inferior vesical artery	**34** Trigone of bladder
10 External oblique aponeurosis	**21** Internal iliac artery	**35** Ureter
and inguinal ligament	**22** Internal oblique	**36** Ureteral orifice
11 Femoral artery	**23** Internal urethral orifice	
12 Femoral branch of	**24** Obturator artery	
genitofemoral nerve	**25** Obturator nerve	

 Carcinoma of the rectum, cytoscopy, see p. 281.

Ⓐ Bladder and prostate

from behind

1 Base of bladder
2 Ductus deferens
3 Left ejaculatory duct
4 Posterior surface of prostate
5 Seminal vesicle
6 Ureter

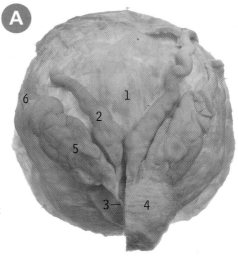

Ⓑ Left side of the male pelvis

from the right

In this midline sagittal section, the prostate (24) is enlarged, lengthening the prostatic urethra (25) and accentuating the trabeculae of the bladder. The mucous membrane of the bladder (whose trigone is labelled at 36) has been removed to show muscular trabeculae in the wall. Variations in the branches of the internal iliac artery (14) are common, and here the obturator artery (22) gives origin to the superior vesical (34) and inferior vesical (13) as well as the middle rectal (20).

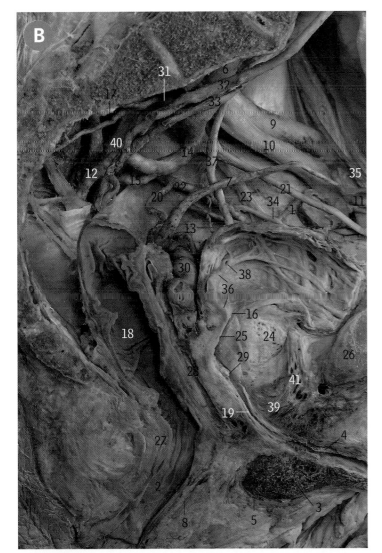

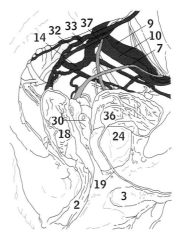

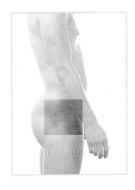

1 Accessory obturator vein
2 Anal canal
3 Bulb of penis
4 Bulbar part of spongy urethra
5 Bulbospongiosus
6 Common iliac artery
7 Ductus deferens
8 External anal sphincter
9 External iliac artery
10 External iliac vein
11 Inferior epigastric vessels
12 Inferior gluteal artery
13 Inferior vesical artery
14 Internal iliac artery
15 Internal pudendal artery
16 Internal urethral orifice
17 Lateral sacral artery
18 Lower end of rectum
19 Membranous part of urethra
20 Middle rectal artery
21 Obliterated umbilical artery
22 Obturator artery
23 Obturator nerve
24 Prostate (enlarged)
25 Prostatic part of urethra
26 Pubic symphysis
27 Puborectalis part of levator ani
28 Rectovesical fascia
29 Seminal colliculus
30 Seminal vesicle
31 Superior gluteal artery
32 Superior rectal artery
33 Superior rectal vein
34 Superior vesical artery
35 Testicular vessels and deep inguinal ring
36 Trigone of bladder
37 Ureter
38 Ureteral orifice
39 Urogenital diaphragm
40 Ventral ramus of first sacral nerve
41 Vesicoprostatic venous plexus

Benign prostatic hyperplasia, carcinoma of the prostate, transurethral resection of prostate (TURP), see pp 281, 283.

Arteries and nerves of the pelvis *left side*

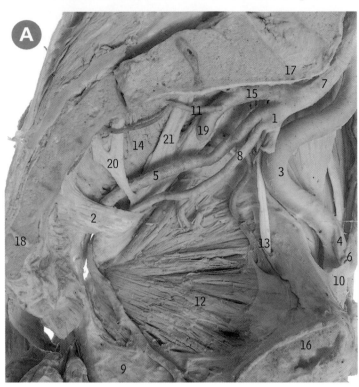

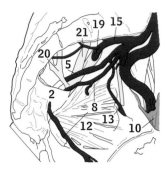

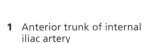

1	Anterior trunk of internal iliac artery
2	Coccygeus and sacrospinous ligament
3	External iliac artery
4	Inferior epigastric artery
5	Inferior gluteal artery
6	Inguinal ligament
7	Internal iliac artery
8	Internal pudendal artery
9	Ischial tuberosity
10	Lacunar ligament
11	Lateral sacral artery
12	Obturator internus
13	Obturator nerve and artery
14	Piriformis
15	Posterior trunk of internal iliac artery
16	Pubic symphysis
17	Sacral promontory
18	Sacrococcygeal joint
19	Superior gluteal artery piercing lumbosacral trunk
20	Union of ventral rami of second and third sacral nerves
21	Ventral ramus of first sacral nerve

In this left half section of the pelvis, all peritoneum, fascia, veins and visceral arteries have been removed together with the left levator ani, so displaying the whole of the internal surface of obturator internus (12). On the posterior pelvic wall, the vessels in general lie superficial to the nerves.

In this specimen the external iliac artery (3) is unusually tortuous, and the anterior trunk of the internal iliac artery (1) has divided unusually high up into its terminal branches, the internal pudendal (8) and the inferior gluteal (5). The superior gluteal artery (19) has perforated the lumbosacral trunk.

Left inferior hypogastric plexus *from the right*

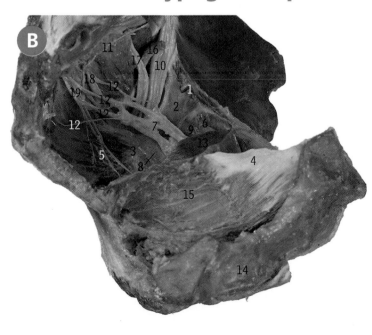

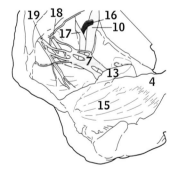

1	Arcuate line of ilium
2	Fascia overlying obturator internus
3	Ischial spine
4	Lateral surface of fascia overlying right obturator internus
5	Left coccygeus and nerves to levator ani
6	Left ductus deferens
7	Left inferior hypogastric plexus
8	Left levator ani
9	Left seminal vesicle
10	Lumbosacral trunk
11	Part of left sympathetic trunk
12	Pelvic splanchnic nerves (nervi erigentes)
13	Rectum
14	Right ischiopubic ramus
15	Right levator ani and ischio-anal (ischiorectal) fossa
16	Superior gluteal artery
17	Ventral ramus of first sacral nerve
18	Ventral ramus of second sacral nerve
19	Ventral ramus of third sacral nerve

In this view of the left side of the pelvis from the right, the right pelvic wall has been removed but the right levator ani (15) forming part of the pelvic floor (pelvic diaphragm) has been preserved and is seen from its right (perineal) side. Pelvic splanchnic nerves (12) arise from the ventral rami of the second and third sacral nerves (18 and 19) and contribute to the inferior hypogastric plexus (7).

Pelvic skeleton and ligaments *left side*

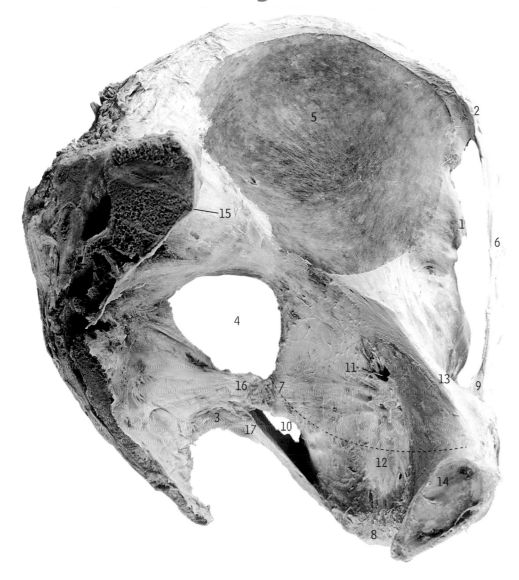

1 Anterior inferior iliac spine and origin of straight head of rectus femoris
2 Anterior superior iliac spine
3 Falciform process of sacrotuberous ligament
4 Greater sciatic foramen
5 Iliac fossa
6 Inguinal ligament
7 Ischial spine
8 Ischial tuberosity
9 Lacunar ligament
10 Lesser sciatic foramen
11 Obturator foramen with obturator nerve and vessels
12 Obturator membrane
13 Pectineal ligament
14 Pubic symphysis
15 Sacral promontory
16 Sacrospinous ligament
17 Sacrotuberous ligament

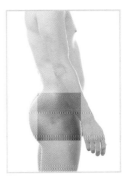

The ligaments classified as 'the ligaments of the pelvis' (vertebropelvic ligaments) are the sacrotuberous (17), sacrospinous (16) and iliolumbar (seen in the posterior view on page 325, C7).

The lacunar ligament (9) passes backwards from the medial end of the inguinal ligament (6) to the medial end of the pectineal line of the pubis, to which the pectineal ligament (13) is attached.

In this mid-sagittal section, viewed from slightly above the midline, most soft tissues except ligaments have been removed.

Female pelvis *left half of a midline sagittal section*

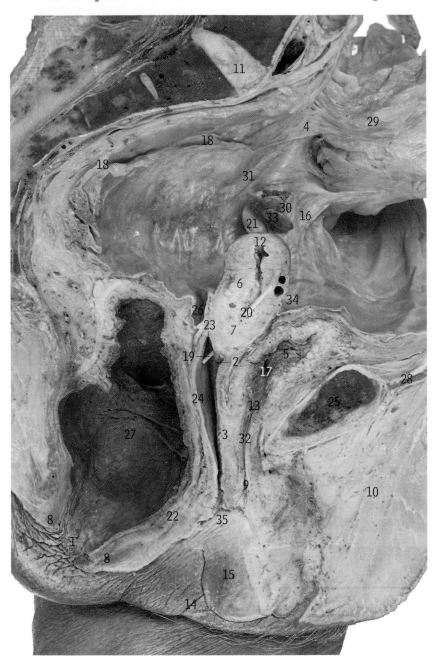

1 Anal canal
2 Anterior fornix of vagina
3 Anterior wall of vagina
4 Apex of sigmoid mesocolon
5 Bladder
6 Body of uterus
7 Cervix of uterus
8 External anal sphincter
9 External urethral orifice
10 Fat of mons pubis
11 Fifth lumbar intervertebral disc
12 Fundus of uterus
13 Internal urethral orifice
14 Labium majus
15 Labium minus
16 Left limb of sigmoid mesocolon overlying external iliac vessels
17 Left ureteral orifice
18 Line of attachment of right limb of sigmoid mesocolon
19 Marker in external os
20 Marker in internal os
21 Ovary
22 Perineal body
23 Posterior fornix of vagina
24 Posterior wall of vagina
25 Pubic symphysis
26 Recto-uterine pouch (of Douglas)
27 Rectum
28 Rectus abdominis (turned forwards)
29 Sigmoid colon (reflected to left and upwards)
30 Suspensory ligament of ovary containing ovarian vessels
31 Ureter underlying peritoneum
32 Urethra
33 Uterine tube
34 Vesico-uterine pouch
35 Vestibule of vagina

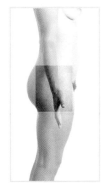

The lower end of the rectum (27) is dilated, and the bladder (5), uterus (6) and vagina (3 and 24) are contracted. The section has opened up the whole length of the urethra (32), but the cervix of the uterus (7) is rarely exactly in the midline and the line of the cervical canal is indicated by the marker in the internal and external os (20 and 19). Compare features in the MR image in A, opposite, with the section.

 Faecal continence, haemorrhoids, rectal examination, see pp 282, 283.

Female pelvis

Ⓐ *sagittal MR image during menstruation* **Ⓑ** *coronal MR image*

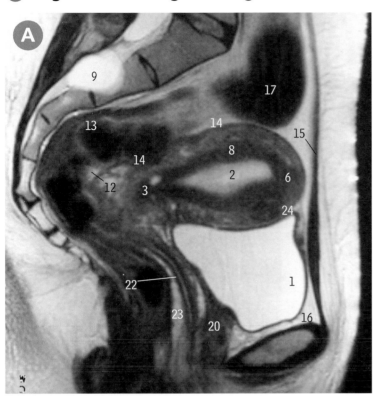

1 Bladder
2 Blood clot in endometrial cavity
3 Cervix of uterus
4 Corpus luteum
5 Endometrial cavity
6 Fundus of uterus
7 Levator ani
8 Myometrium
9 Nerve root cyst (Tarlov)
10 Ovary
11 Perineal muscles
12 Posterior fornix of vagina
13 Rectosigmoid junction
14 Recto-uterine pouch (Douglas)
15 Rectus abdominis muscle
16 Retropubic space (Retzius)
17 Sigmoid colon
18 Small intestine
19 Trigone
20 Urethra
21 Uterine (Fallopian) tube
22 Vaginal cavity
23 Vaginal wall
24 Vesico-uterine pouch

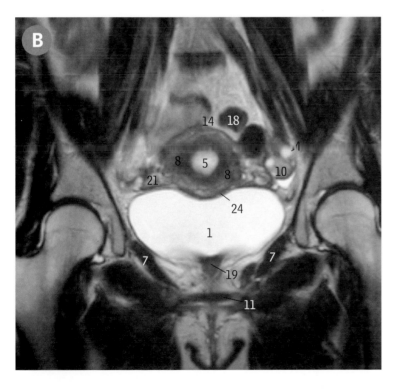

Looking down into the pelvis from the front, the fundus of the uterus (5, 8) overlies the bladder (1) with the peritoneum of the vesico-uterine pouch (24) intervening. These relationships are seen in this MR image.

Cervical smear (Pap smear), cystitis (inflammation of the bladder), urinary continence, vaginal examination (PV), see pp 281, 283.

Female pelvis

A *uterus and ovaries, from above and in front*   **B** *hysterosalpingogram*

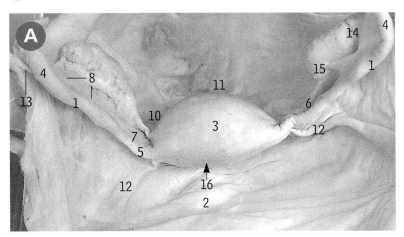

1	Ampulla of uterine tube	**10**	Posterior surface of broad ligament
2	Bladder	**11**	Recto-uterine pouch
3	Fundus of uterus	**12**	Round ligament of uterus
4	Infundibulum of uterine tube	**13**	Suspensory ligament of ovary with ovarian vessels
5	Isthmus of uterine tube	**14**	Tubal extremity of ovary
6	Ligament of ovary	**15**	Uterine extremity of ovary
7	Mesosalpinx	**16**	Vesico-uterine pouch
8	Mesovarium		
9	Overspill of contrast into recto-uterine pouch		

Looking down into the pelvis from the front in A, the fundus of the uterus (3) overlies the bladder (2) with the peritoneum of the vesico-uterine pouch (16) intervening. In B, contrast medium has filled the uterus and tubes (3, 5, 1 and 4) and spilled out into the peritoneal cavity (9).

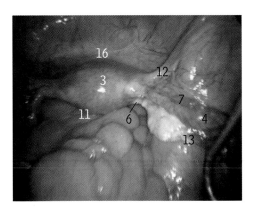

Laparoscopic view of female pelvis

Carcinoma of the ovary, ectopic pregnancy rupture, intrauterine contraceptive devices (IUCD), see pp 281, 282.

Female pelvis *left half, obliquely from the front*

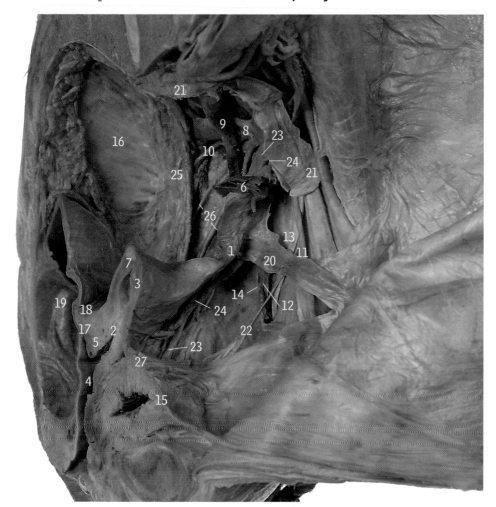

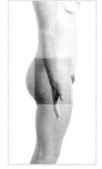

1 Ampulla of uterine tube
2 Anterior fornix of vagina
3 Body of uterus
4 Cavity of vagina
5 Cervix of uterus
6 Fimbriated end of uterine tube
7 Fundus of uterus
8 Internal iliac artery
9 Internal iliac vein
10 Middle rectal artery
11 Obliterated umbilical artery
12 Obturator artery
13 Obturator nerve
14 Obturator vein
15 Peritoneum overlying bladder
16 Peritoneum overlying piriformis
17 Posterior fornix of vagina
18 Recto-uterine pouch (of Douglas)
19 Rectum
20 Round ligament of uterus
21 Sigmoid mesocolon
22 Superior vesical artery
23 Ureter
24 Uterine artery
25 Uterosacral ligament
26 Vaginal artery (double)
27 Vesico-uterine pouch

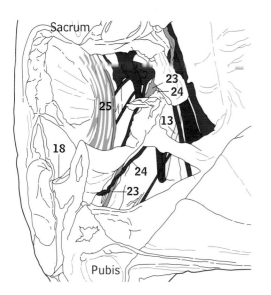

Looking obliquely into the left half of the pelvis from the front, with the anterior abdominal wall turned forwards, the peritoneum of the vesico-uterine pouch (27) has been incised and the uterus (3) displaced backwards. This shows the ureter (23) running towards the bladder and being crossed by the uterine artery (24). The uterosacral ligament (25) passes backwards at the side of the rectum (19) towards the pelvic surface of the sacrum. The root of the sigmoid mesocolon (21) has been left in place to emphasize that the left ureter (23) passes from the abdomen into the pelvis beneath it.

 Anal and rectal abscesses, carcinoma of the uterus, supports of pelvic viscera, see pp 281, 283.

Female perineum Ⓐ *surface features*
Ⓑ *left ischio-anal fossa, from below* Ⓒ *left ischio-anal fossa, from behind*

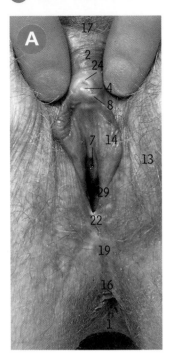

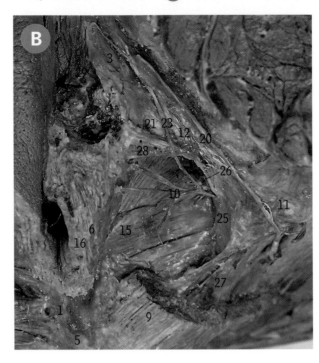

1 Anococcygeal body
2 Anterior commissure
3 Bulbospongiosus overlying bulb of vestibule
4 Clitoris
5 Coccyx
6 External anal sphincter
7 External urethral orifice
8 Frenulum of clitoris
9 Gluteus maximus
10 Inferior rectal nerve
11 Ischial tuberosity
12 Ischiocavernosus overlying crus of clitoris
13 Labium majus
14 Labium minus
15 Levator ani
16 Margin of anus
17 Mons pubis
18 Obturator internus and fascia
19 Perineal body
20 Perineal branch of posterior femoral cutaneous nerve
21 Perineal membrane
22 Posterior commissure
23 Posterior labial nerve
24 Prepuce of clitoris
25 Pudendal canal
26 Pudendal nerve
27 Sacrotuberous ligament
28 Superficial transverse perineal muscle overlying posterior border of perineal membrane
29 Vagina

In A the labia minora (14) have been separated to show the orifice of the vagina (29) with the urethra (7) opening into the vestibule anteriorly, 2.5 cm (1 in) behind the clitoris (4). In B and C fat and vessels have been removed from the ischio-anal fossa to show the pudendal canal (25) in the lateral wall, with levator ani (15) sloping downwards and medially to the external anal sphincter (6). The inferior rectal nerve (10) leaves the pudendal nerve (26) by piercing the wall of the pudendal canal (25) and crosses the fossa to reach the external anal sphincter (6).

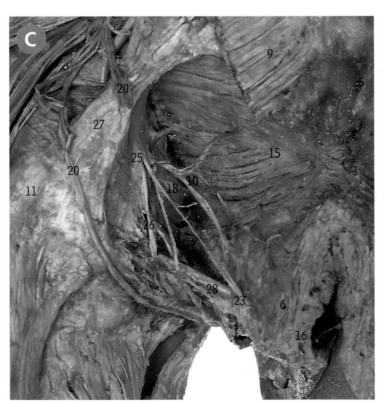

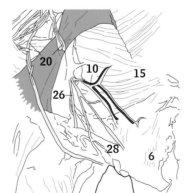

The ischiorectal fossa is now properly and more correctly called the ischio-anal fossa; the anal canal (B and C16), not the rectum, is its lower medial boundary. The walls and contents are similar in both sexes.

 Episiotomy, pudendal block, see pp 282, 283.

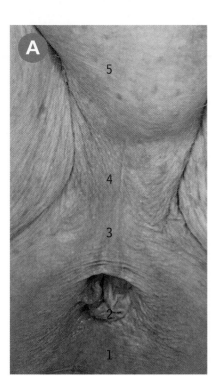

Ⓐ Male perineum

The central area is shown, with the scrotum (5) pulled upwards and forwards.

1 Anococcygeal body
2 Margin of anus, with skin tags
3 Perineal body
4 Raphe overlying bulb of penis
5 Scrotum overlying left testis

> Skin tags are often the remnants of previous haemorrhoids.

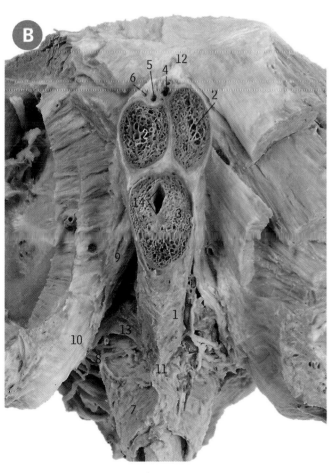

Ⓑ Root of the penis
from below and in front

The front part of the penis has been removed to show the root, formed by the two corpora cavernosa dorsally (2) and the single corpus spongiosum ventrally (3) containing the urethra (14).

1 Bulbospongiosus
2 Corpus cavernosum
3 Corpus spongiosum
4 Deep dorsal vein of penis
5 Dorsal artery of penis
6 Dorsal nerve of penis
7 External anal sphincter
8 Inferior rectal vessels and nerve crossing ischio-anal fossa
9 Ischiocavernosus
10 Ischiopubic ramus
11 Perineal body
12 Pubic symphysis
13 Superficial transverse perineal muscle overlying perineal membrane
14 Urethra

Chordee of the penis, haemorrhoids, hypospadias, priapism, see pp 281, 282, 283.

Male perineum and ischio-anal (ischiorectal) fossae

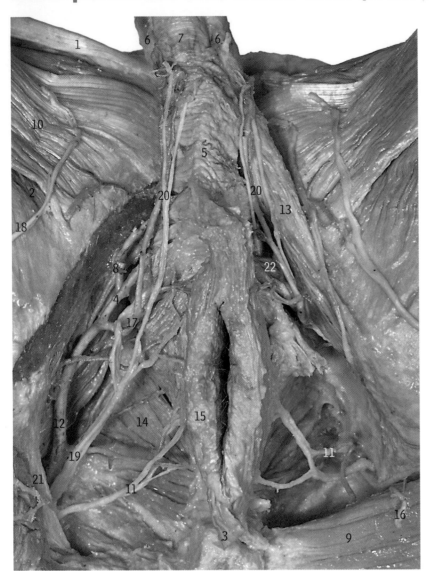

All the fat has been removed from the ischio-anal fossae so that a clear view is obtained of the perineal surface of levator ani (14) and of the vessels and nerves within the fossae. On the left side (right of the picture) the perineal membrane (22) is intact but on the right side it, and the underlying muscle (urogenital diaphragm), have been removed.

1 Adductor longus
2 Adductor magnus
3 Anococcygeal body
4 Artery to bulb
5 Bulbospongiosus overlying bulb of penis
6 Corpus cavernosum of penis
7 Corpus spongiosum of penis
8 Dorsal nerve and artery of penis
9 Gluteus maximus
10 Gracilis
11 Inferior rectal vessels and nerve in ischio-anal fossa
12 Internal pudendal artery
13 Ischiocavernosus overlying crus of penis
14 Levator ani
15 Margin of anus
16 Perforating cutaneous nerve
17 Perineal artery
18 Perineal branch of posterior femoral cutaneous nerve
19 Perineal nerve
20 Posterior scrotal vessels and nerves
21 Sacrotuberous ligament
22 Superficial transverse perineal muscle overlying posterior border of perineal membrane

In both sexes the ischio-anal (ischiorectal) fossa has the pudendal canal in its lateral wall. The canal has been opened up to display its contents: the internal pudendal artery (12) and the terminal branches of the pudendal nerve – the perineal nerve (19) and the dorsal nerve of the penis (8) or clitoris.

Ejaculation, erection, see p. 282.

Abdomen and pelvis
Clinical notes

Abdominal aortic aneurysm. This ballooning of the lower abdominal aorta may extend distally to involve both external iliac arteries and proximally as far as the renal arteries causing renal insufficiency. Treatment is surgical replacement of this section of the aorta with a graft or stent. (page 259)

Abdominal paracentesis is a procedure that drains fluid (ascites) from the abdomen through a cannula inserted through the anterior abdominal wall lateral to the rectus sheath to avoid injury to the epigastric vessels. (page 221)

Anal and rectal abscesses can drain centrally into the lumen or laterally into the ischio-anal fossae (below the level of the levator ani muscle) or pelvis (above this muscle). Successful treatment requires an understanding of these anatomical relationships. (page 277)

Appendicitis. Classically this condition starts as a para-umbilical pain (visceral peritoneum of midgut) which then moves to the region of McBurney's point in the right iliac fossa owing to parietal peritoneal irritation. (page 252)

Aortic bruits are audible rhythmic sounds on auscultation of the abdomen, often due to atherosclerotic narrowing (stenosis) of the aorta. (page 254)

Ascites is the accumulation of fluid within the peritoneal cavity due to a variety of causes, including malignancy, inflammation and portal hypertension. (page 234)

Benign prostatic hyperplasia. In most males over the age of 60 this is a common occurrence and is normally diagnosed on a rectal examination where prostate enlargement can be felt easily. The patient usually complains of getting up at night to pass urine, difficulty in voiding and is unable to empty the bladder. It is the commonest cause of bladder outflow obstruction. (page 271)

Bowel ischaemia. Areas of bowel predisposed to this condition are the 'watershed area' between the superior and inferior mesenteric arterial supply and, following a twisting (volvulus) of the bowel, in the sigmoid colon. (page 240)

Caput medusae. Dilated para-umbilical veins resembling the hair of Medusa of Greek mythology, are often a clinical sign of cirrhosis. (page 227)

Carcinoma of the ovary. The ovary drains to the para-aortic lymph nodes and although carcinoma of the ovary is rare in the young, it is a common cause of peritoneal metastases in older women. (page 276)

Carcinoma of the pancreas. Occurring most commonly at the head of the pancreas, this is an important cause of extrahepatic obstruction of the biliary tree, resulting in jaundice. (page 237)

Carcinoma of the prostate. This common condition in men over the age of 70 is usually diagnosed on a rectal examination by the absence of a median prostatic sulcus and a hard palpable mass. Further spread from within the pelvis is often via the vertebral venous plexus and metastases to bone are common. (page 271)

Carcinoma of the rectum. Carcinomata at the lower end of the hindgut tend to present relatively early, owing to a change in bowel habit, a sensation of incomplete evacuation or rectal bleeding. Surgical treatments (anterior resection and abdominoperineal excision) tend to have a good prognosis. (page 270)

Carcinoma of the uterus. Found normally in the elderly, often in those who have not had children; this condition may spread within the pelvis or, very occasionally, to the superficial inguinal lymph nodes along the round ligament of the uterus which is carrying its accompanying lymphatics. (page 277)

Cervical smear (Pap smear). Named after Dr George N. Papanicolaou, who developed it, this is a simple test to examine epithelial cells from the uterine cervix. Cells are removed by gently scraping, placing on a slide and examining microscopically for abnormalities of shape and size, to detect early uterine/cervical cancer. (page 275)

Cholecystectomy. Surgical removal of the gall bladder was classically performed by Kocher's incision parallel to the right costal margin but is now commonly performed laparoscopically. (page 231)

Cholecystitis is acute inflammation of the gall bladder most commonly associated with stones in the biliary system. Pain occurs over the right hypochondrial region near the tip of the ninth rib and the linea semilunaris. (page 248)

Chordee of the penis is an abnormal downwards bend in the erect penis, often associated with hypospadias. (page 279)

Colostomy is the creation of a temporary or permanent exit (stoma) for the colon through the anterior abdominal wall, and is commonly performed following a left colectomy or an abdominoperineal excision of the rectum. Faeces are collected in a disposable bag stuck to the anterior abdominal wall. (page 241)

Cremasteric reflex tests nerve roots L1 and L2 in males and involves contraction of the cremaster muscle raising the testis after stroking the ipsilateral, medial thigh. (page 266)

Cystitis (inflammation of the bladder) often presents as pain on passing urine. Owing to the shortness of the female urethra it is much more common in young girls and women than in men, as organisms can enter the bladder more easily. (page 275)

Cystoscopy is a transurethral examination of the inner lining of the bladder surface often using a (flexible) fibre-optic cystoscope. (page 270)

Direct inguinal hernia is a protrusion, often of peritoneum and bowel, through the anterior abdominal wall lying medial to the inferior epigastric vessels, in the inguinal (Hesselbach's) triangle. (page 228)

Drainage of peritoneal abscesses. Pus within the peritoneal cavity collects in supine individuals in one of the recesses or pouches within the peritoneal cavity. These include the subphrenic spaces, paracolic gutters and the recto-uterine pouch (of Douglas). Different drainage procedures are used for each space. (page 235)

Ectopic pregnancy rupture occurs most commonly about 6–8 weeks after conception and is an acute medical emergency normally presenting as vaginal bleeding and acute abdominal pain due to rupture of the uterine tube and bleeding into the peritoneal cavity. Occasionally, this may present as shoulder pain from diaphragmatic irritation, an excellent example of referred pain. (page 276)

Ejaculation. The expulsion of semen through the urethra is the result of at least three mechanisms: closure of the bladder neck; contraction of the urethral musculature (sympathetic control); and contraction of the bulbospongiosus muscle (pudendal nerve). A major factor is the sympathetic supply from L1 and L2. (page 280)

Episiotomy is a small incision in the posterolateral vaginal wall, performed in the final stages of childbirth to enlarge the vaginal canal. It is usually performed after a pudendal nerve block has anaesthetized the S2, 3 and 4 dermatomes – the skin of that region. This procedure minimizes labour-induced lacerations in the midline that may damage the central tendon of the perineum or extend into the rectal mucosa. (page 278)

Erection. When stimulated, the pelvic parasympathetics S2–S4 cause relaxation of the coiled arteries of the penis and clitoris and engorgement of the cavernous spaces. The bulbospongiosus and ischiocavernosus muscles compress the venous caverns of these spaces and impede the venous return, causing erection. (page 280)

Extravasation of urine. If the urethra is damaged only in its membranous part, urine will drain into the urogenital diaphragm and into the pelvis extraperitoneally. Much more commonly, the damage and leakage is from the spongy, penile urethra. In this situation the urine first fills up the superficial perineal pouch and then continues up the anterior abdominal wall, because this fascial layer is continuous with the superficial perineal membrane. Urine does not track down the thighs because the superficial abdominal fascia is fused with the deep fascia (lata) of the thigh just below the inguinal ligament. (page 268)

Faecal continence is dependent on a complex mechanism involving both the internal and external anal sphincters and the anorectal angle, maintained by the puborectalis fibres of the levator ani muscle. This angle is normally about 90°; if it is altered to over 100°, incontinence ensues. (page 274)

Haematoma of the rectus sheath. Direct trauma to the anterior abdominal wall or a violent forced expiratory effort, such as at childbirth, may cause tearing of the inferior or superior epigastric vessels, extravasating blood into one or both sheaths of the rectus abdominis muscles. (page 222)

Haemorrhoids (dilatations of the veins in the lower rectum and upper anal regions) are varicosities of the superior rectal veins which may protrude through the external anal sphincter or into the rectum. Haemorrhoids are a common cause of bleeding on defaecation. (pages 274, 279)

Hernia repair. In the inguinal region, the most common area for herniae, manufactured fibres are often used to patch over large hernia openings. The pectineal and lacunar ligaments are often used as anchor points for sutures. (page 225)

Hiatus hernia. Commonly of two varieties, sliding or rolling, these herniae are protrusions of the proximal stomach into the thorax and often produce a burning sensation in the midsternal region. (pages 243, 261)

Hydrocele is an accumulation of fluid around the testis between the parietal and visceral layers of the tunica vaginalis. (page 266)

Hypospadias is a developmental abnormality of the penis in which the external urethral opening appears somewhere along its ventral surface. (page 279)

Indirect inguinal hernia is a protrusion that follows the course of the vas deferens or round ligament. The neck of the hernia lies in the deep inguinal ring lateral to the inferior epigastric vessels. (page 228)

Intrauterine contraceptive devices (IUCDs) are small plastic or metal tubes inserted into the uterine cavity which prevent implantation of fertilized eggs. (page 276)

Laparoscopy is a technique of minimal invasive surgery to examine, remove or repair abdominal or pelvic organs/tissue using small tubes inserted through the abdominal wall. (page 231)

Liver abscess. In tropical countries these are often very large and due to amoebic disease. In other areas they are more commonly related to malignancy. (page 246)

Liver biopsy. Liver tissue samples can be obtained using a needle passed through the ninth or tenth right intercostal space in the axillary line during full expiration to reduce the size of the costodiaphragmatic recess and the risk of pneumothorax. (page 230)

Lumbar sympathectomy is selective transection of the sympathetic trunk to reduce vasoconstriction in the lower limbs, for patients with poor circulation. Usually performed at the L2 level, it is easier to perform on the left than the right, where the inferior vena cava is immediately anterior. (page 263)

McBurney's point (11) is a site on the surface of the anterior abdominal wall indicating the usual location of the base of the appendix internally. It lies one-third of the way along a line from the right anterior superior iliac spine to the umbilicus. (page 226)

Nephrectomy is the surgical removal of a kidney (for malignancy, stones etc.) and takes advantage of the renal fasciae for access to, and closure of, the site. (page 258)

Oesophageal varices are dilatations of left gastric vein tributaries that can cause serious bleeding (haematemesis). (page 242)

Peritoneal dialysis. The peritoneum, being a semipermeable membrane, can be used for dialysis in renal disease. Fluid is introduced into the peritoneal cavity, allowed to mix with the contents and then withdrawn, removing with it most circulating toxins. This procedure, frequently repeated, can be a satisfactory way of controlling uraemia. (page 232)

Peritoneal lavage. A procedure that washes peritoneal surfaces by inserting and removing fluid from the abdominal cavity, it is most commonly used to clean infection, or as peritoneal dialysis for renal disease. Diagnostic peritoneal lavage can be performed in cases of abdominal trauma to detect intraperitoneal bleeding. (page 232)

Peritoneal pain. The visceral peritoneum is sensitive only to stretch and pressure and these are experienced as a dull ache. The parietal peritoneum, however, is sensitive to pain and is innervated by the spinal nerves. (page 227)

Portocaval shunt. Portal vein obstruction from any cause produces varices at sites of portosystemic venous anastomoses. Direct anastomotic connection of parts of the portal vein into the inferior vena cava reduces portal hypertension and some of the potential consequences of varicosities. (page 237)

Portosystemic anastomoses are connections between the portal venous and systemic venous systems which become clinically important when the portal vein is blocked; they are most commonly seen with liver disease. Varicosities develop in anastomotic regions, especially the oesophagus, anus and bare area of the liver. (page 246)

Priapism is a permanent painful erection, often due to thrombosis within the cavernous tissue of the penis. (page 279)

Psoas sign. The psoas major muscle passes from the posterior abdominal wall to the lesser trochanter of the femur. Infections or haemorrhage of the posterior vertebral column (i.e. tuberculosis) drain laterally into the psoas, allowing pus to travel down the muscle and present as a swelling in the groin below the inguinal ligament. (page 262)

Pudendal block produces anaesthesia of the perineum by injecting an anaesthetic agent around the ischial spine and thus affecting the pudendal nerve (S2, 3 and 4) as it travels over this structure. (page 278)

Rectal examination (PR). Examination per rectum is obviously different in male and female patients. The major structures palpable in the male are the median sulcus of the prostate gland, the sacral concavity and coccyx, and in the female the sacrum, coccyx and cervix. This examination may

be used during labour as a way of assessing the dilatation of the cervix, and in acute appendicitis a tender pelvic appendix may be reached by the examining finger. (page 274)

Renal biopsy is a procedure that is best performed only at the lower pole of the kidney because upper pole biopsies may damage the pleura (an immediate posterior relation of the upper part of the kidney) and cause a pneumothorax. (page 260)

Rupture of the liver, commonly caused by trauma, may require removal of a hepatic segment to control bleeding. (page 245)

Sigmoidoscopy. Direct visualization of the internal surfaces of the anus (proctoscopy), rectum and sigmoid colon (sigmoidoscopy) using a sigmoidoscope. (page 268)

Splenectomy. Removal of the spleen may be indicated following trauma or in cases of certain blood disorders and is easily accomplished after clamping its pedicle, taking care not to cut through the tail of the pancreas, which lies across the hilum of the spleen. (page 250)

Splenomegaly. The most common causes of splenic enlargement are tropical diseases and blood diseases such as haemolytic anaemias. The normal spleen is the size of a clenched fist and is not palpable below the left costal margin. (page 250)

Superior mesenteric artery syndrome causes increased pressure in the left renal vein and potentially renal disease by reducing the lumen of this vein as it is sandwiched between the aorta and the superior mesenteric artery (nutcracker effect). (page 258)

Supports of pelvic viscera. Pelvic structures are supported by various parts of the levator ani, sphincter urethrae, sphincter vaginae and puborectalis muscles and the ligamentous supports of the uterus and vagina. (page 277)

Transurethral resection of prostate (TURP) is basically a 'coring out' operation of the hypertrophied prostate which has caused obstruction of urine flow. Care has to be taken not to damage the distal urethral sphincter mechanism. (page 271)

Umbilical hernia is an anterior abdominal hernia at the umbilicus which is often congenital and frequently disappears by the second or third year. (page 227)

Ureteric calculi. Stones within the ureter descend from the kidney towards the bladder and may lodge at the pelvi-ureteric junction, the brim of the pelvis, or at the entrance to the bladder where the ureter traverses the bladder wall, causing excruciating pain. (page 259)

Urinary continence has a complex, poorly understood mechanism involving both the bladder neck and the distal urethral mechanism, which includes the sphincter urethrae. The major control is by the pelvic splanchnic nerves, which are motor to the detrusor muscle and inhibitory to the internal sphincter. When these fibres are stimulated by a full bladder, the bladder contracts, the sphincter relaxes and urine flows into the urethra. (page 275)

Vaginal examination (PV). Often performed in the lithotomy position and preceded by a speculum examination, PV examination is used to assess the state of the cervix, uterus and ovaries. This examination combined with a hand on the abdominal wall (bimanual examination) reveals that the normal uterus is in an anteverted and anteflexed position; however, approximately one-fifth of normal women have a retroverted or retroflexed uterus. The non-pregnant cervix feels firm, like the end of the nose: the pregnant cervix feels warm and softer, rather like warm lips. When feeling the lateral fornices, occasionally one can detect an ovary, or (theoretically) a stone in the ureter. (page 275)

Vagotomy is surgical interruption of the vagus nerve performed selectively to reduce acid secretion in the stomach and relieve peptic ulceration. It has been superseded by pharmacological intervention. (page 242)

Varicoceles are enlarged varicose gonadal veins (pampiniform plexus of either the ovary or testis). (page 266)

Vasectomy is a surgical procedure that aims to produce infertility in males by removal of a section of the ductus deferens between sutured/clipped ends. (page 266)

Volvulus, twisting of the bowel on its mesentery, causes ischaemia of the rotated section. It is most commonly seen in the sigmoid colon in those on a high fibre diet, especially in Africa where this condition replaces the acute appendix as the commonest cause of an 'acute abdomen'. (page 235)

Lower limb

Lower limb Ⓐ *surface anatomy, from the front*
Ⓑ *dissection, from the front* Ⓒ *dissection, from behind*
Ⓓ *dissection, from the lateral side* Ⓔ *skeleton, from the lateral side*

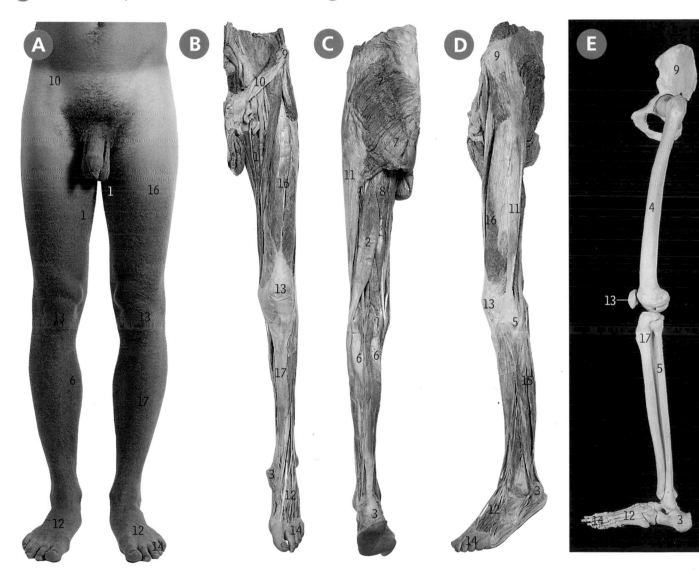

1 Adductors	**5** Fibula	**9** Hip bone	**12** Metatarsal bones	**15** Peroneus (fibularis)
2 Biceps femoris	**6** Gastrocnemius	**10** Inguinal ligament	**13** Patella	**16** Quadriceps
3 Calcaneus	**7** Gluteus maximus	**11** Iliotibial tract	**14** Phalanges of toes	**17** Tibia
4 Femur	**8** Hamstrings			

Left hip bone *lateral surface*

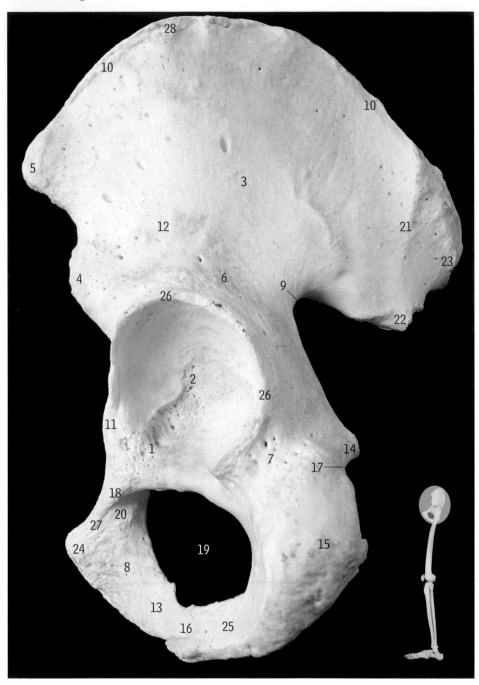

1   Acetabular notch
2   Acetabulum
3   Anterior gluteal line
4   Anterior inferior iliac spine
5   Anterior superior iliac spine
6   Body of ilium
7   Body of ischium
8   Body of pubis
9   Greater sciatic notch
10 Iliac crest
11 Iliopubic eminence
12 Inferior gluteal line
13 Inferior ramus of pubis
14 Ischial spine
15 Ischial tuberosity
16 Junction of 25 and 13
17 Lesser sciatic notch
18 Obturator crest
19 Obturator foramen
20 Obturator groove
21 Posterior gluteal line
22 Posterior inferior iliac spine
23 Posterior superior iliac spine
24 Pubic tubercle
25 Ramus of ischium
26 Rim of acetabulum
27 Superior ramus of pubis
28 Tubercle of iliac crest

The hip (innominate) bone is formed by the union of the ilium (6), ischium (7) and pubis (8).

The two hip bones articulate in the midline anteriorly at the pubic symphysis; posteriorly they are separated by the sacrum, forming the sacro-iliac joints. The two hip bones with the sacrum and coccyx constitute the pelvis (see page 102).

Left hip bone *attachments, lateral surface*

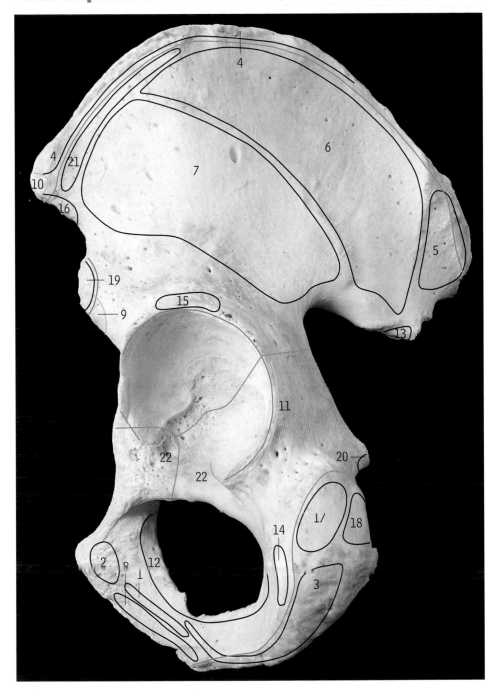

Blue lines = epiphysial lines; green lines = capsular attachment of hip joint; pale green lines = ligament attachments

1 Adductor brevis
2 Adductor longus
3 Adductor magnus
4 External oblique
5 Gluteus maximus
6 Gluteus medius
7 Gluteus minimus
8 Gracilis
9 Iliofemoral ligament
10 Inguinal ligament
11 Ischiofemoral ligament
12 Obturator externus
13 Piriformis
14 Quadratus femoris
15 Reflected head of rectus femoris
16 Sartorius
17 Semimembranosus
18 Semitendinosus and long head of biceps
19 Straight head of rectus femoris
20 Superior gemellus
21 Tensor fasciae latae
22 Transverse ligament

Left hip bone *medial surface*

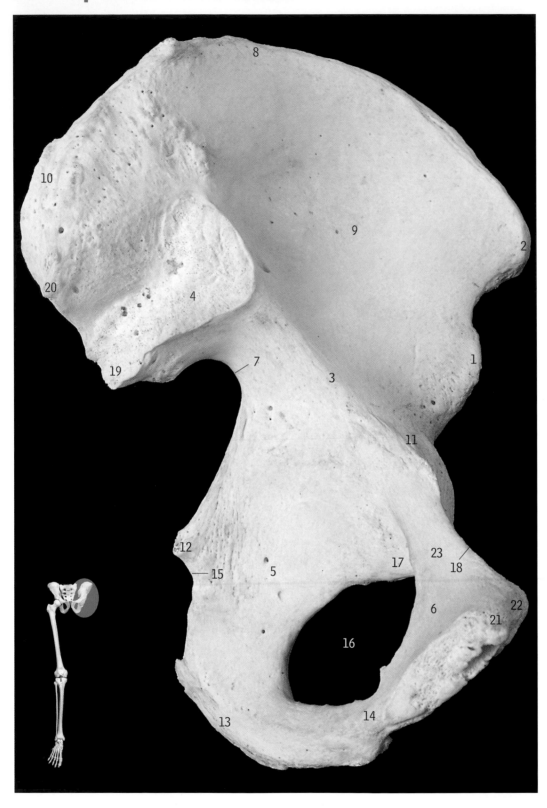

1 Anterior inferior iliac spine
2 Anterior superior iliac spine
3 Arcuate line
4 Auricular surface
5 Body of ischium
6 Body of pubis
7 Greater sciatic notch
8 Iliac crest
9 Iliac fossa
10 Iliac tuberosity
11 Iliopubic eminence
12 Ischial spine
13 Ischial tuberosity
14 Ischiopubic ramus
15 Lesser sciatic notch
16 Obturator foramen
17 Obturator groove
18 Pecten of pubis
   (pectineal line)
19 Posterior inferior iliac spine
20 Posterior superior iliac spine
21 Pubic crest
22 Pubic tubercle
23 Superior ramus of pubis

The auricular surface of
the ilium (4) is the articular
surface for the sacro-iliac
joint.

The greater sciatic notch (7)
is more hooked (J-shaped)
in the male, whereas the
female notch is more
right-angled (L-shaped).

Left hip bone *attachments, medial surface*

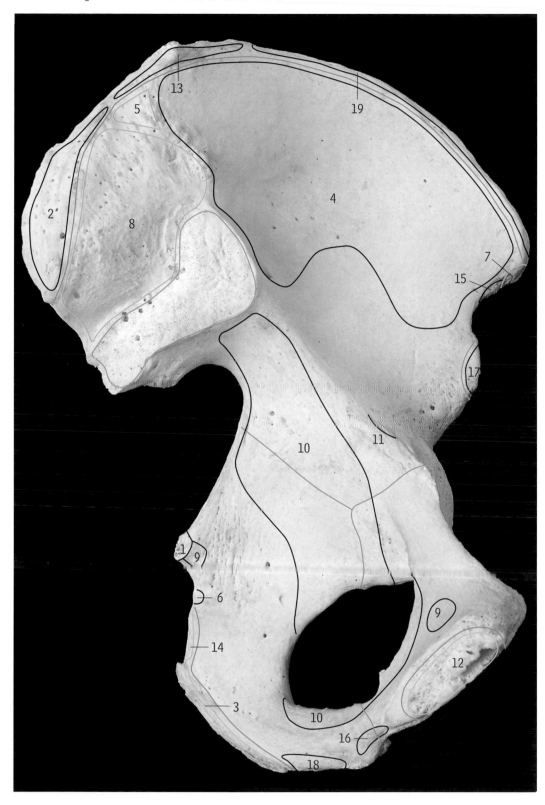

Blue lines = epiphysial lines; green line = capsular attachment of sacro-iliac joint; pale green lines = ligament attachments

1 Coccygeus and sacrospinous ligament
2 Erector spinae
3 Falciform process of sacrotuberous ligament
4 Iliacus
5 Iliolumbar ligament
6 Inferior gemellus
7 Inguinal ligament
8 Interosseous sacro-iliac ligament
9 Levator ani
10 Obturator internus
11 Psoas minor
12 Pubic symphysis
13 Quadratus lumborum
14 Sacrotuberous ligament
15 Sartorius
16 Sphincter urethrae
17 Straight head of rectus femoris
18 Superficial transverse perineal and ischiocavernosus
19 Transversus abdominis

Left hip bone *from above*

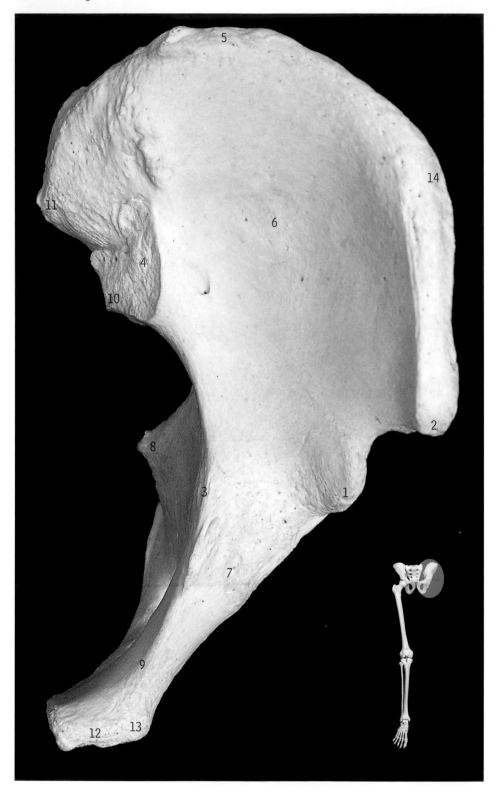

1 Anterior inferior iliac spine
2 Anterior superior iliac spine
3 Arcuate line
4 Auricular surface
5 Iliac crest
6 Iliac fossa
7 Iliopubic eminence
8 Ischial spine
9 Pecten of pubis (pectineal line)
10 Posterior inferior iliac spine
11 Posterior superior iliac spine
12 Pubic crest
13 Pubic tubercle
14 Tubercle of iliac crest

The arcuate line on the ilium (3) and the pecten and crest of the pubis (9 and 12) form part of the brim of the pelvis (the rest of the brim being formed by the promontory and upper surface of the lateral part of the sacrum – see pages 100 and 102).

The pecten of the pubis (9) is more commonly called the pectineal line.

Left hip bone *attachments, from above*

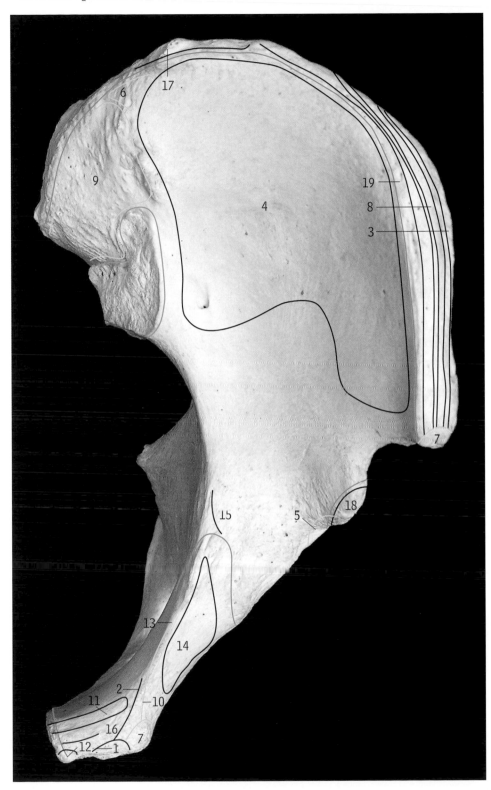

1 Anterior wall of rectus sheath
2 Conjoint tendon
3 External oblique
4 Iliacus
5 Iliofemoral ligament
6 Iliolumbar ligament
7 Inguinal ligament
8 Internal oblique
9 Interosseous sacro-iliac ligament
10 Lacunar ligament
11 Lateral head of rectus abdominis
12 Medial head of rectus abdominis
13 Pectineal ligament
14 Pectineus
15 Psoas minor
16 Pyramidalis
17 Quadratus lumborum
18 Straight head of rectus femoris
19 Transversus abdominis

The inguinal ligament (7) is formed by the lower border of the aponeurosis of the external oblique muscle, and extends from the anterior superior iliac spine to the pubic tubercle.

The lacunar ligament (10, sometimes called the pectineal part of the inguinal ligament) is the part of the inguinal ligament that extends backwards from the medial end of the inguinal ligament to the pecten of the pubis.

The pectineal ligament (13) is the lateral extension of the lacunar ligament along the pecten. It is not classified as a part of the inguinal ligament, and must not be confused with the alternative name for the lacunar ligament, i.e. with the pectineal part of the inguinal ligament.

The conjoint tendon (2) is formed by the aponeuroses of the internal oblique and transversus muscles, and is attached to the pubic crest and the adjoining part of the pecten, blending medially with the anterior wall of the rectus sheath.

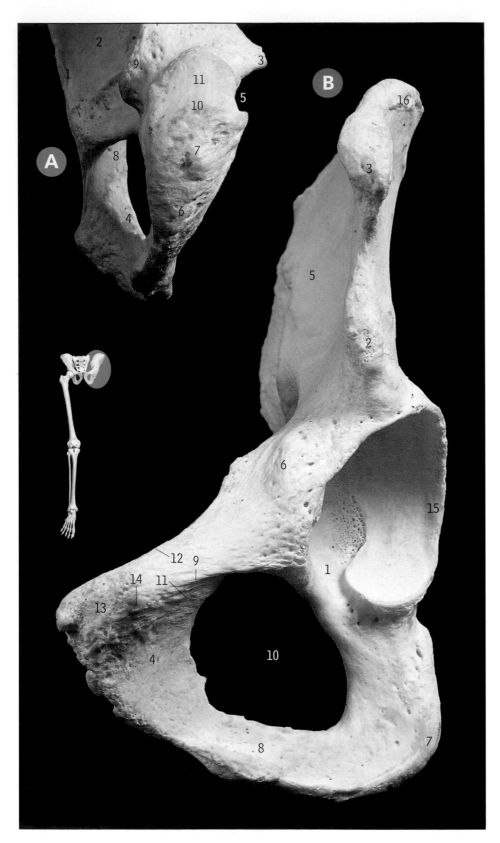

Left hip bone
ischial tuberosity,
from behind and below

1   Acetabular notch
2   Acetabulum
3   Ischial spine
4   Ischiopubic ramus
5   Lesser sciatic notch
6   Longitudinal ridge
7   Lower part of tuberosity
8   Obturator groove
9   Rim of acetabulum
10 Transverse ridge
11 Upper part of tuberosity

Ⓑ **Left hip bone**
from the front

1   Acetabular notch
2   Anterior inferior iliac spine
3   Anterior superior iliac spine
4   Body of pubis
5   Iliac fossa
6   Iliopubic eminence
7   Ischial tuberosity
8   Ischiopubic ramus
9   Obturator crest
10 Obturator foramen
11 Obturator groove
12 Pecten of pubis (pectineal line)
13 Pubic crest
14 Pubic tubercle
15 Rim of acetabulum
16 Tubercle of iliac crest

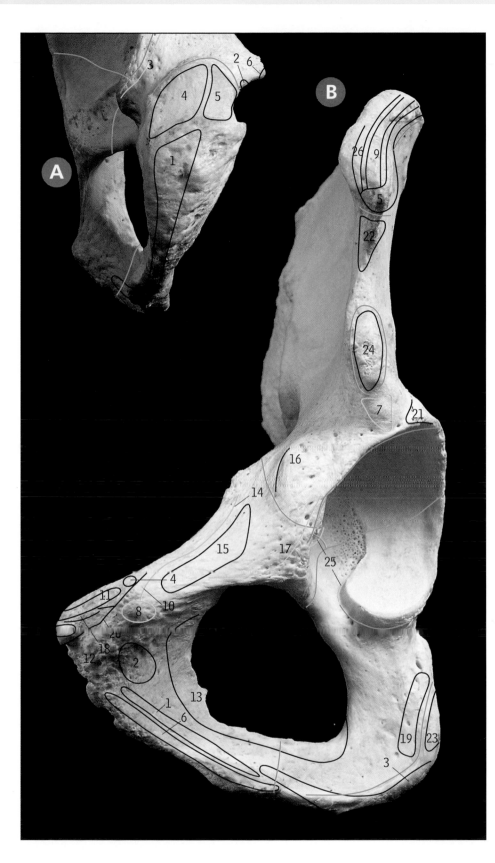

ⓐ Left hip bone
*attachments,
ischial tuberosity,
from behind and below*

Blue lines = epiphysial lines; green line = capsular attachment of hip joint; pale green lines = ligament attachments

1   Adductor magnus
2   Inferior gemellus
3   Ischiofemoral ligament
4   Semimembranosus
5   Semitendinosus and long head of biceps
6   Superior gemellus

> The area on the ischial tuberosity medial to the adductor magnus attachment (1) is covered by fibrofatty tissue and the ischial bursa underlying gluteus maximus.

ⓑ Left hip bone
*attachments,
from the front*

Blue lines = epiphysial lines; green line = capsular attachment of hip joint; pale green lines = ligament attachments

1   Adductor brevis
2   Adductor longus
3   Adductor magnus
4   Conjoint tendon
5   External oblique and inguinal ligament
6   Gracilis
7   Iliofemoral ligament
8   Inguinal ligament
9   Internal oblique
10 Lacunar ligament
11 Lateral head of rectus abdominis
12 Medial head of rectus abdominis
13 Obturator externus
14 Pectineal ligament
15 Pectineus
16 Psoas minor
17 Pubofemoral ligament
18 Pyramidalis
19 Quadratus femoris
20 Rectus sheath
21 Reflected head of rectus femoris
22 Sartorius
23 Semimembranosus
24 Straight head of rectus femoris
25 Transverse ligament
26 Transversus abdominis

Left femur *upper end*

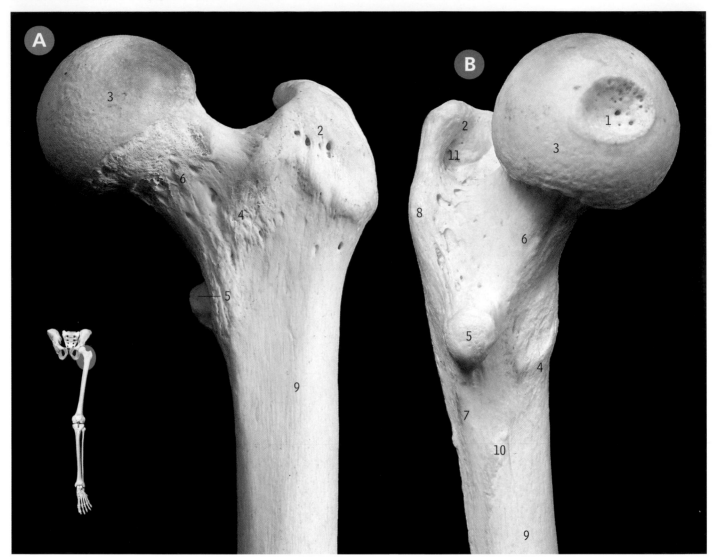

A   **from the front**

B   **from the medial side**

1   Fovea of head
2   Greater trochanter
3   Head
4   Intertrochanteric line
5   Lesser trochanter
6   Neck
7   Pectineal line
8   Quadrate tubercle on
     intertrochanteric crest
9   Shaft
10   Spiral line
11   Trochanteric fossa

The intertrochanteric *line* (4) is at the junction of the neck (6) and shaft (9) on the anterior surface; the intertrochanteric *crest* is in a similar position on the posterior surface (8, and page 296, A5).

The neck makes an angle with the shaft of about 125° in an adult.

The pectineal line of the femur (7) must not be confused with the pectineal line (pecten) of the pubis (page 290), nor with the spiral line of the femur (10) which is usually more prominent than the pectineal line.

Hip fractures, see p. 356.

Left femur *attachments, upper end*

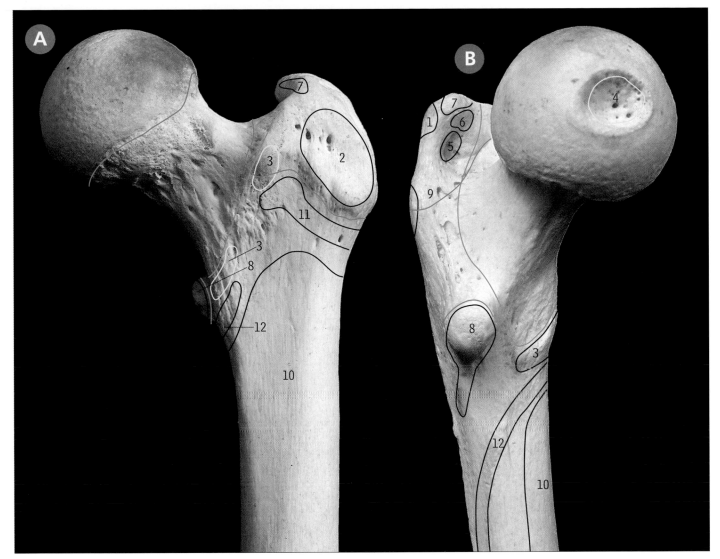

A **from the front**

B **from the medial side**

Blue lines = epiphysial lines;
green line = capsular
attachment of hip joint;
pale green lines = ligament
attachments

1 Gluteus medius
2 Gluteus minimus
3 Iliofemoral ligament
4 Ligament of head of femur
5 Obturator externus
6 Obturator internus and gemelli
7 Piriformis
8 Psoas major and iliacus
9 Quadratus femoris
10 Vastus intermedius
11 Vastus lateralis
12 Vastus medialis

The iliofemoral ligament has the shape of an inverted V, with the
stem attached to the anterior inferior iliac spine of the hip bone
(page 293, B7), and the lateral and medial bands attached to the
upper (lateral) and lower (medial) ends of the intertrochanteric
line (3), blending with the capsule of the hip joint.

The tendon of psoas major is attached to the lesser trochanter (8);
many of the muscle fibres of iliacus are inserted into the psoas
tendon but some reach the femur below the trochanter.

Intertrochanteric fracture of the femur, see p. 356.

Left femur *upper end*

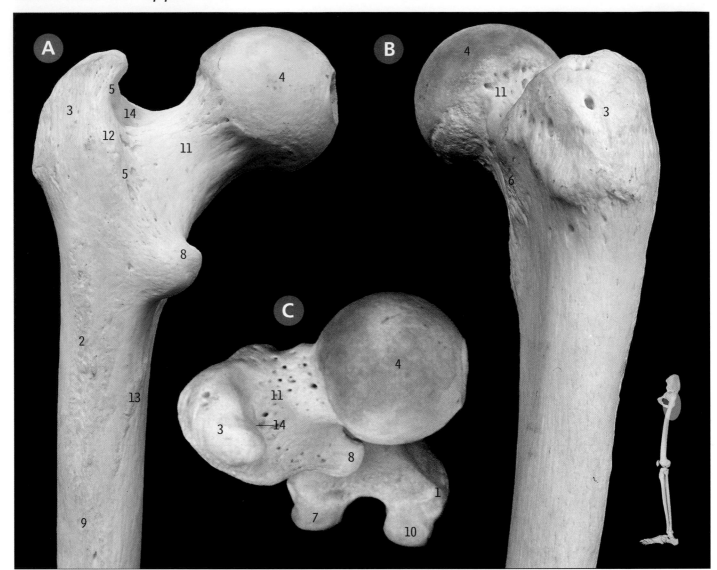

A from behind

B from the lateral side

C from above

1	Adductor tubercle at lower end
2	Gluteal tuberosity
3	Greater trochanter
4	Head
5	Intertrochanteric crest
6	Intertrochanteric line
7	Lateral condyle at lower end
8	Lesser trochanter
9	Linea aspera
10	Medial condyle at lower end
11	Neck
12	Quadrate tubercle
13	Spiral line
14	Trochanteric fossa

The neck of the femur passes forwards as well as upwards and medially (C11), making an angle of about 15° with the transverse axis of the lower end (the angle of femoral torsion).

The lesser trochanter (8) projects backwards and medially.

Subcapital fracture of the femoral neck, see p. 357.

Left femur *attachments, upper end*

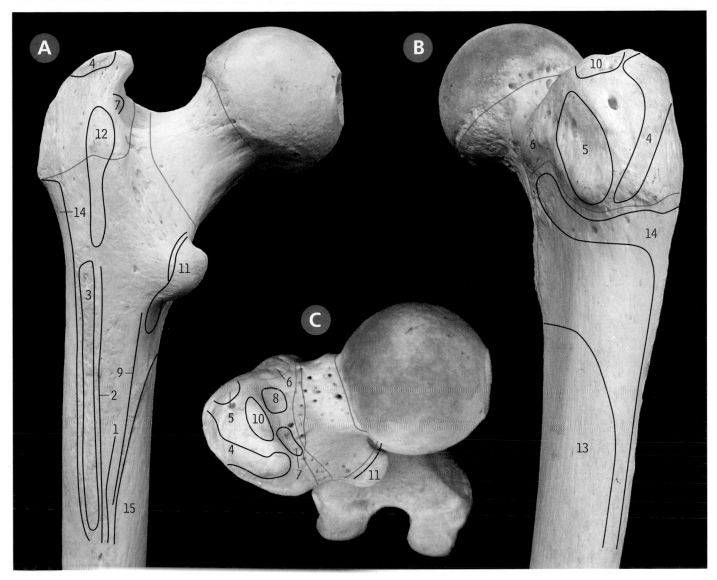

A from behind

B from the lateral side

C from above

Blue lines = epiphysial lines;
green line = capsular attachment
of hip joint; pale green lines =
ligament attachments

1 Adductor brevis
2 Adductor magnus
3 Gluteus maximus
4 Gluteus medius
5 Gluteus minimus
6 Iliofemoral ligament
  (lateral band)
7 Obturator externus
8 Obturator internus
  and gemelli

9 Pectineus
10 Piriformis
11 Psoas major and iliacus
12 Quadratus femoris
13 Vastus intermedius
14 Vastus lateralis
15 Vastus medialis

On the front of the femur
(page 295) the capsule of the
hip joint is attached to the
intertrochanteric line, but at
the back the capsule is attached
to the neck of the femur and
does not extend as far laterally
as the intertrochanteric crest
(page 296, A5).

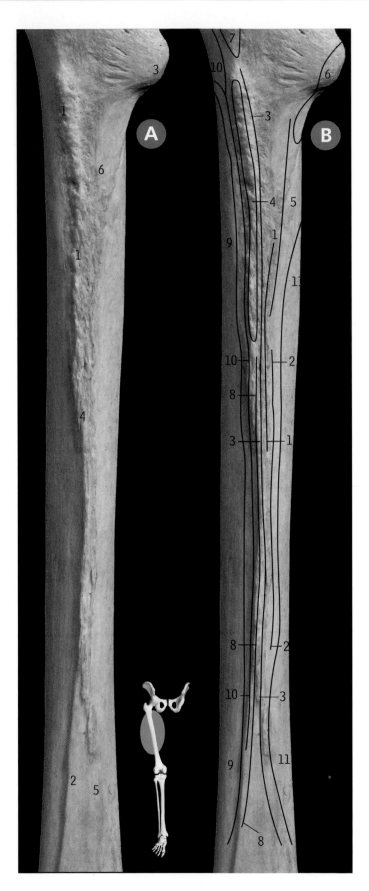

A Left femur *shaft, from behind*

1 Gluteal tuberosity
2 Lateral supracondylar line
3 Lesser trochanter
4 Linea aspera
5 Medial supracondylar line
6 Pectineal line

The rough linea aspera (4) often shows distinct medial and lateral lips; the lateral lip continues upwards as the gluteal tuberosity (1).

B Left femur

attachments, shaft, from behind

1 Adductor brevis
2 Adductor longus
3 Adductor magnus
4 Gluteus maximus
5 Pectineus
6 Psoas and iliacus
7 Quadratus femoris
8 Short head of biceps
9 Vastus intermedius
10 Vastus lateralis
11 Vastus medialis

For diagrammatic clarity the muscle attachments to the linea aspera have been slightly separated.

C Left femur

upper end, from the front

This is the posterior half of a cleared and bisected specimen, to show the major groups of bone trabeculae.

1 Calcar femorale
2 From lateral surface of shaft to greater trochanter
3 From lateral surface of shaft to head
4 From medial surface of shaft to greater trochanter
5 From medial surface of shaft to head
6 Triangular area of few trabeculae

The calcar femorale (1) is a dense concentration of trabeculae passing from the region of the lesser trochanter to the under-surface of the neck.

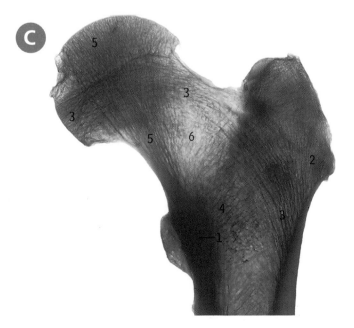

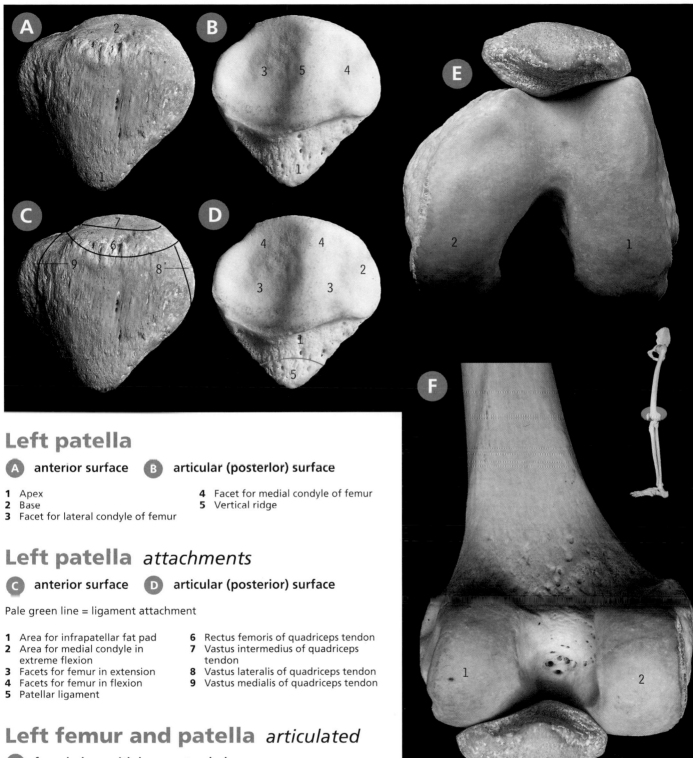

Left patella

A anterior surface   **B** articular (posterior) surface

1 Apex
2 Base
3 Facet for lateral condyle of femur
4 Facet for medial condyle of femur
5 Vertical ridge

Left patella *attachments*

C anterior surface   **D** articular (posterior) surface

Pale green line = ligament attachment

1 Area for infrapatellar fat pad
2 Area for medial condyle in extreme flexion
3 Facets for femur in extension
4 Facets for femur in flexion
5 Patellar ligament
6 Rectus femoris of quadriceps tendon
7 Vastus intermedius of quadriceps tendon
8 Vastus lateralis of quadriceps tendon
9 Vastus medialis of quadriceps tendon

Left femur and patella *articulated*

E from below with knee extended

F from below and behind with knee flexed

In flexion note the increased area of contact between the medial condyle of the femur (2) and the patella.

1 Lateral condyle   **2** Medial condyle

The most medial facet of the patella (D2) only comes into contact with the medial condyle in extreme flexion as in F.

 Dislocation of the patella, see p. 355.

Left femur *lower end*

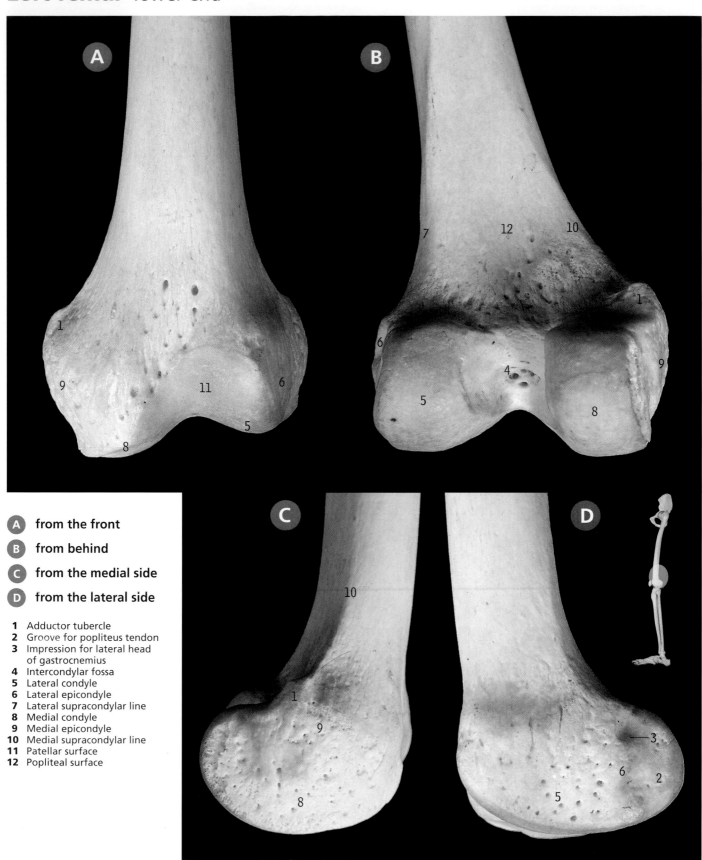

A **from the front**

B **from behind**

C **from the medial side**

D **from the lateral side**

1 Adductor tubercle
2 Groove for popliteus tendon
3 Impression for lateral head
   of gastrocnemius
4 Intercondylar fossa
5 Lateral condyle
6 Lateral epicondyle
7 Lateral supracondylar line
8 Medial condyle
9 Medial epicondyle
10 Medial supracondylar line
11 Patellar surface
12 Popliteal surface

Left femur *attachments, lower end*

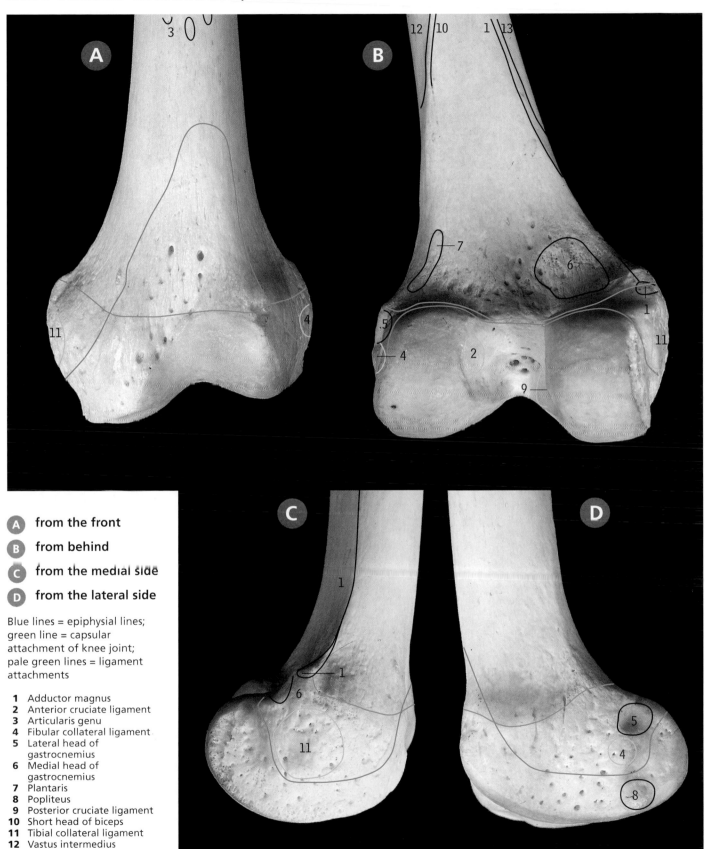

A from the front

B from behind

C from the medial side

D from the lateral side

Blue lines = epiphysial lines; green line = capsular attachment of knee joint; pale green lines = ligament attachments

1 Adductor magnus
2 Anterior cruciate ligament
3 Articularis genu
4 Fibular collateral ligament
5 Lateral head of gastrocnemius
6 Medial head of gastrocnemius
7 Plantaris
8 Popliteus
9 Posterior cruciate ligament
10 Short head of biceps
11 Tibial collateral ligament
12 Vastus intermedius
13 Vastus medialis

Left tibia *upper end*

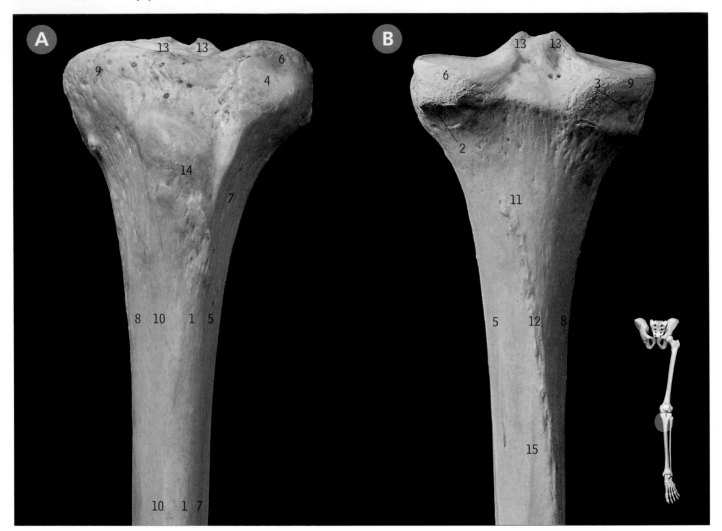

A **from the front**

B **from behind**

1 Anterior border
2 Articular facet for fibula
3 Groove for semimembranosus
4 Impression for iliotibial tract
5 Interosseous border
6 Lateral condyle
7 Lateral surface
8 Medial border
9 Medial condyle
10 Medial surface
11 Posterior surface
12 Soleal line
13 Tubercles of intercondylar eminence
14 Tuberosity
15 Vertical line

The shaft of the tibia has three borders – anterior (1), medial (8) and interosseous (5) – and three surfaces – medial (10), lateral (7) and posterior (11).

Much of the anterior border (1) forms a slightly curved crest commonly known as the shin. Most of the smooth medial surface (10) is subcutaneous. The posterior surface contains the soleal and vertical lines (12 and 15).

The tuberosity (14) is at the upper end of the anterior border.

Left tibia *attachments, upper end*

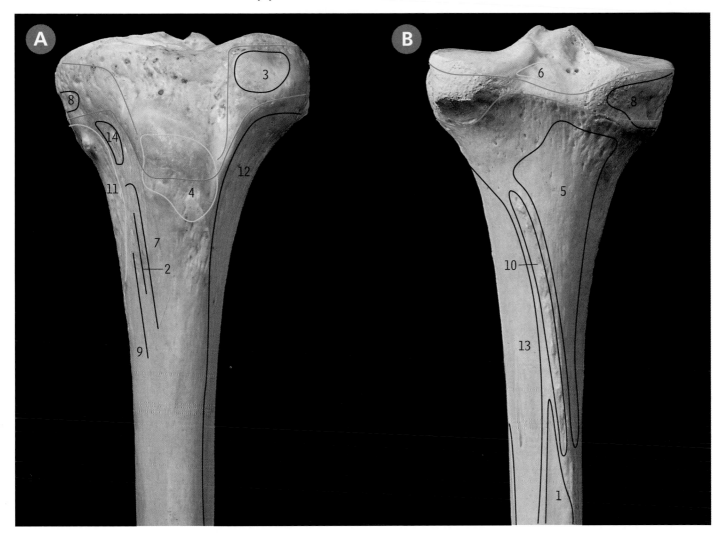

Blue lines = epiphysial lines;
green line = capsular
attachment of knee joint;
pale green lines = ligament
attachments

1 Flexor digitorum longus	**8** Semimembranosus
2 Gracilis	**9** Semitendinosus
3 Iliotibial tract	**10** Soleus
4 Patellar ligament	**11** Tibial collateral ligament
5 Popliteus	**12** Tibialis anterior
6 Posterior cruciate ligament	**13** Tibialis posterior
7 Sartorius	**14** Vastus medialis

Left tibia *upper end*

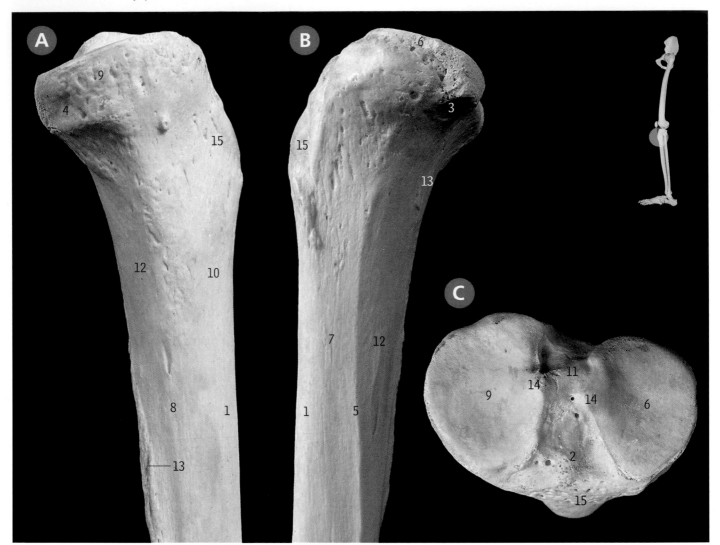

A from the medial side

B from the lateral side

C from above

1 Anterior border	**9** Medial condyle
2 Anterior intercondylar area	**10** Medial surface
3 Articular facet for fibula	**11** Posterior intercondylar area
4 Groove for semimembranosus	**12** Posterior surface
5 Interosseous border	**13** Soleal line
6 Lateral condyle	**14** Tubercles of intercondylar eminence
7 Lateral surface	**15** Tuberosity
8 Medial border	

The medial condyle (C9) is larger than the lateral condyle (C6).

The articular facet for the fibula is on the postero-inferior aspect of the lateral condyle (B3).

Avulsion of the tibial tuberosity, see p. 355.

Left tibia *attachments, upper end*

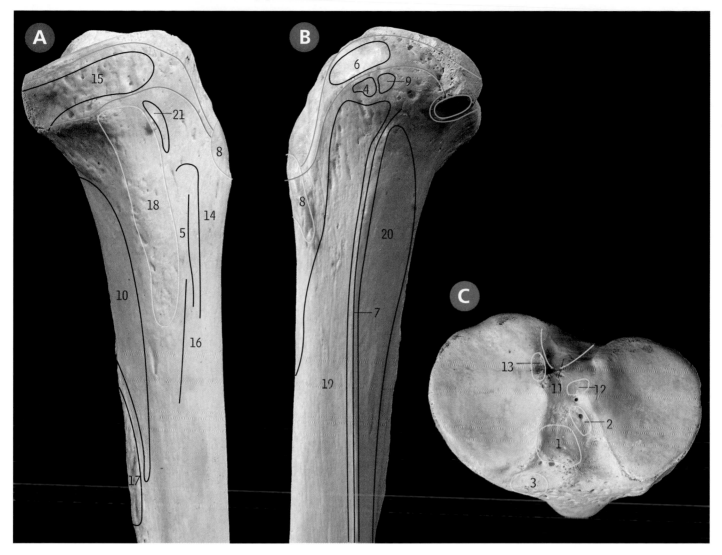

Blue lines = epiphysial lines, green lines = capsular attachments of knee joint and superior tibiofibular joint; pale green lines = ligament attachments

1 Anterior cruciate ligament
2 Anterior horn of lateral meniscus
3 Anterior horn of medial meniscus
4 Extensor digitorum longus
5 Gracilis
6 Iliotibial tract
7 Interosseous membrane
8 Patellar ligament
9 Peroneus longus
10 Popliteus
11 Posterior cruciate ligament
12 Posterior horn of lateral meniscus
13 Posterior horn of medial meniscus
14 Sartorius
15 Semimembranosus
16 Semitendinosus
17 Soleus
18 Tibial collateral ligament
19 Tibialis anterior
20 Tibialis posterior
21 Vastus medialis

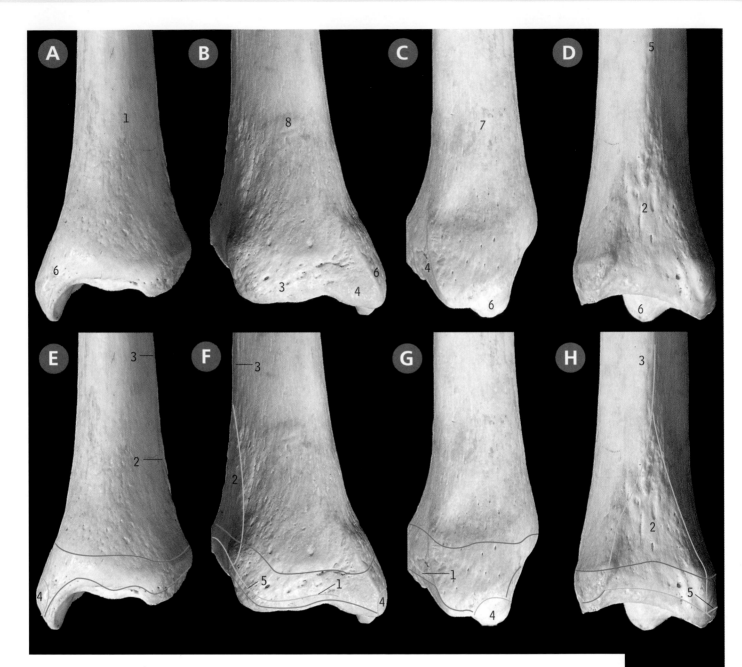

Left tibia *lower end*

A from the front

B from behind

C from the medial side

D from the lateral side

1 Anterior surface
2 Fibular notch
3 Groove for flexor hallucis longus
4 Groove for tibialis posterior
5 Interosseous border
6 Medial malleolus
7 Medial surface
8 Posterior surface

Left tibia *attachments, lower end*

E from the front

F from behind

G from the medial side

H from the lateral side

Blue line = epiphysial line; green line = capsular attachment of ankle joint; pale green lines = ligament attachments

1 Inferior transverse ligament
2 Interosseous ligament
3 Interosseous membrane
4 Medial collateral ligament
5 Posterior tibiofibular ligament

The medial collateral ligament (G4) is commonly known as the deltoid ligament.

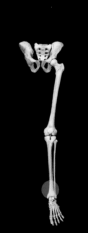

Left tibia and fibula *articulated*

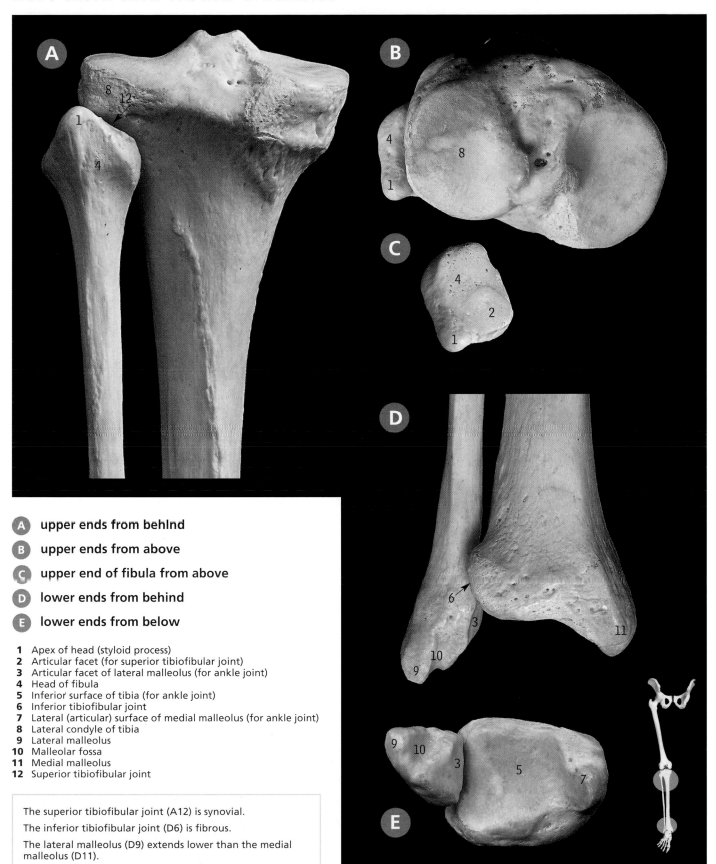

A upper ends from behind

B upper ends from above

C upper end of fibula from above

D lower ends from behind

E lower ends from below

1 Apex of head (styloid process)
2 Articular facet (for superior tibiofibular joint)
3 Articular facet of lateral malleolus (for ankle joint)
4 Head of fibula
5 Inferior surface of tibia (for ankle joint)
6 Inferior tibiofibular joint
7 Lateral (articular) surface of medial malleolus (for ankle joint)
8 Lateral condyle of tibia
9 Lateral malleolus
10 Malleolar fossa
11 Medial malleolus
12 Superior tibiofibular joint

The superior tibiofibular joint (A12) is synovial.

The inferior tibiofibular joint (D6) is fibrous.

The lateral malleolus (D9) extends lower than the medial malleolus (D11).

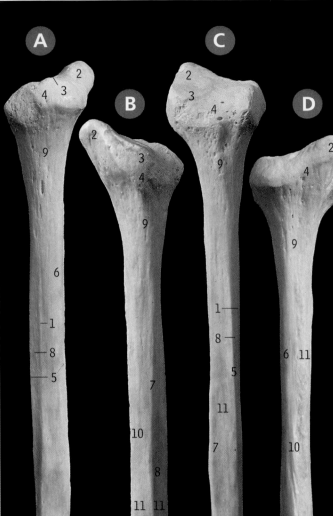

Left fibula *upper end*

A from the front   **C** from the medial side

B from behind   **D** from the lateral side

1 Anterior border
2 Apex (styloid process)
3 Articular facet on upper surface
4 Head
5 Interosseous border
6 Lateral surface
7 Medial crest
8 Medial surface
9 Neck
10 Posterior border
11 Posterior surface

The fibula has three borders – anterior (A1), interosseous (A5) and posterior (B10) – and three surfaces – medial (A8), lateral (A6) and posterior (B11).

At first sight much of the shaft appears to have four borders and four surfaces, but this is because the posterior surface (B11) is divided into two parts (medial and lateral) by the medial crest (B7).

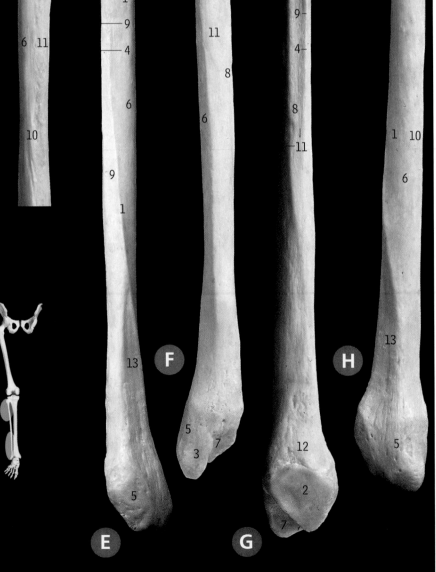

Left fibula *lower end*

E from the front

F from behind

G from the medial side

H from the lateral side

1 Anterior border
2 Articular surface of lateral malleolus
3 Groove for peroneus brevis
4 Interosseous border
5 Lateral malleolus
6 Lateral surface
7 Malleolar fossa
8 Medial crest
9 Medial surface
10 Posterior border
11 Posterior surface
12 Surface for interosseous ligament
13 Triangular subcutaneous area

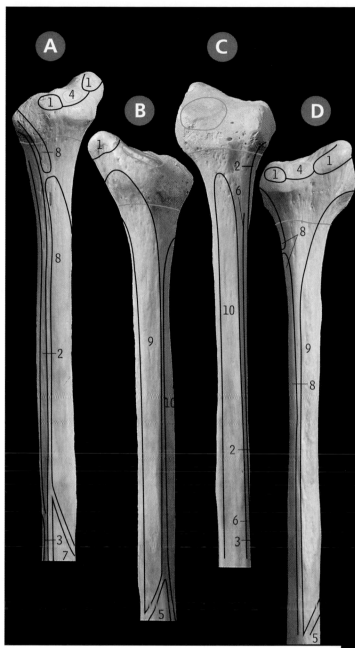

Left fibula

attachments, upper end

A from the front   **C** from the medial side

B from behind   **D** from the lateral side

Blue line = epiphysial line; green line = capsular attachment of superior tibiofibular joint; pale green lines = ligament attachments

1 Biceps
2 Extensor digitorum longus
3 Extensor hallucis longus
4 Fibular collateral ligament
5 Flexor hallucis longus
6 Interosseous membrane
7 Peroneus brevis
8 Peroneus longus
9 Soleus
10 Tibialis posterior

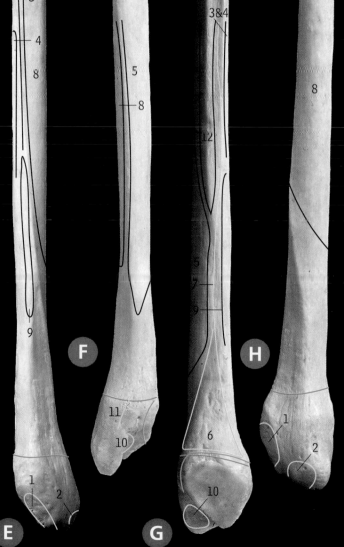

Left fibula

attachments, lower end

E from the front   **G** from the medial side

F from behind   **H** from the lateral side

Blue line = epiphysial line; green line = capsular attachment of ankle joint; pale green lines = ligament attachments

1 Anterior talofibular ligament
2 Calcaneofibular ligament
3 Extensor digitorum longus
4 Extensor hallucis longus
5 Flexor hallucis longus
6 Interosseous ligament
7 Interosseous membrane
8 Peroneus brevis
9 Peroneus tertius
10 Posterior talofibular ligament
11 Posterior tibiofibular ligament
12 Tibialis posterior

Bones of the left foot

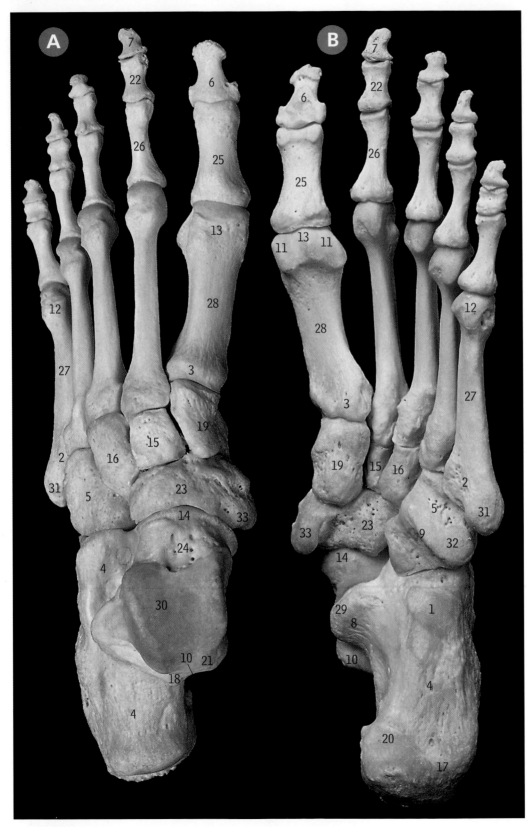

Hallux valgus, see p. 356.

A from above (dorsum)

B from below (plantar surface)

1 Anterior tubercle of calcaneus
2 Base of fifth metatarsal
3 Base of first metatarsal
4 Calcaneus
5 Cuboid
6 Distal phalanx of great toe
7 Distal phalanx of second toe
8 Groove on calcaneus for flexor hallucis longus
9 Groove on cuboid for peroneus longus
10 Groove on talus for flexor hallucis longus
11 Grooves for sesamoid bones in flexor hallucis brevis
12 Head of fifth metatarsal
13 Head of first metatarsal
14 Head of talus
15 Intermediate cuneiform
16 Lateral cuneiform
17 Lateral process of calcaneus
18 Lateral tubercle of talus
19 Medial cuneiform
20 Medial process of calcaneus
21 Medial tubercle of talus
22 Middle phalanx of second toe
23 Navicular
24 Neck of talus
25 Proximal phalanx of great toe
26 Proximal phalanx of second toe
27 Shaft of fifth metatarsal
28 Shaft of first metatarsal
29 Sustentaculum tali of calcaneus
30 Trochlear surface of body of talus
31 Tuberosity of base of fifth metatarsal
32 Tuberosity of cuboid
33 Tuberosity of navicular

Bones of the left foot *attachments*

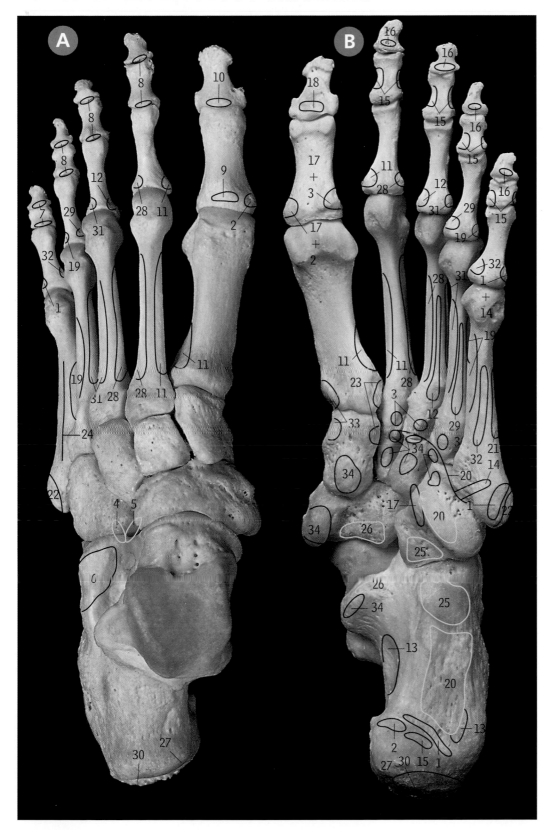

Metatarsal fractures, see p. 356.

A from above

B from below

Joint capsules and minor ligaments have been omitted.

Pale green lines = ligament attachments

1   Abductor digiti minimi
2   Abductor hallucis
3   Adductor hallucis
4   Calcaneocuboid part of bifurcate ligament
5   Calcaneonavicular part of bifurcate ligament
6   Extensor digitorum brevis
7   Extensor digitorum longus
8   Extensor digitorum longus and brevis
9   Extensor hallucis brevis
10   Extensor hallucis longus
11   First dorsal interosseous
12   First plantar interosseous
13   Flexor accessorius
14   Flexor digiti minimi brevis
15   Flexor digitorum brevis
16   Flexor digitorum longus
17   Flexor hallucis brevis
18   Flexor hallucis longus
19   Fourth dorsal interosseous
20   Long plantar ligament
21   Opponens digiti minimi (part of 14)
22   Peroneus brevis
23   Peroneus longus
24   Peroneus tertius
25   Plantar calcaneocuboid (short plantar) ligament
26   Plantar calcaneonavicular (spring) ligament
27   Plantaris
28   Second dorsal interosseous
29   Second plantar interosseous
30   Tendo calcaneus (Achilles tendon)
31   Third dorsal interosseous
32   Third plantar interosseous
33   Tibialis anterior
34   Tibialis posterior

Bones of the left foot

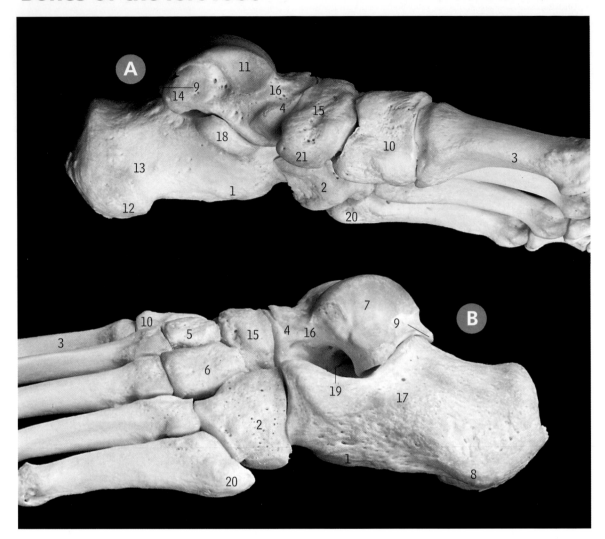

A from the medial side   **B** from the lateral side

1 Anterior tubercle of calcaneus	
2 Cuboid	
3 First metatarsal	
4 Head of talus	
5 Intermediate cuneiform	
6 Lateral cuneiform	
7 Lateral malleolar surface of talus	
8 Lateral process of calcaneus	

9 Lateral tubercle of talus
10 Medial cuneiform
11 Medial malleolar surface of talus
12 Medial process of calcaneus
13 Medial surface of calcaneus
14 Medial tubercle of talus
15 Navicular
16 Neck of talus

17 Peroneal trochlea of calcaneus
18 Sustentaculum tali of calcaneus
19 Tarsal sinus
20 Tuberosity of base of fifth metatarsal
21 Tuberosity of navicular

Fracture of the fifth metatarsal, see p. 356.

Bones of the left foot

Left calcaneus

A from above   **B** from behind

Left talus

C from below

1   Anterior calcanean articular surface of talus
2   Anterior talal articular surface of calcaneus
3   Groove for flexor hallucis longus of calcaneus
4   Groove for flexor hallucis longus of talus
5   Head of talus
6   Medial process of calcaneus
7   Middle calcanean articular surface of talus
8   Middle talal articular surface of calcaneus
9   Posterior calcanean articular surface of talus
10 Posterior surface of calcaneus
11 Posterior talal articular surface of calcaneus
12 Sulcus of calcaneus
13 Sulcus of talus
14 Surface for plantar calneonavicular (spring) ligament of talus
15 Sustentaculum tali of calcaneus

Left calcaneus, attachments

D from above   **E** from behind

Left talus, attachments

F from below

Curved lines indicate corresponding articular surfaces: green = capsular attachment of talocalcanean (subtalar) and talocalcaneonavicular joints; pale green lines = ligament attachments

1   Area for bursa
2   Area for fibrofatty tissue
3   Calcaneocuboid part of bifurcate ligament
4   Calcaneofibular ligament
5   Calcaneonavicular part of bifurcate ligament
6   Cervical ligament
7   Extensor digitorum brevis
8   Inferior extensor retinaculum
9   Interosseous talocalcanean ligament
10 Lateral talocalcanean ligament
11 Medial talocalcanean ligament
12 Plantaris
13 Tendo calcaneus (Achilles tendon)
14 Tibiocalcanean part of deltoid ligament

The interosseous talocalcanean ligament (9) is formed by thickening of the adjacent capsules of the talocalcanean and talocalcaneonavicular joints.

For different interpretations of the term 'subtalar joint' see the notes on page 348.

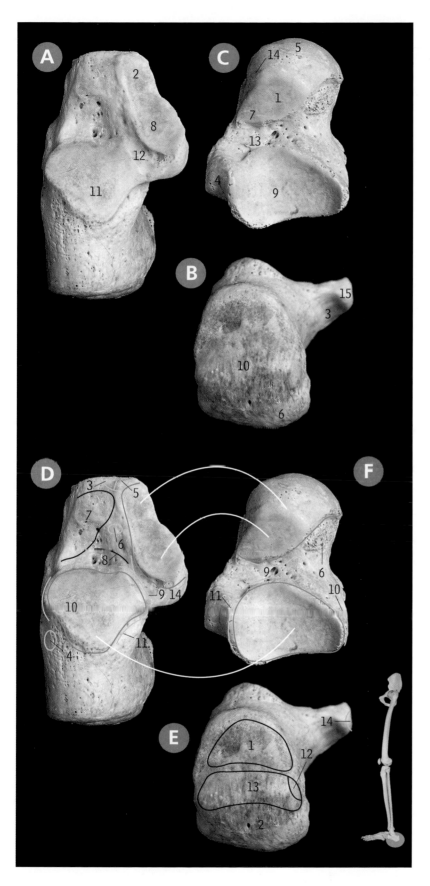

Left lower limb bones *secondary centres of ossification*

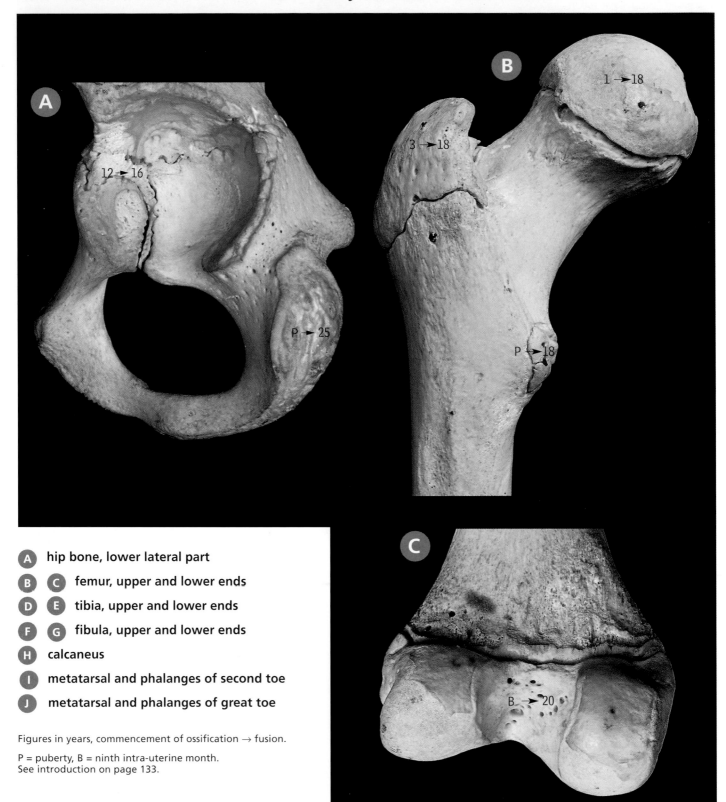

A   hip bone, lower lateral part

B   C   femur, upper and lower ends

D   E   tibia, upper and lower ends

F   G   fibula, upper and lower ends

H   calcaneus

I   metatarsal and phalanges of second toe

J   metatarsal and phalanges of great toe

Figures in years, commencement of ossification → fusion.

P = puberty, B = ninth intra-uterine month.
See introduction on page 133.

Slipped upper femoral epiphysis, see p. 357.

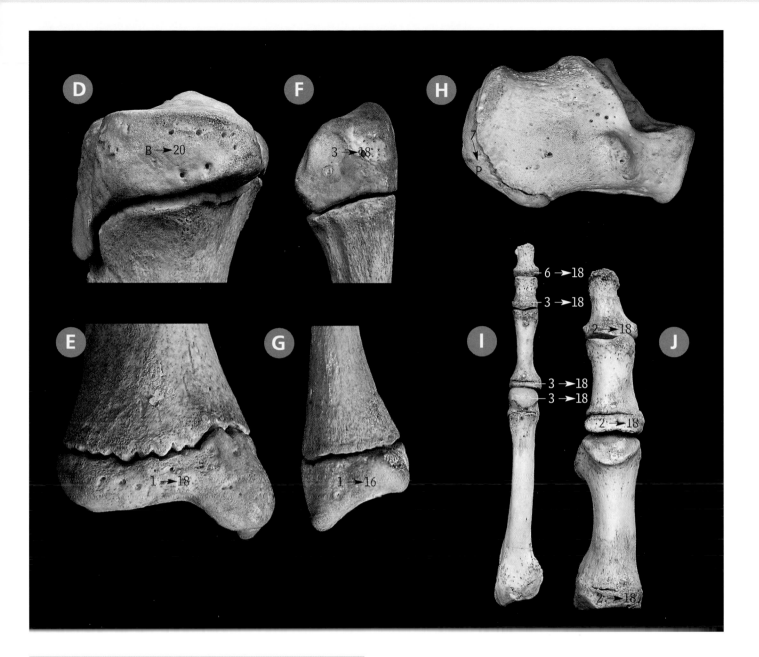

In the hip bone (A) one or more secondary centres appear in the Y-shaped cartilage between ilium, ischium and pubis. Other centres (not illustrated) are usually present for the iliac crest, anterior inferior iliac spine, and (possibly) the pubic tubercle and pubic crest (all P → 25).

The patella (not illustrated) begins to ossify from one or more centres between the third and sixth year.

All the phalanges, and the first metatarsal, have a secondary centre at their proximal ends; the other metatarsals have one at their distal ends.

Of the tarsal bones, the largest, the calcaneus, begins to ossify in the third intra-uterine month and the talus about three months later. The cuboid may begin to ossify either just before or just after birth, with the lateral cuneiform in the first year, medial cuneiform at two years and the intermediate cuneiform and navicular at three years.

The calcaneus (H) is the only tarsal bone to have a secondary centre.

Right gluteal region *surface features*

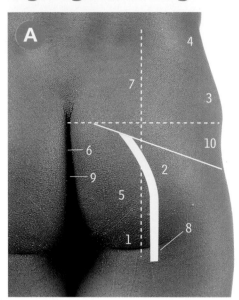

The interrupted lines divide the gluteal region into quadrants (see the note below). The iliac crest (4) with the posterior superior iliac spine (7), the tip of the coccyx (9), the ischial tuberosity (5) and the tip of the greater trochanter of the femur (10) are palpable landmarks. A line drawn from a point midway between the posterior superior iliac spine (7) and the tip of the coccyx (9) to the tip of the greater trochanter (10) marks the lower border of piriformis (solid white line) which is a key feature of the gluteal region, where the most important structure is the sciatic nerve (indicated here in yellow, 8; see dissections and notes opposite).

 1 Fold of buttock
 2 Gluteus maximus
 3 Gluteus medius
 4 Iliac crest
 5 Ischial tuberosity
 6 Natal cleft
 7 Posterior superior iliac spine
 8 Sciatic nerve
 9 Tip of coccyx
10 Tip of greater trochanter of femur

Right gluteal region *superficial nerves*

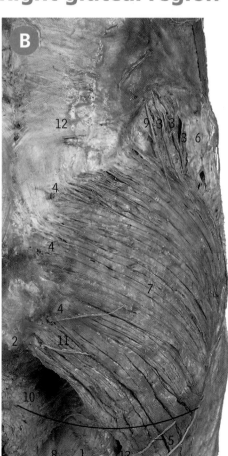

Skin and subcutaneous tissue have been removed, preserving cutaneous branches from the first three lumbar (3) and first three sacral (4) nerves, the cutaneous branches of the posterior femoral cutaneous nerve (5) and the perforating cutaneous nerve (11). The curved line near the bottom of the picture indicates the position of the gluteal fold (fold of the buttock). The muscle fibres of gluteus maximus (7) run downwards and laterally, and its lower border does not correspond to the gluteal fold.

 1 Adductor magnus
 2 Coccyx
 3 Cutaneous branches of dorsal rami of first three lumbar nerves
 4 Gluteal branches of dorsal rami of first three sacral nerves
 5 Gluteal branches of the posterior femoral cutaneous nerve
 6 Gluteal fascia overlying gluteus medius
 7 Gluteus maximus
 8 Gracilis
 9 Iliac crest
10 Ischio-anal fossa and levator ani
11 Perforating cutaneous nerve
12 Posterior layer of lumbar fascia overlying erector spinae
13 Semitendinosus

The gluteal region or buttock is sometimes used as a site for intramuscular injections. The correct site is in the upper outer quadrant of the buttock, and for delimiting this quadrant it is essential to remember that the upper boundary of the buttock is the uppermost part of the iliac crest. The lower boundary is the fold of the buttock. Dividing the area between these two boundaries by a vertical line midway between the midline and the lateral side of the body indicates that the upper outer quadrant is well above and to the right of the label 7 in B, and this is the safe site for injection – well above and to the right of the sciatic nerve which is displayed in the dissections opposite.

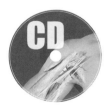

Sciatica, see p. 357.

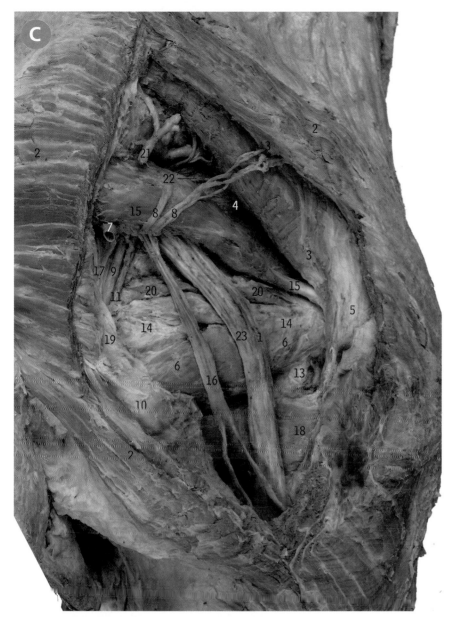

Right gluteal region

C with most of gluteus maximus removed

D with the sciatic trunk displaced

1 Common peroneal part of sciatic nerve
2 Gluteus maximus
3 Gluteus medius
4 Gluteus minimus
5 Greater trochanter of femur
6 Inferior gemellus
7 Inferior gluteal artery
8 Inferior gluteal nerve
9 Internal pudendal artery
10 Ischial tuberosity
11 Nerve to obturator internus
12 Nerve to quadratus femoris
13 Obturator externus
14 Obturator internus
15 Piriformis
16 Posterior femoral cutaneous nerve
17 Pudendal nerve
18 Quadratus femoris
19 Sacrotuberous ligament
20 Superior gemellus
21 Superior gluteal artery
22 Superior gluteal nerve
23 Tibial part of sciatic nerve

The two parts of the sciatic trunk (common peroneal (fibular) and tibial, 1 and 23) usually divide from one another at the top of the popliteal fossa (page 330B) but are sometimes separate as they emerge beneath piriformis, and the common peroneal (fibular) may even perforate piriformis.

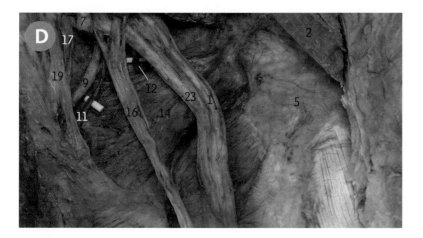

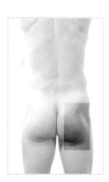

Gluteal nerve paralysis, sciatic trunk paralysis, see pp 356, 357.

Right thigh *posterior view*

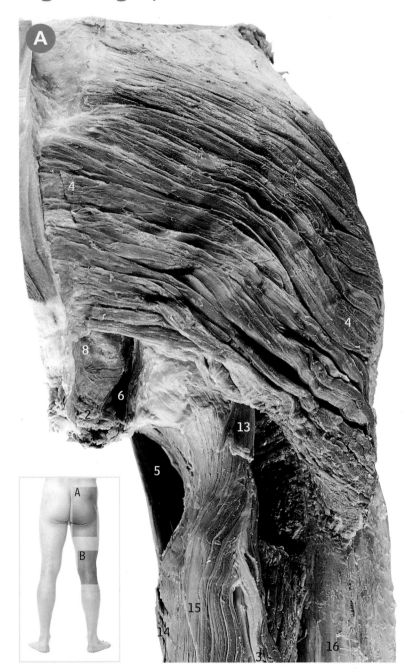

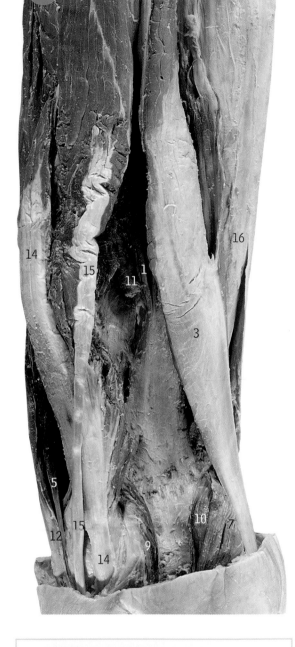

A   muscles in the proximal part

B   muscles in the distal popliteal parts

1	Adductor magnus	**9**	Medial head of gastrocnemius
2	Anal sphincter	**10**	Plantaris
3	Biceps femoris, long head	**11**	Popliteal artery
4	Gluteus maximus	**12**	Sartorius
5	Gracilis	**13**	Sciatic nerve trunk
6	Ischio-anal fossa	**14**	Semimembranosus
7	Lateral head of gastrocnemius	**15**	Semitendinosus
8	Levator ani	**16**	Vastus lateralis

The long head of biceps (the part seen in B, 3), semimembranosus (14) and semitendinosus (15) are commonly called the hamstrings. The short head of biceps, which is under cover of the long head and arises from the back of the shaft of the femur and not from the ischial tuberosity (as the other muscles do), is not classified as a hamstring. The true hamstrings span both the hip and knee joint; they extend the hip and flex the knee.

Torn hamstrings, see p. 357.

Right upper thigh *posterior view*

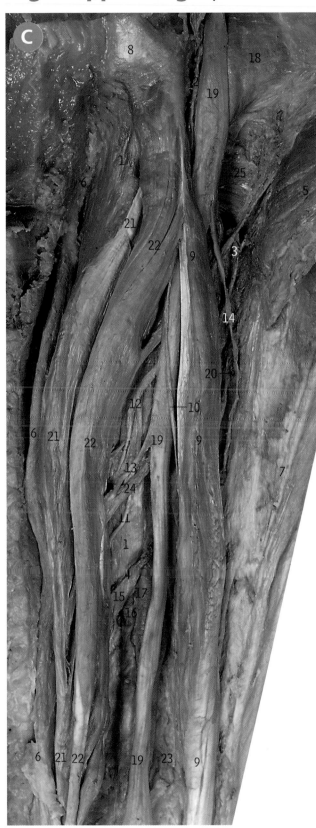

Gluteus maximus (5) has been reflected laterally and the gap between semitendinosus (22) and biceps (9) has been opened up to show the sciatic trunk (19) and its muscular branches.

1 Adductor magnus
2 Anastomotic branch of inferior gluteal artery
3 First perforating artery
4 Fourth perforating artery
5 Gluteus maximus
6 Gracilis
7 Iliotibial tract overlying vastus lateralis
8 Ischial tuberosity
9 Long head of biceps
10 Nerve to long head of biceps
11 Nerve to semimembranosus
12 Nerve to semimembranosus and adductor magnus
13 Nerve to semitendinosus
14 Nerve to short head of biceps
15 Opening in adductor magnus
16 Popliteal artery
17 Popliteal vein
18 Quadratus femoris
19 Sciatic trunk
20 Second perforating artery
21 Semimembranosus
22 Semitendinosus
23 Short head of biceps
24 Third perforating artery
25 Upper part of adductor magnus ('adductor minimus')

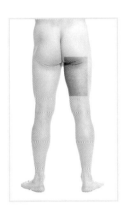

The only muscular branch to arise from the lateral side of the sciatic trunk (i.e. from the common peroneal part of the nerve – 19, uppermost label near the top of the picture), is the nerve to the short head of biceps (14). All the other muscular branches – to the long head of biceps (10), semimembranosus (11), semimembranosus and adductor magnus (12) and semitendinosus (13) – arise from the medial side of the sciatic trunk (19, near the centre of the picture) (i.e. from the tibial part of the nerve).

Femoral arteriogram

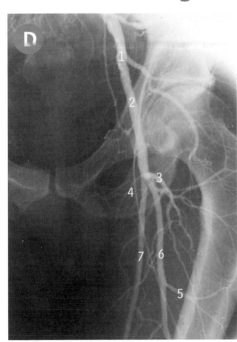

1 Catheter introduced into distal abdominal aorta via left femoral artery
2 Common femoral artery
3 Lateral circumflex femoral artery
4 Medial circumflex femoral artery
5 Perforating artery
6 Profunda femoris artery
7 Superficial femoral artery

Right femoral region

A *femoral vessels and lymphatics* **B** *branches of femoral nerve*

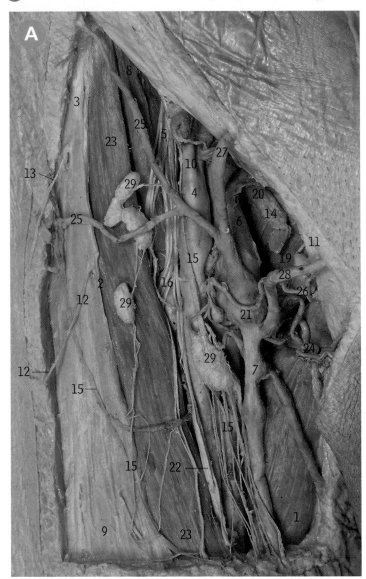

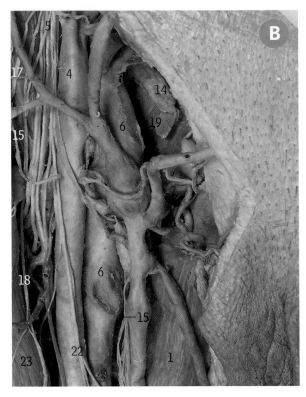

1 Adductor longus
2 Fascia lata, cut edge
3 Fascia lata overlying tensor fasciae latae
4 Femoral artery
5 Femoral nerve
6 Femoral vein
7 Great saphenous vein
8 Iliacus
9 Iliotibial tract overlying vastus lateralis
10 Inferior epigastric vessels
11 Inguinal ligament
12 Intermediate cutaneous nerve of the thigh
13 Lateral cutaneous nerve of the thigh
14 Lymph node (Cloquet)
15 Lymph vessels
16 Muscular branches of femoral nerve overlying lateral circumflex femoral vessels
17 Nerve to sartorius
18 Nerve to vastus lateralis
19 Pectineus
20 Position of femoral canal
21 Saphena varix
22 Saphenous nerve
23 Sartorius
24 Scrotal veins
25 Superficial circumflex iliac vein
26 Superficial external pudendal artery
27 Superficial epigastric vein
28 Superficial external pudendal vein
29 Vertical chain of superficial inguinal lymph nodes

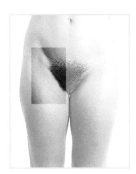

The boundaries of the femoral triangle are the inguinal ligament (11), the medial border of sartorius (23) and the medial border of adductor longus (1).

The femoral canal (20) is the medial compartment of the femoral sheath (removed) which contains in its middle compartment the femoral vein (6), and in the lateral compartment the femoral artery (4). The femoral nerve (5) is lateral to the sheath, not within it.

Femoral hernia (1), the Trendelenburg test, see pp 355, 357.

C Right obturator nerve

In this right femoral region, pectineus (10), adductor longus (2, lower label) and adductor brevis (1) have been detached from their origins and reflected laterally to display obturator externus (9) and the anterior (4) and posterior (11) branches of the obturator nerve.

1 Adductor brevis
2 Adductor longus
3 Adductor magnus
4 Anterior branch of obturator nerve
5 Femoral artery
6 Femoral vein
7 Gracilis
8 Nerve and vessels to gracilis
9 Obturator externus
10 Pectineus
11 Posterior branch of obturator nerve
12 Superior ramus of pubis

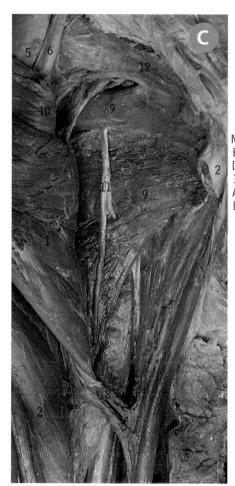

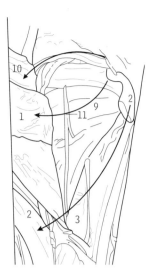

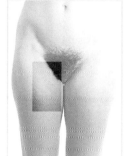

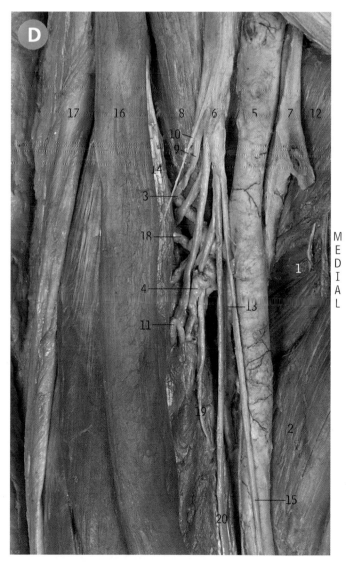

D Right femoral nerve

Sartorius (16) and rectus femoris (14) have been displaced laterally to open up the upper part of the adductor canal and show the lateral circumflex femoral vessels (3, 18 and 4) between branches of the femoral nerve (6).

1 Adductor brevis and nerve
2 Adductor longus
3 Ascending branch of lateral circumflex femoral artery
4 Descending branch of lateral circumflex femoral artery
5 Femoral artery
6 Femoral nerve
7 Femoral vein
8 Iliacus
9 Nerve to rectus femoris
10 Nerve to sartorius
11 Nerve to vastus lateralis
12 Pectineus
13 Profunda femoris artery
14 Rectus femoris
15 Saphenous nerve
16 Sartorius
17 Tensor fasciae latae
18 Transverse branch of lateral circumflex femoral artery
19 Vastus intermedius and nerve
20 Vastus medialis and nerves

 Femoral nerve paralysis, obturator nerve paralysis, see pp 355, 356.

Right femoral artery

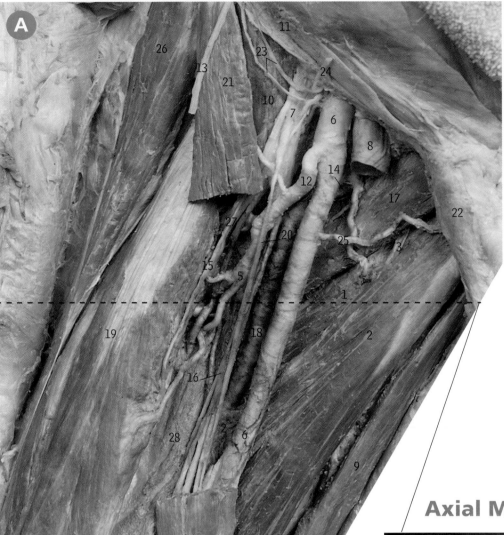

1 Adductor brevis
2 Adductor longus
3 Anterior branch of obturator nerve
4 Ascending branch of lateral circumflex femoral artery
5 Descending branch of lateral circumflex femoral artery
6 Femoral artery
7 Femoral nerve
8 Femoral vein
9 Gracilis
10 Iliacus
11 Inguinal ligament
12 Lateral circumflex femoral artery
13 Lateral femoral cutaneous nerve
14 Medial circumflex femoral artery
15 Nerve to rectus femoris
16 Nerve to vastus medialis
17 Pectineus
18 Profunda femoris artery
19 Rectus femoris
20 Saphenous nerve
21 Sartorius
22 Spermatic cord
23 Superficial circumflex iliac artery (double)
24 Superficial epigastric artery
25 Superficial external pudendal artery (low origin)
26 Tensor fasciae latae
27 Transverse branch of lateral circumflex femoral artery
28 Vastus intermedius
29 Vastus medialis

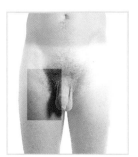

Axial MR image of thigh

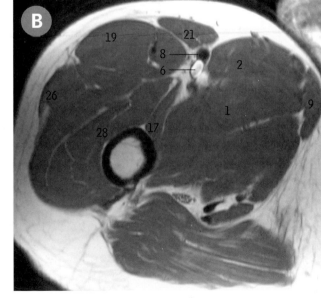

Femoral artery catheterization, femoral hernia (2), femoral vein catheterization, meralgia paraesthetica, see pp 355, 356.

Ⓒ **Right lower thigh**
from the front and medial side

The lower part of sartorius (13) has been displaced medially to open up the lower part of the adductor canal and expose the femoral artery (2) passing through the opening in adductor magnus (7) to enter the popliteal fossa behind the knee and become the popliteal artery (page 330).

1	Adductor magnus	**8**	Patella
2	Femoral artery	**9**	Quadriceps tendon
3	Gracilis	**10**	Rectus femoris
4	Iliotibial tract	**11**	Saphenous branch of
5	Lowest (horizontal) fibres of		descending genicular artery
	vastus medialis	**12**	Saphenous nerve
6	Medial patellar retinaculum	**13**	Sartorius
7	Opening in adductor magnus	**14**	Vastus medialis and nerve

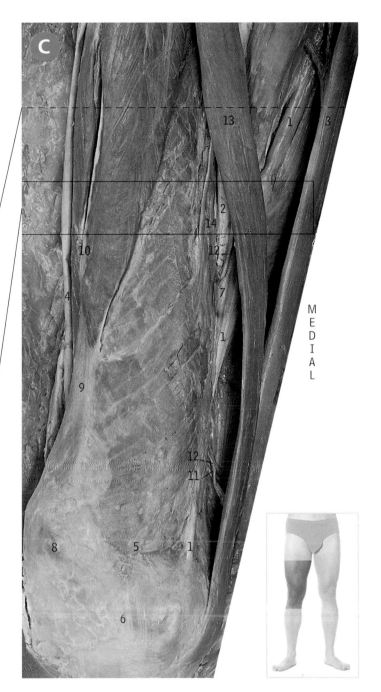

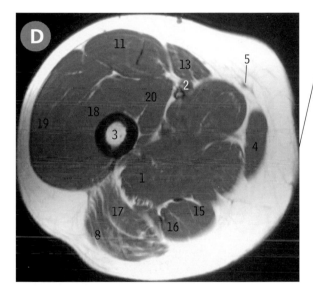

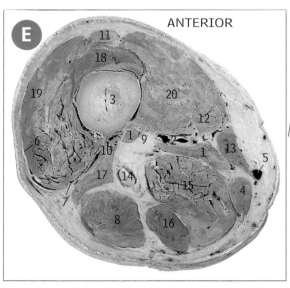

Right lower thigh
Ⓓ *axial MR image* Ⓔ *cross section*

1	Adductor magnus	**11**	Rectus femoris
2	Femoral vessels	**12**	Saphenous nerve
3	Femur	**13**	Sartorius
4	Gracilis	**14**	Sciatic nerve
5	Great saphenous vein	**15**	Semimembranosus
6	Iliotibial tract of fascia lata	**16**	Semitendinosus
7	Lateral intermuscular septum	**17**	Short head of biceps
8	Long head of biceps	**18**	Vastus intermedius
9	Opening in adductor magnus	**19**	Vastus lateralis
10	Profunda femoris vessels	**20**	Vastus medialis

 Femoropopliteal bypass, intermittent claudication, see p. 356.

Right hip joint

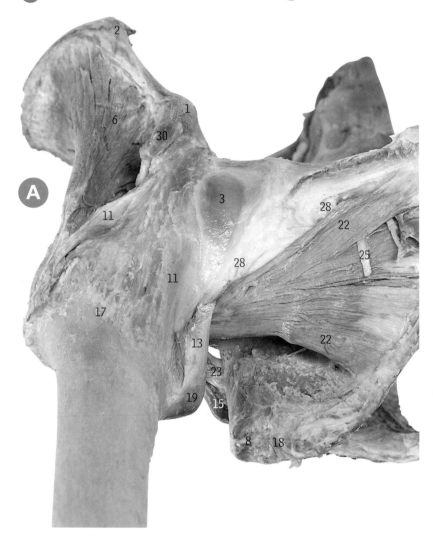 *from the front and below* 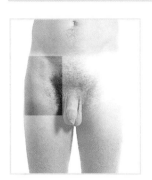 *from the front and above*

Some of the fibres of the ischiofemoral ligament help to form the zona orbicularis – circular fibres of the capsule that form a collar around the neck of the femur.

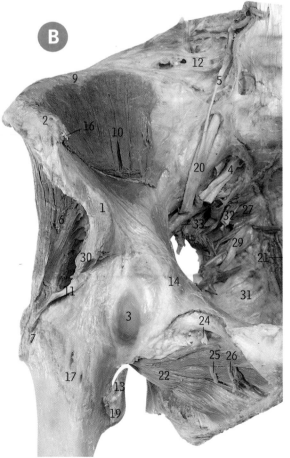

1 Anterior inferior iliac spine	**18** Ischial tuberosity
2 Anterior superior iliac spine	**19** Lesser trochanter
3 Bursa for psoas tendon	**20** Lumbosacral trunk
4 First sacral nerve root	**21** Median sacral artery
5 Fourth lumbar nerve root	**22** Obturator externus
6 Gluteus minimus muscle	**23** Obturator internus tendon
7 Greater trochanter	**24** Obturator nerve, anterior branch
8 Hamstring origin	**25** Obturator nerve, posterior branch
9 Iliac crest	**26** Obturator vessels
10 Iliacus muscle	**27** Piriformis muscle
11 Iliofemoral ligament	**28** Pubofemoral ligament
12 Iliolumbar ligament	**29** Pudendal nerve
13 Iliopsoas tendon	**30** Rectus femoris muscle
14 Iliopubic eminence	**31** Sacrospinous ligament
15 Inferior gemellus muscle	**32** Second sacral nerve root
16 Inguinal ligament	**33** Superior gluteal artery
17 Intertrochanteric line and capsule attachment	

Trendelenburg's sign, see p. 357.

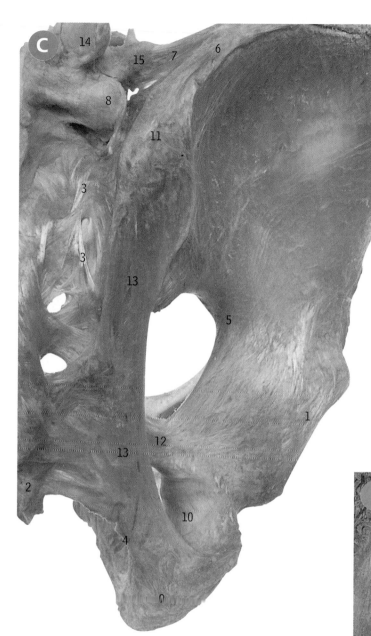

ⓒ Right vertebropelvic and sacro-iliac ligaments *from behind*

1 Acetabular labrum
2 Coccyx
3 Dorsal sacro-iliac ligaments
4 Falciform process of sacrotuberous ligament
5 Greater sciatic notch
6 Iliac crest
7 Iliolumbar ligament
8 Inferior articular process of fifth lumbar vertebra
9 Ischial tuberosity
10 Lesser sciatic notch
11 Posterior superior iliac spine
12 Sacrospinous ligament and ischial spine
13 Sacrotuberous ligament
14 Superior articular process of fifth lumbar vertebra
15 Transverse process of fifth lumbar vertebra

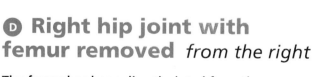

ⓓ Right hip joint with femur removed *from the right*

The femur has been disarticulated from the acetabulum and removed, leaving the acetabular labrum (2), transverse ligament (10) and the ligament teres (5).

1 Acetabular fossa
  (non-articular)
2 Acetabular labrum
3 Adductor longus
4 Articular surface
5 Ligament teres femoris
6 Obturator externus

7 Pectineus
8 Reflected head of rectus femoris
9 Straight head of rectus femoris
10 Transverse ligament

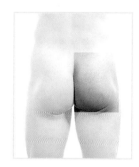

 Avascular necrosis of the head of the femur, see p. 355.

Left hip joint Ⓐ *coronal section, from the front* Ⓑ *coronal MR image*

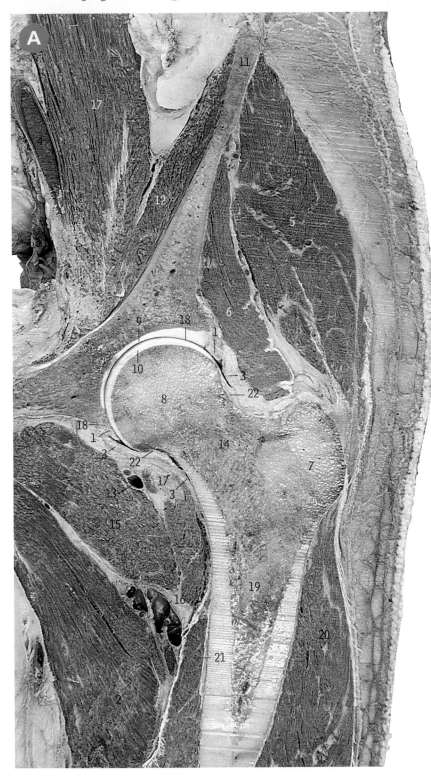

The section has almost passed through the centre of the head (8) of the femur and the centre of the greater trochanter (7). Above the neck of the femur (14), gluteus minimus (6) with gluteus medius (5) above it run down to their attachments to the greater trochanter (7), while below the neck the tendon of psoas major (17) and muscle fibres of iliacus (12) pass backwards towards the lesser trochanter. The circular fibres of the zona orbicularis (22) constrict the capsule (3) around the intracapsular part of the neck of the femur.

 1 Acetabular labrum
 2 Adductor longus
 3 Capsule of hip joint
 4 External iliac artery
 5 Gluteus medius
 6 Gluteus minimus
 7 Greater trochanter
 8 Head of femur
 9 Hyaline cartilage of acetabulum
10 Hyaline cartilage of head
11 Iliac crest
12 Iliacus
13 Medial circumflex femoral vessels
14 Neck of femur
15 Pectineus
16 Profunda femoris vessels
17 Psoas major
18 Rim of acetabulum
19 Shaft of femur
20 Vastus lateralis
21 Vastus medialis
22 Zona orbicularis of capsule

 *   Contrast outlines the joint cavity
**   Ligamentum teres

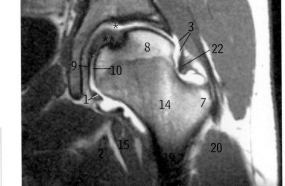

The convergence of gluteus medius and minimus (5 and 6) on to the greater trochanter is well displayed in this section. These muscles are classified as abductors of the femur at the hip joint, but their more important action is in walking, where they act to prevent adduction – preventing the pelvis from tilting to the opposite side when the opposite limb is off the ground (see Trendelenburg's sign).

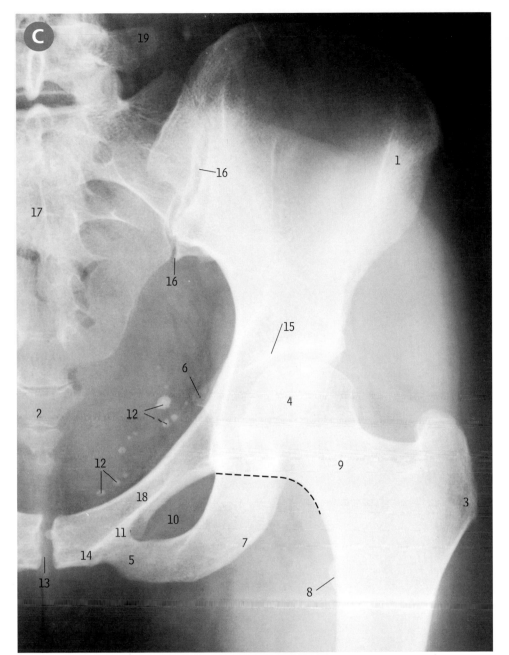

C Left hip and sacro-iliac joint
radiograph

In this standard anteroposterior view of the hip joint (15 and 4), much of the joint line of the sacro-iliac joint can also be seen (16). The dashed line on C is Shenton's line, a guide to diagnosing femoral neck fractures.

1 Anterior superior iliac spine
2 First coccygeal vertebra
3 Greater trochanter of femur
4 Head of femur
5 Inferior pubic ramus
6 Ischial spine
7 Ischial tuberosity
8 Lesser trochanter of femur
9 Neck of femur
10 Obturator foramen
11 Pectineal line
12 Phleboliths in pelvic veins
13 Pubic symphysis
14 Pubic tubercle
15 Rim of acetabulum
16 Sacro-iliac joint
17 Sacrum
18 Superior pubic ramus
19 Transverse process of fifth lumbar vertebra

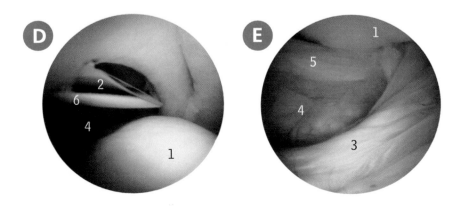

Hip joint
D E *arthroscopic views*

Reproduced with kind permission of Richard N. Villar from *Hip Arthroscopy* (Butterworth Heinemann).

1 Femoral head
2 Irrigation needle
3 Ligamentum teres
4 Synovium
5 Transverse ligament
6 Zona orbicularis

Right knee
partially flexed

A from the lateral side

B from the medial side

1 Biceps femoris
2 Common peroneal (fibular) nerve
3 Head of fibula
4 Iliotibial tract
5 Lateral head of gastrocnemius
6 Margin of condyle of femur
7 Margin of condyle of tibia
8 Patella
9 Patellar ligament
10 Popliteal fossa
11 Semimembranosus
12 Semitendinosus
13 Tuberosity of tibia
14 Vastus medialis

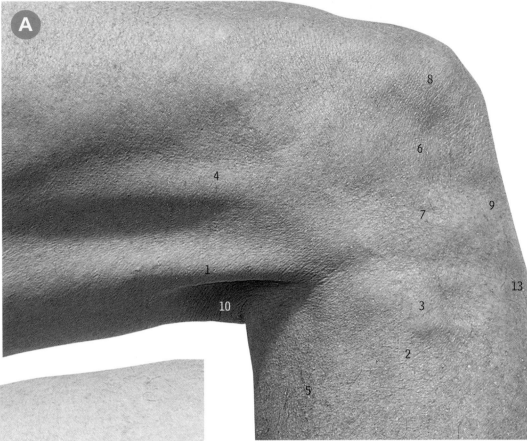

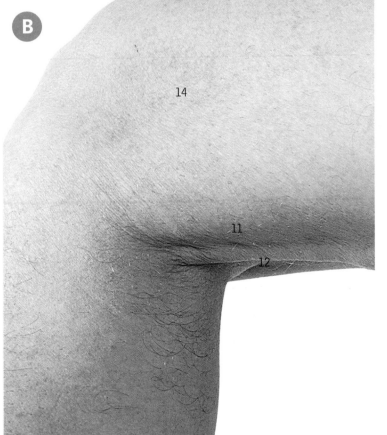

Behind the knee on the lateral side the rounded tendon of biceps (1) can be felt easily, with the broad strap-like iliotibial tract (4) in front of it, with a furrow between them. On the medial side two tendons can be felt – the narrow rounded semitendinosus (12) just behind the broader semimembranosus (11). At the front the patellar ligament (9) keeps the patella (8) at a constant distance from the tibial tuberosity (13), while at the side the adjacent margins of the femoral and tibial condyles (6 and 7) can be palpated.

Patellar tendon reflex, see p. 356.

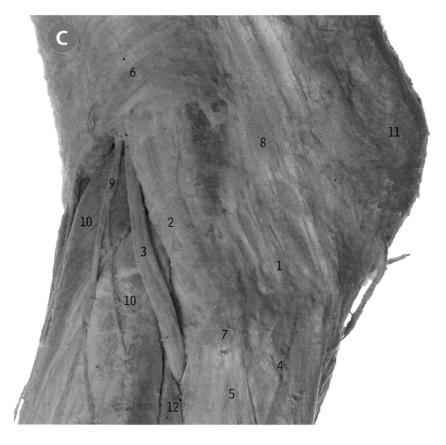

ⓒ Right knee

superficial dissection, from the lateral side

The fascia behind biceps (2) has been removed to show the common peroneal (fibular) nerve (3) passing downwards immediately behind the tendon, and then running between the adjacent borders of soleus (12) and peroneus longus (5), under cover of which it lies against the neck of the fibula. Minor superficial vessels and nerves have been removed.

1   Attachment of iliotibial tract to tibia
2   Biceps
3   Common peroneal (fibular) nerve
4   Deep fascia overlying extensor muscles
5   Deep fascia overlying peroneus (fibularis) longus
6   Fascia lata
7   Head of fibula
8   Iliotibial tract
9   Lateral cutaneous nerve of calf
10 Lateral head of gastrocnemius
11 Patella
12 Soleus

The iliotibial tract (8) is the thickened lateral part of the fascia lata (6). At its upper part the tensor fasciae latae and most of gluteus maximus are inserted into it.

Its subcutaneous position and contact with the neck of the fibula make the common peroneal (fibular) nerve (3) the most commonly injured nerve in the lower limb.

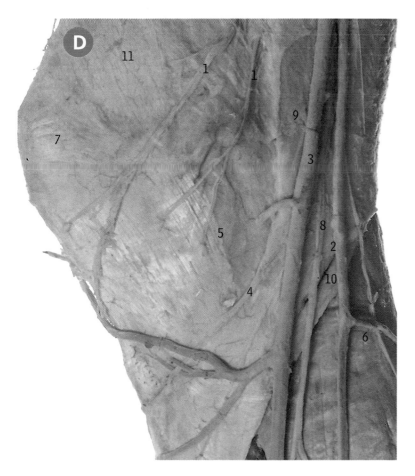

ⓓ Right knee

superficial dissection, from the medial side

The great saphenous vein (3) runs upwards about a hand's breadth behind the medial border of the patella (7). The saphenous nerve (8) becomes superficial between the tendons of sartorius (9) and gracilis (2), and its infrapatellar branch (4) curls forwards a little below the upper margin of the tibial condyle.

1   Branches of medial femoral cutaneous nerve
2   Gracilis
3   Great saphenous vein
4   Infrapatellar branch of saphenous nerve
5   Level of margin of medial condyle of tibia
6   Medial head of gastrocnemius
7   Patella
8   Saphenous nerve
9   Sartorius
10 Semitendinosus
11 Vastus medialis

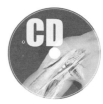

Right popliteal fossa *superficial dissections*

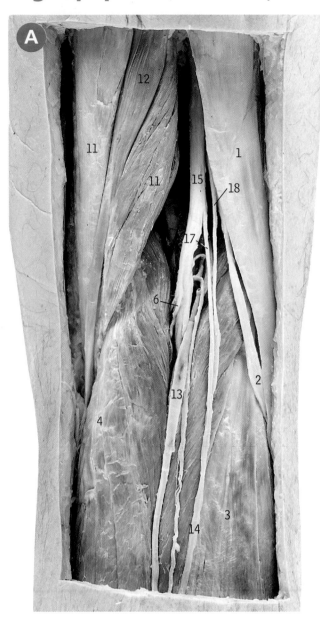

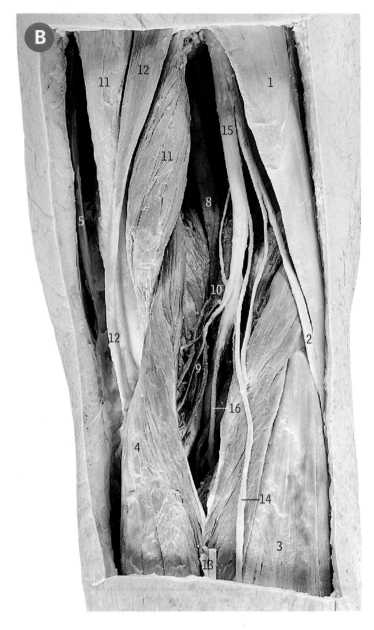

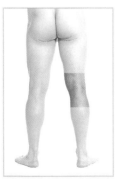

A Skin and fascia forming the roof of the diamond-shaped popliteal fossa and the fat within it have been removed but the small saphenous vein which pierces the fascia has been preserved. A high (proximal) union of the lateral and medial sural cutaneous nerves places the sural nerve in this field.

B Heads of gastrocnemius have been separated to show deeper structures.

1 Biceps femoris
2 Common peroneal (fibular) nerve
3 Gastrocnemius, lateral head
4 Gastrocnemius, medial head
5 Gracilis
6 Nerve to medial head of gastrocnemius
7 Plantaris
8 Popliteal artery
9 Popliteal vascular branches to gastrocnemius
10 Popliteal vein
11 Semimembranosus
12 Semitendinosus
13 Small saphenous vein
14 Sural nerve
15 Tibial nerve
16 Tibial nerve, muscular branches
17 Sural nerve, branch from tibial
18 Sural nerve, branch from common peroneal (fibular)

Popliteal fossa *progressive dissections*

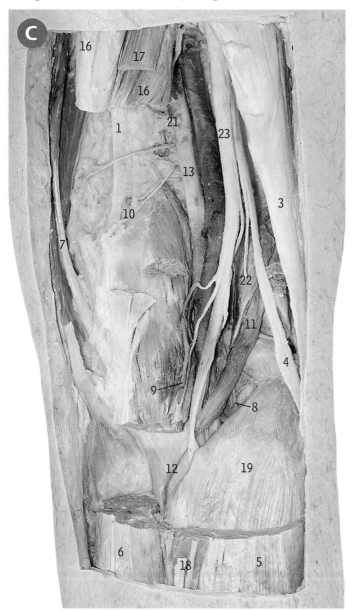

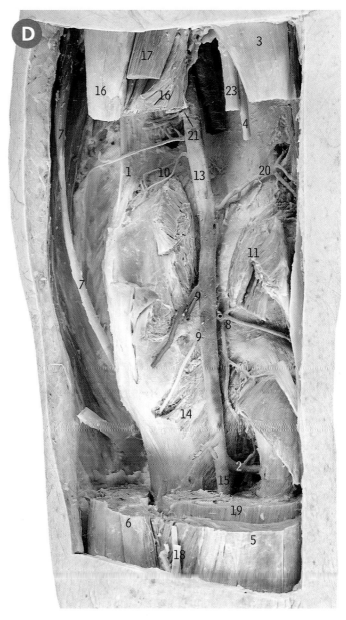

C
Removal of the semitendinosus, semimembranosus and most of the origins of the gastrocnemius reveals the plantaris and branches of the deeply situated popliteal artery and soleus.

D
Removal of the muscular boundaries of the popliteal fossa shows the popliteal artery, its genicular anastomoses and its terminal branches, the anterior and posterior tibial arteries.

1	Adductor magnus	**12**	Plantaris tendon
2	Anterior tibial artery	**13**	Popliteal artery
3	Biceps femoris	**14**	Popliteus
4	Common peroneal (fibular) nerve	**15**	Posterior tibial artery
5	Gastrocnemius, lateral head	**16**	Semimembranosus
6	Gastrocnemius, medial head	**17**	Semitendinosus
7	Gracilis	**18**	Short saphenous vein
8	Inferior lateral genicular artery	**19**	Soleus
9	Inferior medial genicular artery	**20**	Superior lateral genicular artery
10	Middle genicular artery	**21**	Superior medial genicular artery
11	Plantaris muscle	**22**	Sural nerve
		23	Tibial nerve

 Baker's cyst, popliteal aneurysm, see pp 355, 356.

Left knee joint *ligaments*

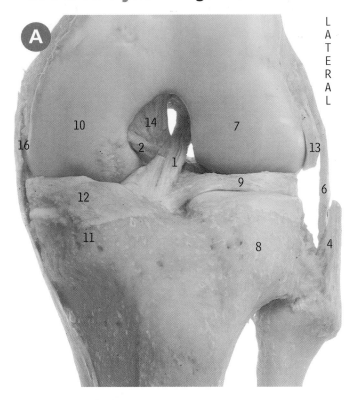

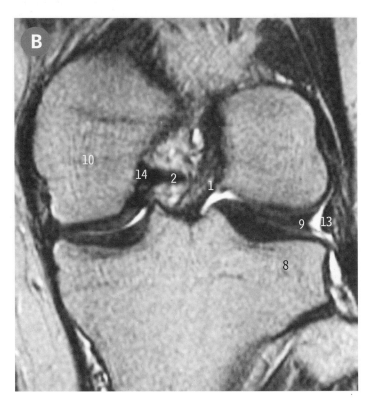

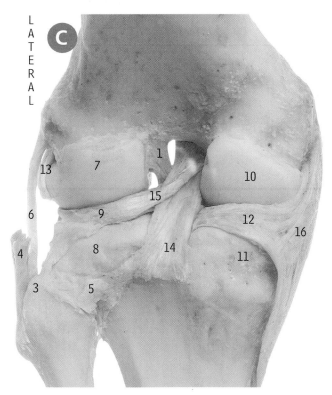

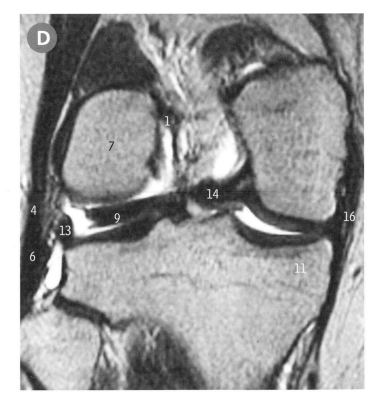

A from the front   **C** from behind

B coronal MR image   **D** coronal MR image

The capsule of the knee joint and all surrounding tissues have been removed, leaving only the ligaments of the joint, which is partially flexed.

A–D label key

1 Anterior cruciate ligament
2 Anterior meniscofemoral ligament
3 Apex of head of fibula
4 Biceps tendon
5 Capsule of superior tibiofemoral joint
6 Fibular collateral ligament (lateral)
7 Lateral condyle of femur
8 Lateral condyle of tibia
9 Lateral meniscus
10 Medial condyle of femur
11 Medial condyle of tibia
12 Medial meniscus
13 Popliteus tendon
14 Posterior cruciate ligament
15 Posterior meniscofemoral ligament
16 Tibial collateral ligament (medial)

The fibular collateral (lateral) ligament (A6) is a rounded cord about 5 cm long, passing from the lateral epicondyle of the femur to the head of the fibula just in front of its apex (C3), largely under cover of the tendon of biceps (C4).

The medial meniscus (E12 and F12) is attached to the deep part of the tibial collateral ligament (E19 and F20). This helps to anchor the meniscus but makes it liable to become trapped and torn by rotatory movements between the tibia and femur.

The lateral meniscus (A9) is not attached to the fibular collateral ligament (A6), but is attached posteriorly to the popliteus muscle (F5).

The tibial collateral (medial) ligament (E19) is a broad flat band about 12 cm long, passing from the medial epicondyle of the femur (E11) to the medial condyle of the tibia (E10) and an extensive area of the medial surface of the tibia below the condyle (as in the lower part of E).

The cruciate ligaments are named from their attachments to the tibia.

The anterior cruciate ligament (A1 and F1) passes upwards, backwards and laterally to be attached to the medial side of the lateral condyle of the femur (C7).

The posterior cruciate ligament (C14 and F13) passes upwards, forwards and medially to be attached to the lateral surface of the medial condyle of the femur (A10).

Left knee joint *ligaments*

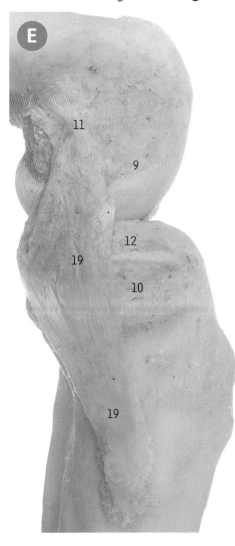

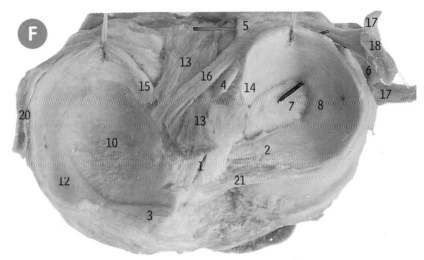

E from the medial side   **F** from above

The same specimen as in A and C is seen from the medial side in E, to show the broad tibial collateral ligament (19). F is the view looking down on the upper surface of the tibia after removing the femur by cutting through the capsule, the collateral ligaments, and the cruciate ligaments. The medial and lateral menisci (12 and 8) remain at the periphery of the articular surfaces of the tibial condyles. The horns of the menisci (3 and 15; 2 and 14) and the cruciate ligaments (1 and 13) are attached to the non-articular intercondylar area of the tibia. Compare with C on page 305.

1 Anterior cruciate ligament
2 Anterior horn of lateral meniscus
3 Anterior horn of medial meniscus
4 Anterior meniscofemoral ligament
5 Attachment of lateral meniscus to popliteus (with underlying marker)
6 Fibular collateral ligament
7 Lateral condyle of tibia
8 Lateral meniscus
9 Medial condyle of femur
10 Medial condyle of tibia
11 Medial epicondyle of femur
12 Medial meniscus
13 Posterior cruciate ligament
14 Posterior horn of lateral meniscus
15 Posterior horn of medial meniscus
16 Posterior meniscofemoral ligament
17 Tendon of biceps
18 Tendon of popliteus
19 Tibial collateral ligament
20 Tibial collateral ligament attached to medial meniscus
21 Transverse ligament

 Anterior cruciate ligament rupture, meniscal tears, see pp 355, 356.

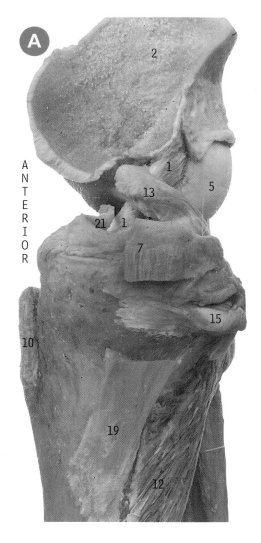

Right knee joint

A from the medial side with the medial femoral condyle removed

B sagittal MR image

Removal of the medial half of the lower end of the femur enables the X-shaped crossover of the cruciate ligaments to be seen; the anterior cruciate (1) is passing backwards and laterally, while the posterior cruciate (13) passes forwards and medially. The MR image in B shows the infrapatellar fat pad (3).

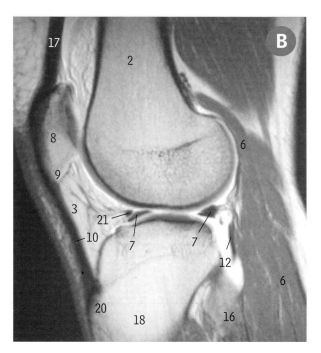

1 Anterior cruciate ligament	**8** Patella	**15** Semimembranosus
2 Femur	**9** Patellar apex	**16** Soleus
3 Infrapatellar fat pad	**10** Patellar ligament (tendon)	**17** Tendon of quadriceps
4 Intercondylar notch	**11** Popliteal artery and vein	**18** Tibia
5 Lateral condyle of femur	**12** Popliteus	**19** Tibial collateral ligament
6 Lateral head of gastrocnemius muscle	**13** Posterior cruciate ligament	**20** Tibial tubercle
7 Meniscus	**14** Posterior meniscofemoral ligament	**21** Transverse ligament (displaced backwards)

Left knee *arthroscopic views*

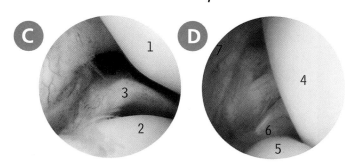

C anterolateral approach

D posteromedial approach

Reproduced with kind permission of David J. Dandy from *Current Problems in Orthopaedics: Arthroscopic Management of the Knee*, 2nd Edition, Churchill Livingstone

1 Lateral condyle of femur	**5** Medial meniscus
2 Lateral condyle of tibia	**6** Posterior cruciate ligament
3 Lateral meniscus	**7** Posterior part of capsule
4 Medial condyle of femur	

Suprapatellar bursitis, see p. 357.

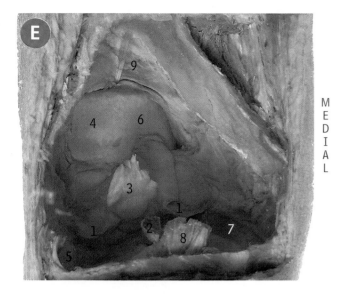

ⓔ Left knee joint

opened from behind with the femur removed

By looking into the joint from behind after removal of the femur, the articular surfaces of the patella (4 and 6) are seen, while below them are the alar and infrapatellar folds (1 and 3).

1　Alar fold
2　Anterior cruciate ligament
3　Infrapatellar fold (ligamentum mucosum)
4　Lateral articular surface of patella
5　Lateral meniscus
6　Medial articular surface of patella
7　Medial meniscus
8　Posterior cruciate ligament
9　Suprapatellar bursa (supported by glass rod)

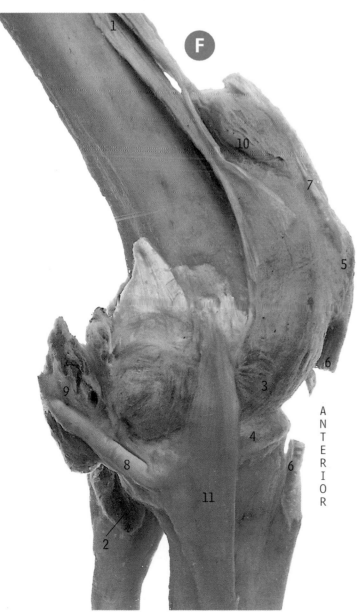

ⓕ Left knee joint

from the medial side, with synovial and bursal cavities injected

The resin injection has distended the synovial cavity of the joint (3) and extends into the suprapatellar bursa (10), the bursa round the popliteus tendon (2) and the semimembranosus bursa (9).

1　Articularis genu
2　Bursa of popliteus tendon
3　Capsule
4　Medial meniscus
5　Patella
6　Patellar ligament
7　Quadriceps tendon
8　Semimembranosus
9　Semimembranosus bursa
10　Suprapatellar bursa
11　Tibial collateral ligament

The suprapatellar bursa (F10) always communicates with the joint cavity. The bursa around the popliteus tendon (F2) usually does so. The semimembranosus bursa (F9) may do so.

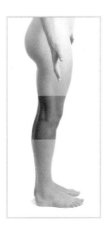

Knee *radiographs and arthroscopic views*

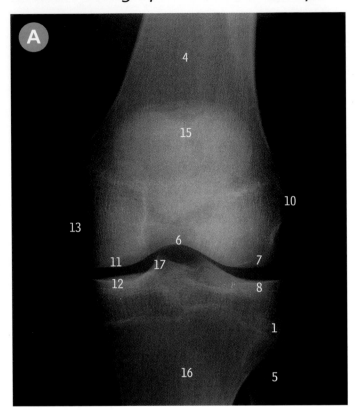

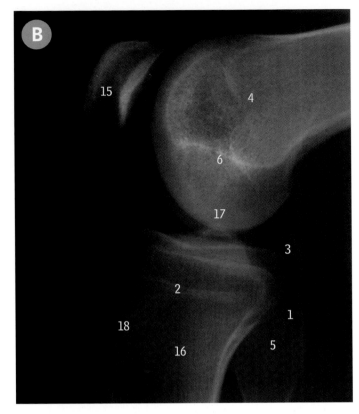

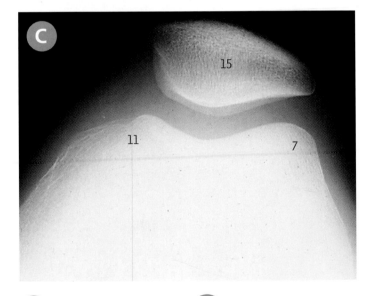

A from the front

B from the lateral side in partial flexion

C skyline view projection

D anterolateral approach

E lateral view of patella

In A the shadow of the patella (15) is superimposed on that of the femur. The regular space between the condyles of the femur and tibia (7 and 8, 11 and 12) is due to the thickness of the hyaline cartilage on the articulating surface, with the menisci at the periphery. In C with the knee flexed, the view should be compared with the bones seen on page 299, E, and the lateral edge of the patella (9) is seen in the arthroscopic view in E. (D and E reproduced with kind permission of David J Dandy from *Current Problems in Orthopaedics: Arthroscopic Management of the Knee*, 2nd Edition, Churchill Livingstone.)

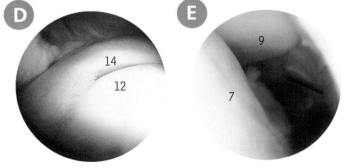

1 Apex (styloid process) of fibula
2 Epiphysial line
3 Fabella
4 Femur
5 Head of fibula
6 Intercondylar fossa
7 Lateral condyle of femur
8 Lateral condyle of tibia
9 Lateral edge of patella

10 Lateral epicondyle of femur
11 Medial condyle of femur
12 Medial condyle of tibia
13 Medial epicondyle of femur
14 Medial meniscus
15 Patella
16 Tibia
17 Tubercles of intercondylar eminence
18 Tuberosity of tibia

A Left leg *from the front and lateral side*

Most of the deep fascia has been removed, and segments of extensor digitorum longus (4) and peroneus (fibularis) longus (9) have been cut out to display the deep (3) and superficial (11) branches of the common peroneal (fibular) nerve just below the head of the fibula (6). The gap between tibialis anterior (12) and extensor digitorum longus (4) has been opened up to show the anterior tibial artery (1).

1 Anterior tibial artery overlying interosseous membrane
2 Branch of deep peroneal (fibular) nerve to tibialis anterior
3 Deep peroneal (fibular) nerve
4 Extensor digitorum longus
5 Extensor hallucis longus
6 Head of fibula
7 Lateral branch of superficial peroneal (fibular) nerve

8 Medial branch of superficial peroneal (fibular) nerve
9 Peroneus longus
10 Recurrent branch of common peroneal (fibular) nerve
11 Superficial peroneal (fibular) nerve
12 Tibialis anterior and overlying fascia
13 Tuberosity of tibia and patellar ligament

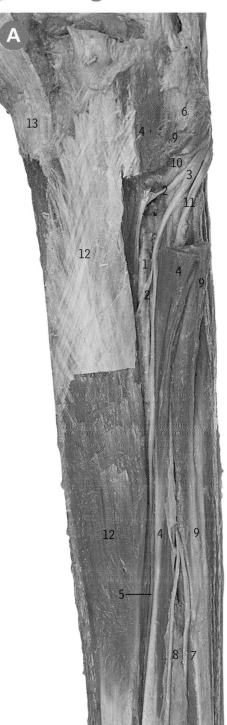

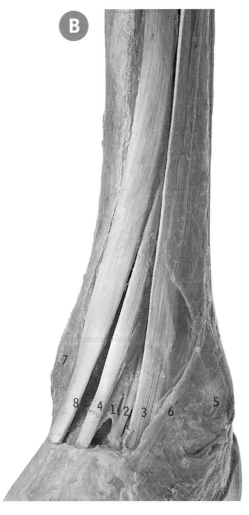

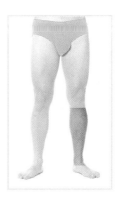

B Left lower leg and ankle

from the front and lateral side

1 Anterior tibial vessels
2 Deep peroneal (fibular) nerve
3 Extensor digitorum longus
4 Extensor hallucis longus
5 Lateral malleolus
6 Medial branch of superficial peroneal (fibular) nerve
7 Medial malleolus
8 Tibialis anterior

Common peroneal (fibular) nerve paralysis, deep peroneal (fibular) nerve paralysis, see p. 355.

Left knee and leg

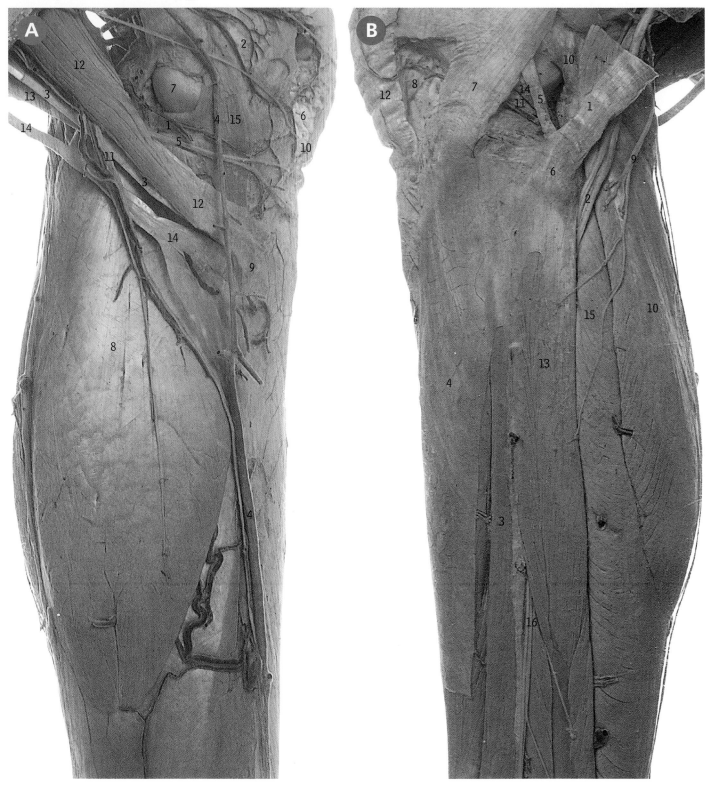

(A) *from the medial side and behind*

A small window has been cut in the capsule of the knee joint to show part of the medial condyle of the femur (7) and the medial meniscus (1).

1   Branch of saphenous artery overlying medial meniscus
2   Branches of superior medial genicular artery
3   Gracilis
4   Great saphenous vein
5   Infrapatellar branch of saphenous nerve
6   Infrapatellar fat pad
7   Medial condyle of femur (part of capsule removed)
8   Medial head of gastrocnemius
9   Medial surface of tibia
10 Patellar ligament
11 Saphenous nerve and artery
12 Sartorius
13 Semimembranosus
14 Semitendinosus
15 Tibial collateral ligament

(B) *from the lateral side*

A small window has been cut in the capsule of the knee joint to show the tendon of popliteus (14) passing deep to the fibular collateral ligament (5). The common peroneal (fibular) nerve (2) runs down behind biceps (1) to pass through the gap between peroneus (fibularis) longus (13) and soleus (15). The superficial peroneal (fibular) nerve becomes superficial between peroneus longus (13) and extensor digitorum longus (3).

1   Biceps
2   Common peroneal (fibular) nerve
3   Extensor digitorum longus
4   Fascia overlying tibialis anterior
5   Fibular collateral ligament
6   Head of fibula
7   Iliotibial tract
8   Infrapatellar fat pad
9   Lateral cutaneous nerve of calf
10 Lateral head of gastrocnemius
11 Lateral meniscus
12 Patellar ligament
13 Peroneus (fibularis) longus
14 Popliteus
15 Soleus
16 Superficial peroneal (fibular) nerve

Below knee level the great saphenous vein (A4) is accompanied by the saphenous nerve (A11).

In the calf the small saphenous vein (C7) is accompanied by the sural nerve (C9).

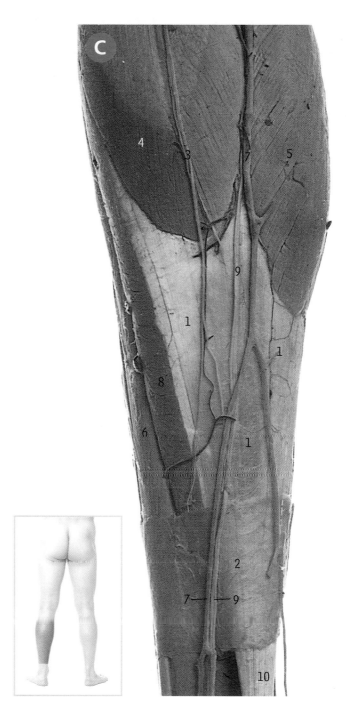

(C) **Left calf**
superficial dissection, from behind

1   Aponeurosis of gastrocnemius
2   Deep fascia
3   Lateral cutaneous nerve of calf
4   Lateral head of gastrocnemius
5   Medial head of gastrocnemius
6   Peroneus (fibularis) longus
7   Small saphenous vein
8   Soleus
9   Sural nerve
10 Tendocalcaneus (Achilles tendon)

Vein harvest for coronary artery bypass grafting (CABG), see p. 357.

Left leg and ankle *superficial veins and nerves*
(A) *from the medial side* (B) *from behind*

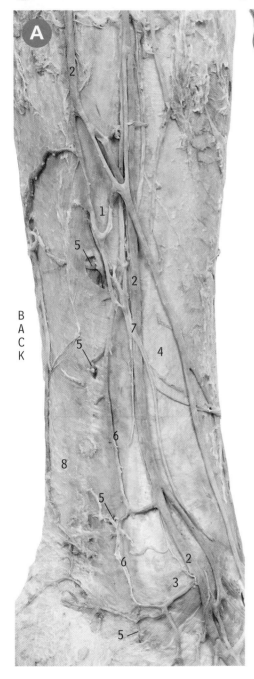

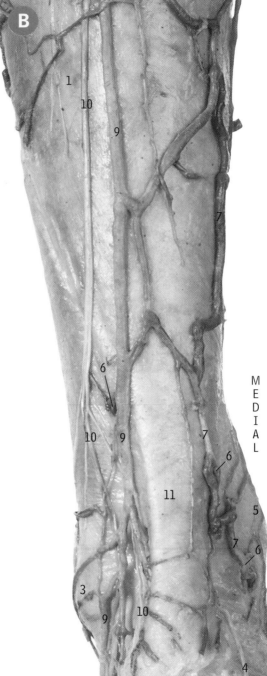

In B (a different specimen from that in A), the posterior arch vein (7) on the medial side is large and becoming varicose.

1 Deep fascia
2 Fibrofatty tissue of heel
3 Lateral malleolus
4 Medial calcanean nerve
5 Medial malleolus
6 Perforating vein
7 Posterior arch vein
8 Posterior surface of calcaneus
9 Small saphenous vein
10 Sural nerve
11 Tendocalcaneus (under fascia)

The perforating veins are communications between the superficial veins (outside the deep fascia) and the deep veins (inside the fascia). The commonest sites for them are just behind the tibia, behind the fibula and in the adductor canal. These communicating vessels possess valves which direct the blood flow from superficial to deep; venous return from the limb is then brought about by the pumping action of the deep muscles (which are all below the deep fascia). If the valves become incompetent or the deep veins blocked, pressure in the superficial veins increases and they become varicose (dilated and tortuous).

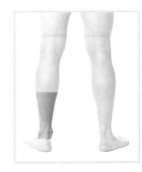

1 Deep fascia over soleus
2 Great saphenous vein
3 Medial malleolus
4 Medial (subcutaneous) surface of tibia
5 Perforating veins
6 Posterior arch vein
7 Saphenous nerve
8 Tendo calcaneus (Achilles tendon)

 Thrombophlebitis, see p. 357.

Left popliteal fossa and upper calf

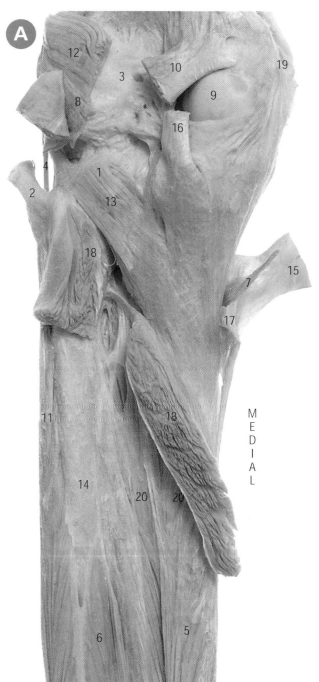

Left lower calf and ankle

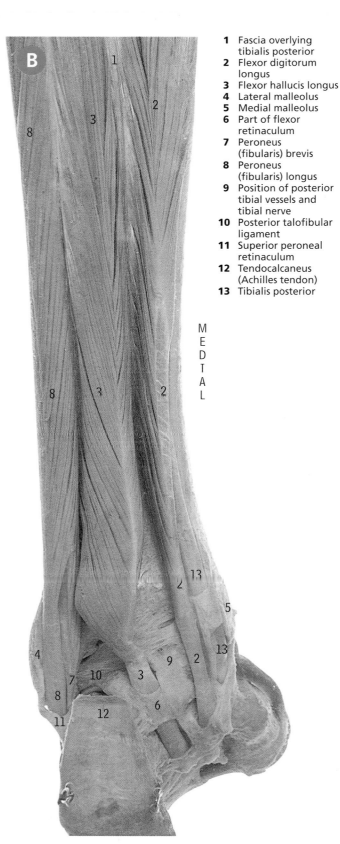

1 Fascia overlying tibialis posterior
2 Flexor digitorum longus
3 Flexor hallucis longus
4 Lateral malleolus
5 Medial malleolus
6 Part of flexor retinaculum
7 Peroneus (fibularis) brevis
8 Peroneus (fibularis) longus
9 Position of posterior tibial vessels and tibial nerve
10 Posterior talofibular ligament
11 Superior peroneal retinaculum
12 Tendocalcaneus (Achilles tendon)
13 Tibialis posterior

1 Attachment of popliteus to lateral meniscus
2 Biceps
3 Capsule of knee joint
4 Fibular collateral ligament
5 Flexor digitorum longus
6 Flexor hallucis longus
7 Gracilis
8 Lateral head of gastrocnemius
9 Medial condyle of femur
10 Medial head of gastrocnemius
11 Peroneus (fibularis) longus
12 Plantaris
13 Popliteus
14 Posterior surface of fibula (soleus removed)
15 Sartorius
16 Semimembranosus
17 Semitendinosus
18 Soleus
19 Tibial collateral ligament
20 Tibialis posterior

Left popliteal fossa and upper calf

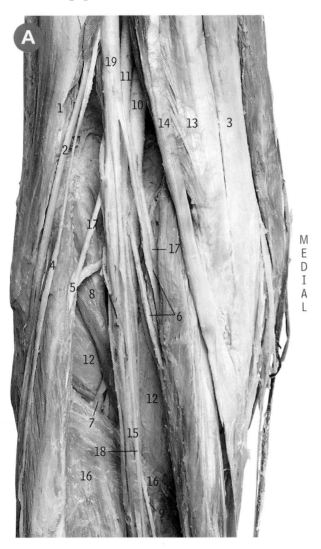

Left calf
deep dissection of muscles and arteries

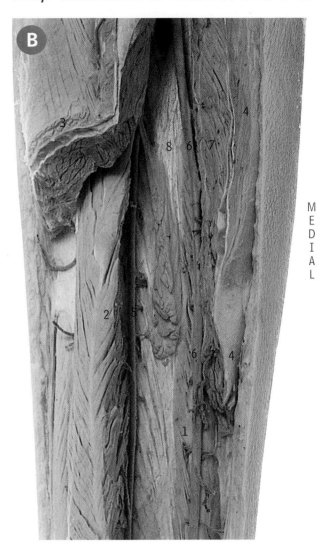

Gastrocnemius has been incised longitudinally and the two heads (6 and 5) split apart to reveal plantaris (8) and its thin tendon (9), popliteus (12) and the upper part of soleus (16).

1 Biceps	**9** Plantaris tendon
2 Common peroneal (fibular) nerve	**10** Popliteal artery
3 Gracilis	**11** Popliteal vein
4 Lateral cutaneous nerve of calf	**12** Popliteus
5 Lateral head of gastrocnemius and nerve	**13** Semimembranosus
6 Medial head of gastrocnemius and nerves	**14** Semitendinosus
7 Nerve to soleus	**15** Small saphenous vein (double)
8 Plantaris	**16** Soleus
	17 Sural artery
	18 Sural nerve
	19 Tibial nerve

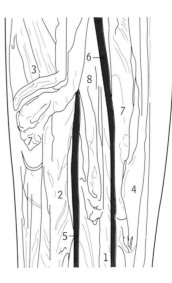

1	Flexor digitorum longus
2	Flexor hallucis longus
3	Lateral head of gastrocnemius
4	Medial head of gastrocnemius
5	Peroneal (fibular) artery
6	Posterior tibial artery
7	Soleus
8	Tibialis posterior

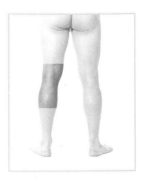

Left popliteal fossa and calf
deep dissection

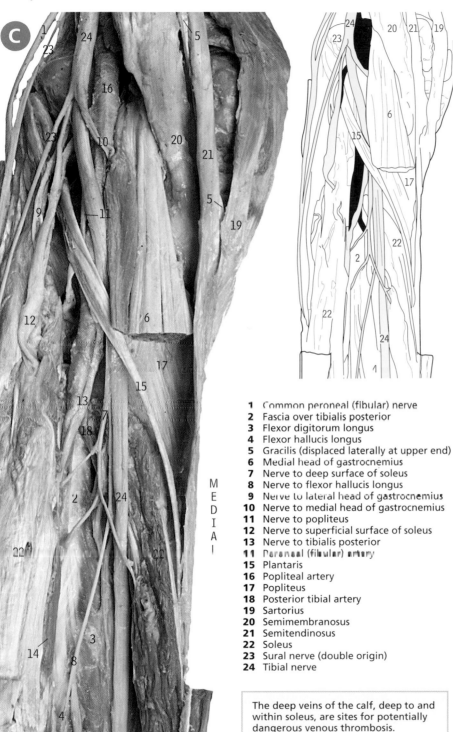

Popliteal arteriogram

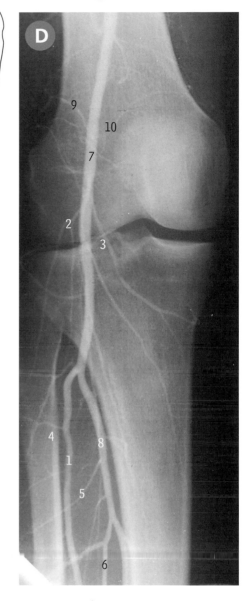

1 Common peroneal (fibular) nerve
2 Fascia over tibialis posterior
3 Flexor digitorum longus
4 Flexor hallucis longus
5 Gracilis (displaced laterally at upper end)
6 Medial head of gastrocnemius
7 Nerve to deep surface of soleus
8 Nerve to flexor hallucis longus
9 Nerve to lateral head of gastrocnemius
10 Nerve to medial head of gastrocnemius
11 Nerve to popliteus
12 Nerve to superficial surface of soleus
13 Nerve to tibialis posterior
14 Peroneal (fibular) artery
15 Plantaris
16 Popliteal artery
17 Popliteus
18 Posterior tibial artery
19 Sartorius
20 Semimembranosus
21 Semitendinosus
22 Soleus
23 Sural nerve (double origin)
24 Tibial nerve

The deep veins of the calf, deep to and within soleus, are sites for potentially dangerous venous thrombosis.

1 Anterior tibial artery
2 Inferior lateral genicular artery
3 Inferior medial genicular artery
4 Muscular branches of anterior tibial artery
5 Muscular branches of posterior tibial artery
6 Peroneal (fibular) artery
7 Popliteal artery
8 Posterior tibial artery
9 Superior lateral genicular artery
10 Superior medial genicular artery

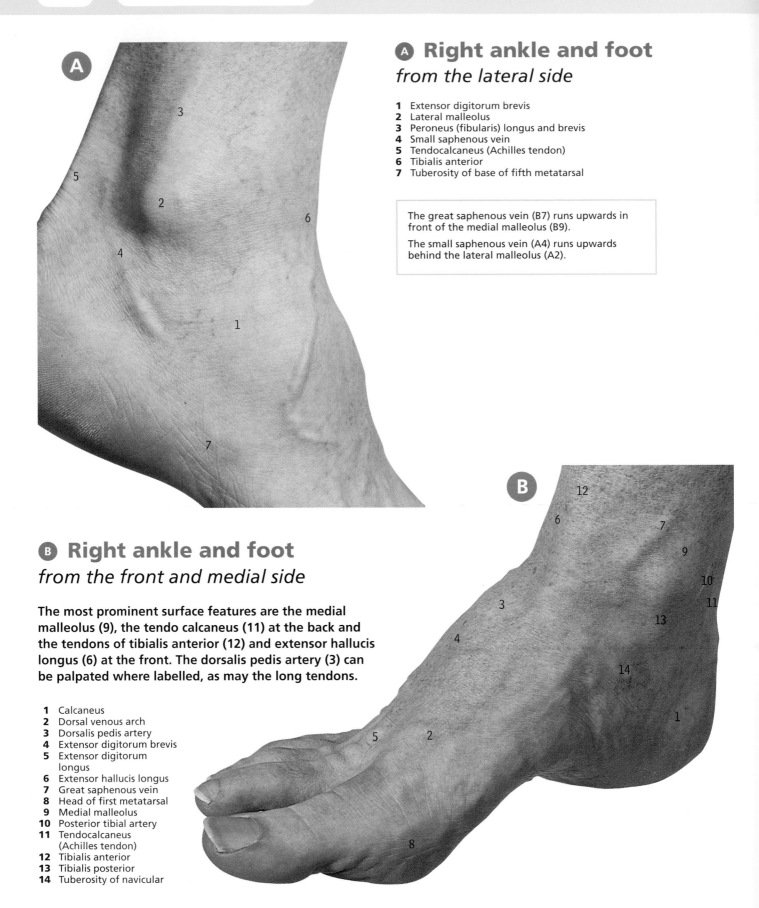

Ⓐ Right ankle and foot
from the lateral side

1 Extensor digitorum brevis
2 Lateral malleolus
3 Peroneus (fibularis) longus and brevis
4 Small saphenous vein
5 Tendocalcaneus (Achilles tendon)
6 Tibialis anterior
7 Tuberosity of base of fifth metatarsal

The great saphenous vein (B7) runs upwards in front of the medial malleolus (B9).

The small saphenous vein (A4) runs upwards behind the lateral malleolus (A2).

Ⓑ Right ankle and foot
from the front and medial side

The most prominent surface features are the medial malleolus (9), the tendo calcaneus (11) at the back and the tendons of tibialis anterior (12) and extensor hallucis longus (6) at the front. The dorsalis pedis artery (3) can be palpated where labelled, as may the long tendons.

1 Calcaneus
2 Dorsal venous arch
3 Dorsalis pedis artery
4 Extensor digitorum brevis
5 Extensor digitorum longus
6 Extensor hallucis longus
7 Great saphenous vein
8 Head of first metatarsal
9 Medial malleolus
10 Posterior tibial artery
11 Tendocalcaneus (Achilles tendon)
12 Tibialis anterior
13 Tibialis posterior
14 Tuberosity of navicular

Achilles tendon reflex, Achilles tendon rupture, venous cutdowns, see pp 355, 357.

ⓒ Right ankle and foot *from the lateral side*

Fascia has been removed but the thickenings that form the superior and inferior extensor retinacula (16 and 6) and the superior and inferior peroneal (fibular) retinacula (17 and 7) have been preserved. The synovial sheaths of tendons have been emphasized by blue tissue.

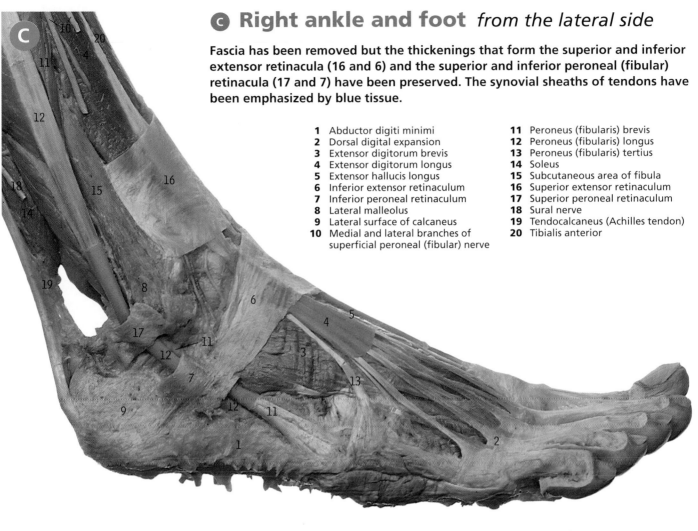

1 Abductor digiti minimi
2 Dorsal digital expansion
3 Extensor digitorum brevis
4 Extensor digitorum longus
5 Extensor hallucis longus
6 Inferior extensor retinaculum
7 Inferior peroneal retinaculum
8 Lateral malleolus
9 Lateral surface of calcaneus
10 Medial and lateral branches of superficial peroneal (fibular) nerve

11 Peroneus (fibularis) brevis
12 Peroneus (fibularis) longus
13 Peroneus (fibularis) tertius
14 Soleus
15 Subcutaneous area of fibula
16 Superior extensor retinaculum
17 Superior peroneal retinaculum
18 Sural nerve
19 Tendocalcaneus (Achilles tendon)
20 Tibialis anterior

ⓓ Right ankle and foot *from the medial side*

1 Abductor hallucis
2 Extensor hallucis longus
3 Flexor digitorum longus
4 Flexor hallucis longus
5 Flexor retinaculum
6 Inferior extensor retinaculum (lower band)
7 Inferior extensor retinaculum (upper band)
8 Medial calcanean nerve
9 Medial malleolus

10 Medial surface of tibia
11 Plantaris tendon
12 Posterior surface of calcaneus
13 Posterior tibial artery and venae comitantes
14 Soleus
15 Tendocalcaneus (Achilles tendon)
16 Tibial nerve
17 Tibialis anterior
18 Tibialis posterior

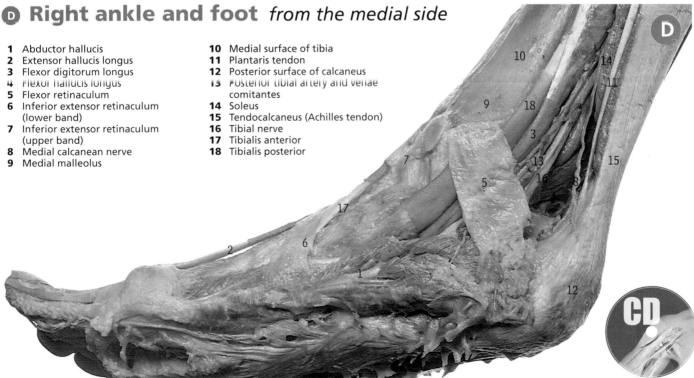

Right lower leg and ankle
from the medial side and behind

Right ankle and sole
from the medial side and below

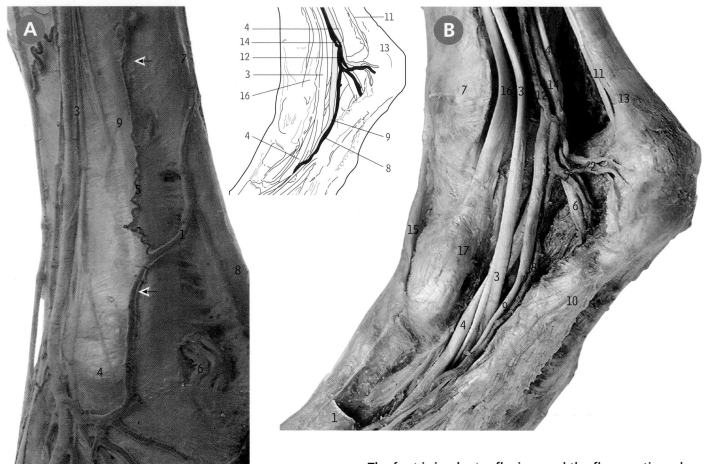

The deep fascia remains intact apart from a small window cut to show the position of the posterior tibial vessels and tibial nerve (6). The great saphenous vein (3) runs upwards in front of the medial malleolus (4) with the posterior arch vein (5) behind it. The arrows indicate common levels for perforating veins (page 340, A5 and B6).

1 Communication with small saphenous vein
2 Dorsal venous arch
3 Great saphenous vein and saphenous nerve
4 Medial malleolus
5 Posterior arch vein
6 Posterior tibial vessels and tibial nerve
7 Small saphenous vein
8 Tendocalcaneus (Achilles tendon)
9 Tibialis posterior and flexor digitorum longus underlying deep fascia

The foot is in plantar flexion, and the flexor retinaculum and most of abductor hallucis (1) have been removed to show how the tendon of flexor hallucis longus (4) passes deep to flexor digitorum longus (3) in the sole to run towards the great toe.

1 Abductor hallucis
2 Calcanean nerves and vessels
3 Flexor digitorum longus
4 Flexor hallucis longus
5 Lateral plantar artery
6 Lateral plantar nerve
7 Medial malleolus
8 Medial plantar artery
9 Medial plantar nerve
10 Plantar aponeurosis overlying flexor digitorum brevis
11 Plantaris tendon
12 Posterior tibial artery
13 Tendocalcaneus (Achilles tendon)
14 Tibial nerve
15 Tibialis anterior
16 Tibialis posterior
17 Tuberosity of navicular

Varicose veins, see p. 357.

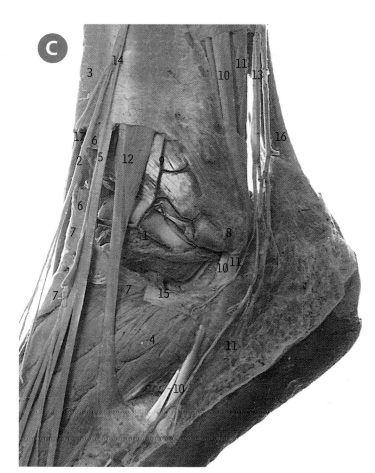

© Left ankle and foot
from the front and lateral side

The foot is plantar flexed and part of the capsule of the ankle joint has been removed to show the talus (1). The tendons of peroneus tertius (12) and extensor digitorum longus (5) lie superficial to extensor digitorum brevis (4). The sural nerve and small saphenous vein (13) pass behind the lateral malleolus (8).

1 Anterior lateral malleolar artery overlying talus (ankle joint capsule removed)
2 Anterior tibial vessels and deep peroneal (fibular) nerve
3 Deep fascia forming superior extensor retinaculum
4 Extensor digitorum brevis
5 Extensor digitorum longus
6 Extensor hallucis longus
7 Inferior extensor retinaculum (partly removed)
8 Lateral malleolus
9 Perforating branch of peroneal artery
10 Peroneus (fibularis) brevis
11 Peroneus (fibularis) longus
12 Peroneus (fibularis) tertius
13 Small saphenous vein and sural nerve
14 Superficial peroneal (fibular) nerve
15 Tarsal sinus
16 Tendocalcaneus (Achilles tendon)
17 Tibialis anterior

Left ankle

Ⓓ cross section
Ⓔ axial MR image

This section, looking down from above, emphasizes the positions of tendons, vessels and nerves in the ankle region. The talus (18) is in the centre, with the medial malleolus (9) on the left of the picture and the lateral malleolus (8) on the right. The great saphenous vein (7) and saphenous nerve (15) are in front of the medial malleolus, with the tendon of tibialis posterior (22) immediately behind it. The small saphenous vein (16) and the sural nerve (17) are behind the lateral malleolus, with the tendons of peroneus (fibularis) longus (11) and peroneus (fibularis) brevis (10) intervening. At the front of the ankle the dorsalis pedis vessels (2) and deep peroneal (fibular) nerve (1) are between the tendons of extensor hallucis longus (4) and extensor digitorum longus (3). Behind the medial malleolus (9) and tibialis posterior (22), the posterior tibial vessels (14) and tibial nerve (20) are between the tendons of flexor digitorum longus (5) and flexor hallucis longus (6).

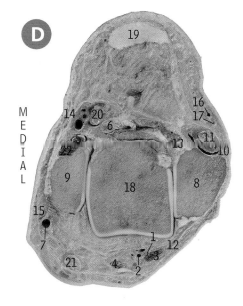

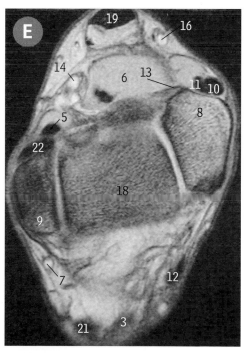

1 Deep peroneal (fibular) nerve
2 Dorsalis pedis artery and venae comitantes
3 Extensor digitorum longus
4 Extensor hallucis longus
5 Flexor digitorum longus
6 Flexor hallucis longus
7 Great saphenous vein
8 Lateral malleolus of fibula
9 Medial malleolus of tibia
10 Peroneus (fibularis) brevis
11 Peroneus (fibularis) longus

12 Peroneus (fibularis) tertius
13 Posterior talofibular ligament
14 Posterior tibial artery and venae comitantes
15 Saphenous nerve
16 Small saphenous vein
17 Sural nerve
18 Talus
19 Tendocalcaneus (Achilles tendon)
20 Tibial nerve
21 Tibialis anterior
22 Tibialis posterior

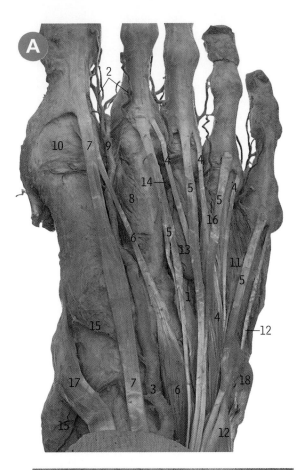

Ⓐ Dorsum of the right foot

1 Arcuate artery	**11** Fourth dorsal interosseous
2 Digital arteries	**12** Peroneus (fibularis) tertius
3 Dorsalis pedis artery	**13** Second dorsal interosseous
4 Extensor digitorum brevis	**14** Second dorsal metatarsal artery
5 Extensor digitorum longus	**15** Tarsal arteries
6 Extensor hallucis brevis	**16** Third dorsal interosseous
7 Extensor hallucis longus	**17** Tibialis anterior
8 First dorsal interosseous	**18** Tuberosity of base of fifth
9 First dorsal metatarsal artery	metatarsal and peroneus brevis
10 First metatarsophalangeal joint	

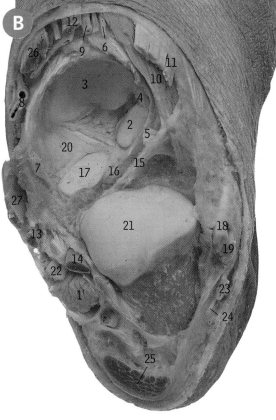

Ⓑ Right talocalcanean and talocalcaneonavicular joints

The talus has been removed to show the articular surfaces of the calcaneus (21, 17 and 2), navicular (3) and plantar calcaneonavicular (spring) ligament (20).

1 Abductor hallucis	**15** Inferior extensor retinaculum
2 Anterior articular surface on calcaneus for talus	**16** Interosseous talocalcanean ligament
3 Articular surface on navicular for talus	**17** Middle articular surface on calcaneus for talus
4 Calcaneonavicular part of bifurcate ligament	**18** Peroneus (fibularis) brevis
5 Cervical ligament	**19** Peroneus (fibularis) longus
6 Deep peroneal (fibular) nerve	**20** Plantar calcaneonavicular (spring) ligament
7 Deltoid ligament	**21** Posterior articular surface on calcaneus for talus
8 Dorsal venous arch	**22** Posterior tibial vessels and medial and lateral plantar nerves
9 Dorsalis pedis artery and vena comitans	**23** Small saphenous vein
10 Extensor digitorum brevis	**24** Sural nerve
11 Extensor digitorum longus	**25** Tendocalcaneus (Achilles tendon)
12 Extensor hallucis longus	**26** Tibialis anterior
13 Flexor digitorum longus	**27** Tibialis posterior
14 Flexor hallucis longus	

Clinicians sometimes use the term subtalar joint as a combined name for both the talocalcanean joint and the talocalcanean part of the talocalcaneonavicular joint, because it is at both these joints beneath the talus that most of the movements of inversion and eversion of the foot occur.

Deltoid ligament rupture, see p. 355.

Left ankle and foot *ligaments*

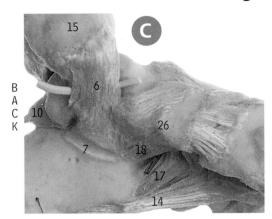

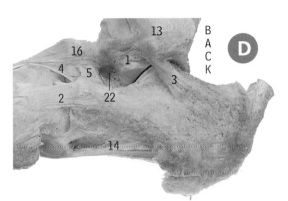

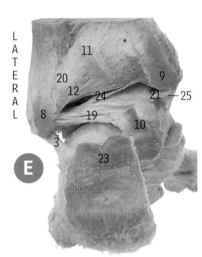

C from the medial side
D from the lateral side
E from behind

In C the marker below the medial malleolus (15) passes between the superficial and deep parts of the deltoid ligament (6). The marker below the tuberosity of the navicular (26) passes between the plantar calcaneonavicular (spring) and calcaneocuboid (short plantar) ligaments (18 and 17).

1 Anterior talofibular ligament
2 Calcaneocuboid part of bifurcate ligament
3 Calcaneofibular ligament
4 Calcaneonavicular part of bifurcate ligament
5 Cervical ligament
6 Deltoid ligament
7 Groove below sustentaculum tali for flexor hallucis longus
8 Groove on lateral malleolus for peroneus (fibularis) brevis
9 Groove on medial malleolus for tibialis posterior
10 Groove on talus for flexor hallucis longus
11 Groove on tibia for flexor hallucis longus
12 Inferior transverse ligament
13 Lateral malleolus
14 Long plantar ligament
15 Medial malleolus
16 Neck of talus
17 Plantar calcaneocuboid (short plantar) ligament
18 Plantar calcaneonavicular (spring) ligament
19 Posterior talofibular ligament
20 Posterior tibiofibular ligament
21 Posterior tibiotalar part of deltoid ligament
22 Tarsal sinus
23 Tendocalcaneus (Achilles tendon)
24 Tibial slip of posterior talofibular ligament
25 Tibiocalcanean part of deltoid ligament
26 Tuberosity of navicular

F Left foot *sagittal section, from the right*

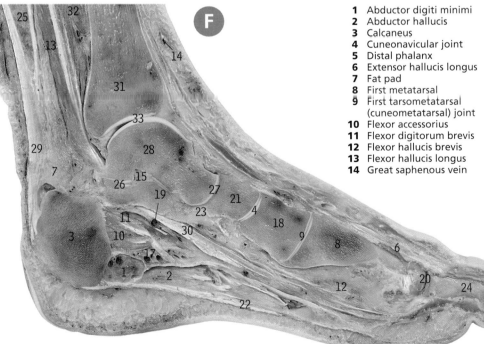

1 Abductor digiti minimi
2 Abductor hallucis
3 Calcaneus
4 Cuneonavicular joint
5 Distal phalanx
6 Extensor hallucis longus
7 Fat pad
8 First metatarsal
9 First tarsometatarsal (cuneometatarsal) joint
10 Flexor accessorius
11 Flexor digitorum brevis
12 Flexor hallucis brevis
13 Flexor hallucis longus
14 Great saphenous vein
15 Interosseous talocalcanean ligament
16 Interphalangeal joint
17 Lateral plantar nerve and vessels
18 Medial cuneiform
19 Medial plantar artery
20 Metatarsophalangeal joint of great toe
21 Navicular
22 Plantar aponeurosis
23 Plantar calcaneonavicular (spring) ligament
24 Proximal phalanx
25 Soleus muscle
26 Talocalcanean (subtalar) joint
27 Talonavicular part of talocalcaneonavicular joint
28 Talus
29 Tendocalcaneus (Achilles tendon)
30 Tendon of flexor hallucis
31 Tibia
32 Tibialis posterior muscle
33 Tibiotalal part of ankle joint

Sprained ankle, see p. 357.

Sole of the left foot

A *plantar aponeurosis* **B** *superficial neuromuscular layer*

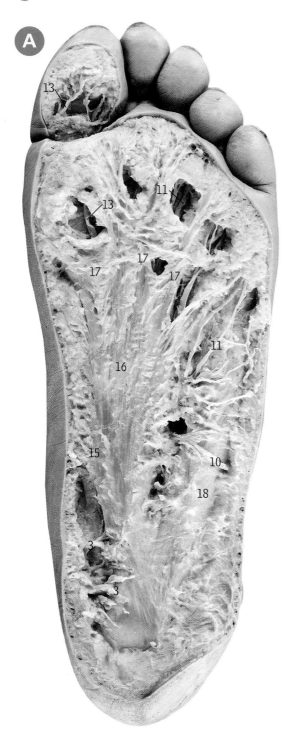

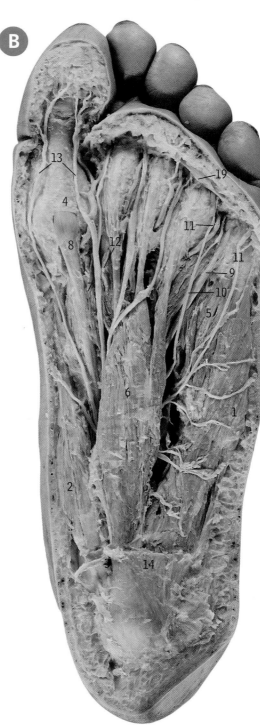

1	Abductor digiti minimi
2	Abductor hallucis
3	Calcaneal neurovascular bundle
4	Fibrous flexor sheath
5	Flexor digiti minimi brevis
6	Flexor digitorum brevis
7	Flexor hallucis brevis
8	Flexor hallucis longus
9	Lateral plantar artery
10	Lateral plantar nerve
11	Lateral plantar nerve, digital branches
12	Lumbrical
13	Medial plantar nerve, digital branches
14	Plantar aponeurosis
15	Plantar aponeurosis, overlying abductor hallucis
16	Plantar aponeurosis, overlying flexor digitorum brevis
17	Plantar aponeurosis, digital slips
18	Plantar aponeurosis, overlying abductor digiti minimi
19	Superficial transverse metatarsal ligament

Removal of the plantar skin reveals the plantar aponeurosis with thick central and digital slips and thin lateral and medial parts.

Deep to the plantar aponeurosis lie the superficial plantar nerves, arteries and muscles.

 Flat foot (pes planus), plantar fasciitis, see p. 356.

Sole of the left foot

C *after removal of flexor digitorum brevis*
D *after removal of flexor digitorum longus*

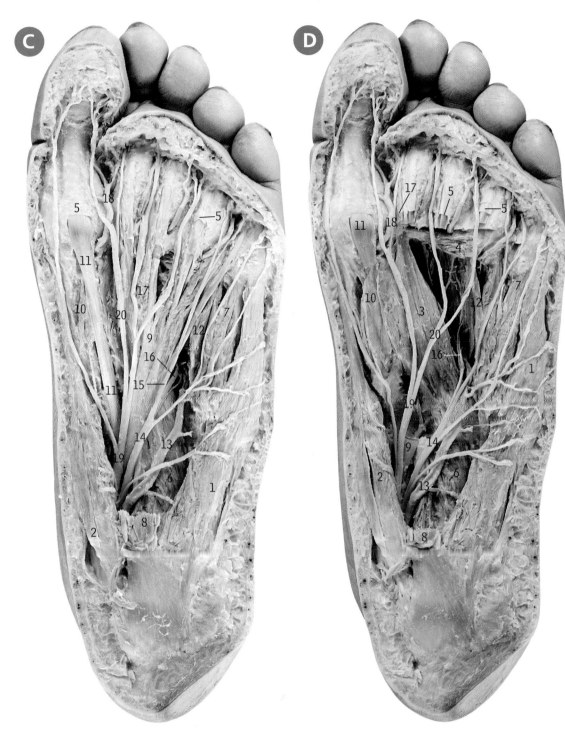

1 Abductor digiti minimi
2 Abductor hallucis
3 Adductor hallucis, oblique head
4 Adductor hallucis, transverse head
5 Fibrous sheath, flexors
6 Flexor accessorius (Quadratus plantae)
7 Flexor digiti minimi brevis
8 Flexor digitorum brevis (cut)
9 Flexor digitorum longus
10 Flexor hallucis brevis
11 Flexor hallucis longus
12 Interossei
13 Lateral plantar artery
14 Lateral plantar nerve
15 Lateral plantar nerve, common digital branch
16 Lateral plantar nerve, deep branch
17 Lumbrical
18 Medial plantar artery
19 Medial plantar nerve
20 Medial plantar nerve, common digital branch

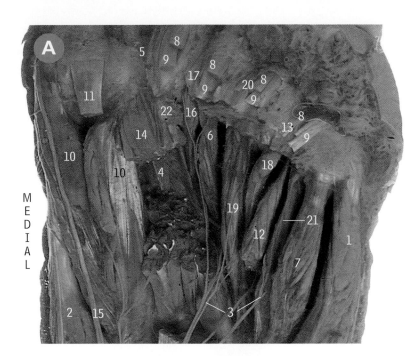

Ⓐ Sole of the left foot
deep muscles, interossei

1 Abductor digiti minimi
2 Abductor hallucis
3 Branches of deep branch of lateral plantar nerve
4 First dorsal interosseous
5 First lumbrical
6 First plantar interosseous
7 Flexor digiti minimi brevis
8 Flexor digitorum brevis
9 Flexor digitorum longus
10 Flexor hallucis brevis
11 Flexor hallucis longus
12 Fourth dorsal interosseous
13 Fourth lumbrical
14 Oblique head of adductor hallucis
15 Plantar digital nerve of great toe
16 Second dorsal interosseous
17 Second lumbrical
18 Second plantar interosseous
19 Third dorsal interosseous
20 Third lumbrical
21 Third plantar interosseous
22 Transverse head of adductor hallucis

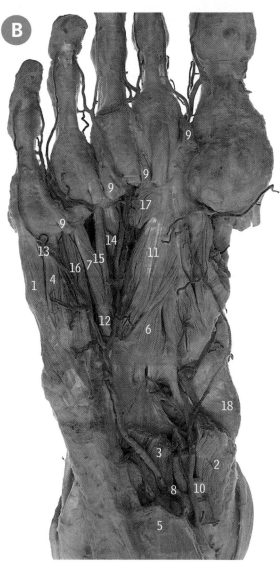

Ⓑ Sole of the right foot
plantar arch

Most of the flexor muscles and tendons have been removed to show the lateral plantar artery (8) crossing flexor accessorius (quadratus plantae) (3) to become the plantar arch (12) which would lie deep to the flexor tendons.

1 Abductor digiti minimi
2 Abductor hallucis
3 Flexor accessorius (quadratus plantae)
4 Flexor digiti minimi brevis
5 Flexor digitorum brevis
6 Flexor hallucis brevis
7 Fourth dorsal interosseous
8 Lateral plantar artery
9 Lumbrical
10 Medial plantar artery and nerve
11 Oblique head of adductor hallucis
12 Plantar arch
13 Plantar digital artery
14 Plantar metatarsal artery
15 Second plantar interosseous
16 Third plantar interosseous
17 Transverse head of adductor hallucis
18 Tuberosity of navicular

Sole of the left foot **C** *ligaments and tendons* **D** *ligaments*

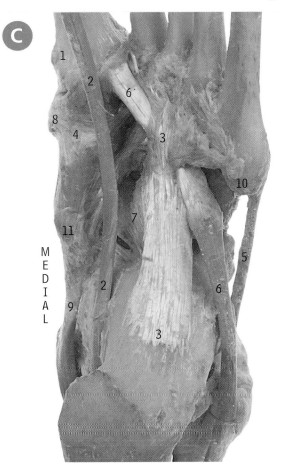

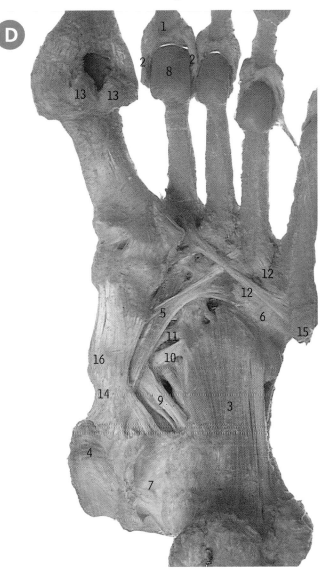

The anterior end of the long plantar ligament (3) forms with the groove of the cuboid (D6) a tunnel for the peroneus (fibularis) longus tendon (6) which runs to the medial cuneiform (4) and the base of the first metatarsal (1).

1 Base of first metatarsal
2 Flexor hallucis longus
3 Long plantar ligament
4 Medial cuneiform
5 Peroneus (fibularis) brevis
6 Peroneus (fibularis) longus
7 Plantar calcaneocuboid (short plantar) ligament
8 Tibialis anterior
9 Tibialis posterior
10 Tuberosity of base of fifth metatarsal
11 Tuberosity of navicular

The plantar calcaneonavicular ligament (D9), commonly called the spring ligament, is one of the most important in the foot. It stretches between the sustentaculum tali (D7) and the tuberosity of the navicular (D16), blending on its medial side with the deltoid ligament of the ankle joint and supporting on the upper surface part of the head of the talus.

The anterior end of the long plantar ligament (3) has been removed to show the groove for peroneus longus on the cuboid (6).

1 Base of proximal phalanx
2 Collateral ligament of metatarsophalangeal joint
3 Deep fibres of long plantar ligament
4 Deltoid ligament
5 Fibrous slip from tibialis posterior
6 Groove on cuboid for peroneus longus
7 Groove on sustentaculum tali for flexor hallucis longus
8 Head of second metatarsal
9 Plantar calcaneonavicular (spring) ligament
10 Plantar cuboideonavicular ligament
11 Plantar cuneonavicular ligament
12 Plantar metatarsal ligament
13 Sesamoid bone
14 Tibialis posterior
15 Tuberosity of base of fifth metatarsal
16 Tuberosity of navicular

Ankle Ⓐ *anteroposterior projection* Ⓑ *calcaneus, axial projection*

1 Calcaneus
2 Cuboid
3 Fibula
4 Head of talus
5 Lateral cuneiform
6 Lateral malleolus of fibula
7 Lateral tubercle of talus
8 Medial malleolus
9 Medial malleolus of tibia
10 Medial tubercle of talus
11 Navicular
12 Region of inferior tibiofibular joint
13 Sustentaculum tali of calcaneus
14 Talus
15 Tibia
16 Tuberosity of base of fifth metatarsal

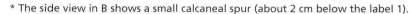

* The side view in B shows a small calcaneal spur (about 2 cm below the label 1).

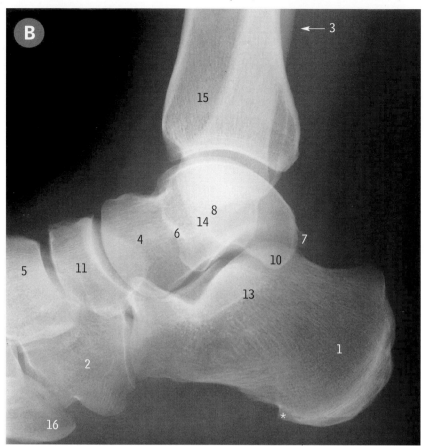

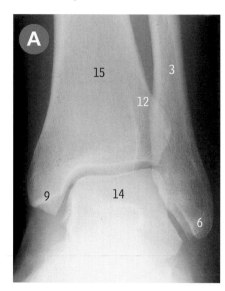

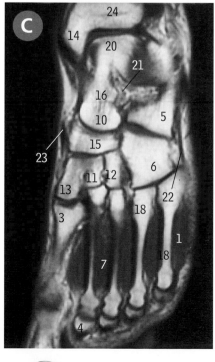

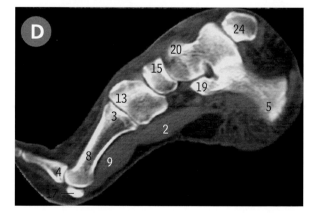

Foot

Ⓒ *oblique axial MR image*

Ⓓ *sagittal CT through hallux*

1 Abductor digiti minimi muscle
2 Abductor hallucis
3 Base of metatarsal
4 Base of proximal phalanx
5 Calcaneus
6 Cuboid
7 Dorsal interossei muscle
8 First metatarsal
9 Flexor digitorum brevis
10 Head of talus
11 Intermediate cuneiform
12 Lateral cuneiform
13 Medial cuneiform
14 Medial malleolus
15 Navicular
16 Neck of talus
17 Sesamoid bone in flexor hallucis brevis
18 Shaft of metatarsal
19 Sustentaculum tali of calcaneus
20 Talus
21 Tarsal sinus
22 Tendon of peroneus brevis muscle
23 Tendon of tibialis anterior muscle
24 Tibia

 Pott's fracture (ankle), see p. 356.

Lower limb
Clinical notes

Achilles tendon reflex (ankle jerk) is elicited by tapping the Achilles tendon with a patellar hammer and noting plantar flexion, a good test of the S1 segment of the spinal cord. (page 344)

Achilles tendon rupture. The Achilles tendon / tendocalcaneus (the weak point in Achilles' anatomy, as he was held by the heel when dipped in the River Styx) is the combined calcaneal insertion of the gastrocnemius and soleus muscles and occasionally the plantaris tendon. Rupture is usually due to an acute contraction in an unexercised muscle. Rupture may be partial or complete; conservative treatment is adequate for the partial tears but surgery is normally required for complete rupture. (page 344)

Anterior cruciate ligament rupture may occur after violent abduction and twisting of the knee (sliding tackle in soccer) which tears the medial meniscus and the anterior cruciate ligament. This is tested clinically by the 'drawer test', moving the tibia with respect to the femur – excessive anterior movement is indicative of an anterior cruciate ligament tear. (page 333)

Avascular necrosis of the head of the femur can occur following subcapital fractures of the femoral neck or less commonly with transcervical fractures. In the young the femoral head receives an abundant blood supply from the ligamentum teres and the obturator artery. In old age this supply is insufficient to maintain the head of the femur, most of the blood coming from anastomoses along the retinacular fibres of the capsule of the neck which are interrupted in these fractures. (page 325)

Avulsion of the tibial tuberosity (Osgood–Schlatter disease) is seen in late childhood when a small part of the upper tibial epiphysis to which the ligamentum patellae is attached is pulled superiorly. (page 304)

Baker's cyst is a large swelling in the popliteal fossa due to herniation of synovial membrane from the knee joint. It can be mistaken for a popliteal aneurysm and on occasions may rupture, allowing fluid to track down the calf muscles where it may be mistaken for deep venous thrombosis of the calf. (page 331)

Common peroneal (fibular) nerve paralysis is normally the result of trauma or pressure on the neck of the fibula, often following a fracture when the lower leg is put in a cast. Pressure on the common peroneal (fibular) nerve will denervate the anterior and lateral compartments of the lower leg, causing sensory loss on the lateral shin and dorsum of the foot and motor loss which makes it impossible to evert and dorsiflex the foot (foot drop). Patients with foot drop scuff their toes on the ground, so this nerve lesion can often be diagnosed by looking at the patient's shoes or gait. (page 337)

Deep peroneal (fibular) nerve paralysis. The deep peroneal (fibular) nerve supplies the anterior tibial compartment and damage is often due to trauma or compression in this compartment. The result is numbness over the dorsum of the foot in the region of the first web space and an inability to dorsiflex the foot with extensor digitorum longus. (page 337)

Deltoid ligament rupture. The strong deltoid ligament attaches the medial malleolus to the talus, navicular and calcaneus and also connects to the spring ligament to maintain the medial longitudinal arch. It is occasionally torn in severe twisting injuries, such as when a ballerina or ski jumper falls from a normally controlled position. (page 348)

Dislocation of the patella is most commonly seen as a lateral dislocation in young women or overweight young boys who have a wide pelvis. Anatomically, it is often due to a flat lateral femoral condyle, an abnormality of the knee (genu valgum) or weakness in the vastus medialis (lower fibres). (page 299)

Femoral artery catheterization. The femoral artery lies in the midinguinal region just below the inguinal ligament. It is here that catheters are passed into the femoral artery for catheterization of abdominopelvic and thoracic structures and it is a site where arterial blood can be obtained for gas analysis. (page 322)

Femoral hernia (1) is a protrusion of peritoneum and/or abdominal contents through the femoral ring into the thigh. The swelling usually lies inferior and lateral to the pubic tubercle. (page 320)

Femoral hernia (2), a protrusion through the femoral canal, has the lacunar ligament medially, the inguinal ligament anteriorly, the pectineal ligament posteriorly and the femoral vein laterally. It is a common cause of a strangulated hernia and tends to be seen more commonly in women, who have a wider pelvis and a slightly larger femoral canal. The swelling usually lies lateral and inferior to the pubic tubercle. (page 322)

Femoral nerve paralysis, the result of pressure on the roots of the femoral nerve in high lumbar disc lesions or compression beneath the inguinal ligament by a tumour or swelling within the psoas muscle, presents clinically as quadriceps weakness or atrophy and makes walking downstairs extremely difficult. Weakness in these muscles may lead to instability of the knee joint. Quadriceps exercises are the most important physiotherapy for any knee pathology or femoral nerve damage. (page 321)

Femoral vein catheterization. Lying just medial to the femoral artery is the femoral vein which is easily catheterized. Medial to this point of puncture lies the femoral canal, a site of herniation. (page 322)

Femoropopliteal bypass is a common vascular operation in the lower limb. The blockage nearly always occurs where the femoral artery passes through the adductor hiatus and following occlusion it is common to find that a superior genicular arterial branch, part of the knee anastomosis, is enlarged. Nowadays, instead of a complete bypass, various balloon or stent techniques are being used to enlarge stenotic arteries. (page 323)

Flat foot (pes planus) is due to flattening of the longitudinal arch. Often congenital, it may be associated with minor structural anomalies of the tarsal bones. This condition can be seen in wet footprints where the medial arch (normally raised) is visible. Treatment may be assisted by intensive foot exercises or by arch supports worn in the shoes. Occasionally, surgery is needed in the form of arthrodesis (fusion of the tarsal bones). (page 350)

Fracture of the fifth metatarsal is a common foot fracture; the styloid process of the fifth metatarsal is often avulsed, owing to attachment of the peroneus (fibularis) brevis muscle at this site. (page 312)

Gluteal nerve paralysis. Superior gluteal nerve damage affects the three abductor muscles (tensor fasciae latae, gluteus medius and gluteus minimus), resulting in a waddling gait (sometimes called a Trendelenburg gait) seen in patients with congenital dislocation of the hip. Inferior gluteal nerve damage, which affects only gluteus maximus, is a disabling condition because gluteus maximus is the strongest muscle used in extending the leg on the trunk, such as in running or in climbing stairs. These nerves may also be damaged during intramuscular injections into the buttock. (page 317)

Hallux valgus, lateral displacement of the great toe, usually presents as pain over a prominent metatarsal head due to rubbing from shoes and it may be associated with deformity of the second toe which tends to override the great toe. (page 310)

Hip fractures occur at the upper end of the femur and result from an indirect twisting force, most commonly in the frail and elderly, and the most common are considered under separate titles. (page 294)

Intermittent claudication is limping due to pain, usually experienced in the calf muscles, due to a generalized ischaemia of the lower limb. The patient may be able to walk a fixed distance before this pain occurs. Commonly it is due to atherosclerosis in the region of the adductor hiatus where the femoral artery becomes the popliteal artery. (page 323)

Intertrochanteric fracture of the femur is commonly seen in old people of both sexes and often is associated with an avulsion of the lesser trochanter due to pull of the iliopsoas tendon. (page 295)

Meniscal tears. Both the medial and lateral menisci are subject to rotational injuries and may be torn. The medial is much more liable to injury as it is attached to the medial collateral ligament, whereas the lateral meniscus or semilunar cartilage is separated from the fibular collateral ligament. Commonly seen in footballers' knees, these injuries are nowadays diagnosed by MR imaging or on direct arthroscopy. Presenting symptoms may be pain and swelling of the knee or locking of the knee when a partly detached cartilage wedges between the tibia and femur. Sometimes a momentary click may be heard in flexion/extension movements of the knee. Meniscectomy is a successful operation but nowadays there is greater emphasis on repairing small tears. (page 333)

Meralgia paraesthetica, sensory loss confined to the lateral, proximal thigh, occurs when the lateral femoral cutaneous nerve is trapped, usually just deep to the inguinal ligament near the anterior superior iliac spine. It may be due to increased size of the psoas muscle, such as in professional cyclists, bleeding into that muscle or a complication of laparoscopic hernia repair. (page 322)

Metatarsal fractures. Following a 'sprained ankle', occasionally the peroneus (fibularis) brevis tendon pulls off the base of the fifth metatarsal. However, much more common are stress fractures of the middle metatarsals, often known as 'march fractures'. (page 311)

Obturator nerve paralysis is a rare condition causing pain down the medial side of the upper thigh and weakness of the adductor group of muscles. It is seen in lateral pelvic wall pathology, often related to malignancy. (page 321)

Patellar tendon reflex (knee jerk) is elicited by tapping the patellar tendon with a patellar hammer and noting the quadriceps muscle contraction. This tests the L3 segment of the spinal cord. (page 328)

Plantar fasciitis is inflammation of the plantar aponeurosis, an important structure in maintaining the longitudinal arches of the foot. Inflammation of these strong fibrous bands may be extremely painful at the calcaneal end and is particularly common in people who have been walking in thin-soled shoes over rough ground. (page 350)

Popliteal aneurysm. The popliteal pulse is difficult to feel because the popliteal artery is the deepest structure in the popliteal fossa, lying against the oblique popliteal ligament – the reinforcement of the posterior capsule of the knee. To feel the pulse it is often necessary to flex the knee and press all fingers into the popliteal fossa hard against the bone. Owing to the constant bending and stretching of this artery with flexion of the knee, it is a site where aneurysms develop. A popliteal aneurysm may not be palpated until fairly large and may be mistaken for a Baker's cyst. (page 331)

Pott's fracture (ankle). External rotation injuries to the ankle are often associated with fractures. Identified in 1769 by Sir Percival Pott, they are more commonly described as first-degree, second-degree and third-degree ankle injuries. In a first-degree fracture a single structure – the lateral malleolus – is damaged. In a second-degree fracture the two structures damaged are the lateral malleolus (obliquely fractured and displaced) and the medial malleolus (fractured transversely and usually moved laterally with the talus). In a third-degree fracture the talus is displaced both outwards and backwards, in addition to being externally rotated, and three structures are damaged – lateral malleolus, the medial malleolus with displacement of the talus and a vertical fracture through the tibial articular surface. (page 354)

Sciatica is a clinical condition presenting as pain down the leg anywhere from the buttock to the heel and may be from any cause irritating the sciatic trunk or its nerve roots. Commonly it is due to intervertebral disc pathology in the L4/L5 or L5/S1 level. In the younger patient, back problems are the most common cause of this presenting symptom; however, in the older patient it is important to exclude neoplastic pathology within the pelvis, such as spread from rectal, uterine or prostate malignancies. A useful test for its diagnosis is the straight leg raising test or Achilles tendon reflex (see page 355), which tests the S1/2 nerve root. (page 316)

Sciatic trunk paralysis may be the unfortunate result of a badly placed intramuscular injection. When injecting into the buttock it is important to remember the surface markings of the sciatic trunk which passes through the middle of the buttock swelling. Injections should be placed in the upper outer quadrant of the buttock above a line joining the greater trochanter and the posterior superior iliac spine. Injections are often given in the lateral thigh instead of the buttock because of this potential complication. A complete sciatic trunk lesion will paralyse the hamstrings and all the muscles below the knee, as well as causing sensory loss below the knee except for the area supplied by the saphenous nerve. (page 317)

Slipped upper femoral epiphysis, also known as adolescent coxa vara, tends to occur in children (boys) between the ages of 10 and 15 who are often overweight, and presents as displacement of the upper femoral epiphysis causing a rotational twist to the limb which may be in external rotation and slightly shortened. This condition may present as referred pain to the knee. (page 314)

Sprained ankle. Because the normal range of inversion is greater than that of eversion, the lateral ligaments of the ankle tend to suffer most in inversion rotational injuries. The lateral ligament has three components – the anterior talofibular ligament, the calcaneofibular ligament and the posterior talofibular ligament; the most commonly torn is the anterior talofibular ligament. Clinically, there is tenderness and swelling over the lateral side of the ankle and a particularly tender spot just anterior to the tip of the lateral malleolus. (page 349)

Subcapital fracture of the femoral neck, commonly seen in frail osteoporotic women, can be impacted when the head of the femur is driven into the neck (sometimes with no pain or shortening of the leg) or unimpacted (severe pain with the affected leg shortened, and externally rotated and no active movement of the hip). If untreated, avascular necrosis of the femoral head may occur. (page 296)

Suprapatellar bursitis. The suprapatellar bursa lies a hand's breadth superior to the upper border of the patella and communicates with the knee joint. A knee joint effusion can therefore be 'milked' into the suprapatellar region and a patellar tap may be an indication of increased fluid within the whole knee joint complex. (page 334)

Thrombophlebitis, inflammation of the veins with resultant thrombosis, may occur in either the deep or the superficial veins. In the superficial veins, serious complications are rare. However, if the deep veins of the leg are blocked there is risk of a thrombus breaking off and causing a pulmonary embolism. Diagnosis is made using venography or colour Doppler ultrasound and the treatment usually involves pharmacological thinning of the blood. (page 340)

Torn hamstrings is a common injury seen when the unwarmed muscles are suddenly put into violent contraction, tearing fibres within one of the four major hamstrings (adductor magnus, biceps femoris, semitendinosus or semimembranosus). Stretching exercises are often the best treatment, though occasionally surgery is indicated. (page 318)

Trendelenburg's sign occurs when a patient stands on one leg, and the contralateral hip droops. The causes are numerous but any damage to the abductors (tensor fasciae latae, gluteus medius and gluteus minimus), the superior gluteal nerve, or an abnormality of the hip joint (congenital dislocation) will give this positive sign. It is often associated with a 'waddling' gait as the person is unable to raise the pelvis on the swing-through leg during normal walking. (page 324)

The Trendelenburg test for varicose veins checks the competence of the valves in the superficial venous system, especially at the saphenofemoral junction just before the great saphenous vein pierces the cribriform fascia of the leg to enter the femoral vein. Lack of competence of this valve may lead to severe varicosities throughout the great saphenous system. (page 320)

Varicose veins. Normally, the superficial venous supply below the knee drains via numerous perforators into the deep system. If the valves controlling this flow are damaged, which is often a congenital weakness, then the blood will flow from the deep system to the superficial system and many dilated, tortuous veins will be seen in the calf region. These unsightly veins may be cosmetically unacceptable; physiologically, the leg may begin to swell and eventually ulceration may occur in the region of the medial malleolus. Removal (stripping) or injection of these veins will improve the vascular physiology of the lower extremity. (page 346)

Vein harvest for coronary artery bypass grafting (CABG). This procedure has become a routine practice in cardiovascular units that are carrying out CABG – known as a 'cabbage' operation. During removal of the long saphenous vein for use by the cardiac surgeon, the saphenous nerve (the terminal branch, L4, of the femoral nerve) which lies entwined with the branches of the long saphenous vein may be damaged and result in loss of sensation on the medial side of the foot and ankle. (page 339)

Venous cutdowns. The most reliable site for a venous cutdown is just anterior to the medial malleolus of the ankle where the great saphenous vein is found. Prior to the advent of central venous catheterization in the 1960s this was, and in many parts of the world still is; the most common access to a vein in an emergency. (page 344)

Appendix I *Skull foramina*

PRINCIPAL FORAMINA AND CONTENTS

Supra-orbital foramen
Supra-orbital nerve and vessels

Infra-orbital foramen
Infra-orbital nerve and vessels

Mental foramen
Mental nerve and vessels

Mandibular foramen
Inferior alveolar nerve and vessels

Optic canal
Optic nerve
Ophthalmic artery

Superior orbital fissure
Ophthalmic nerve and veins
Oculomotor, trochlear and abducent
    nerves

Inferior orbital fissure
Maxillary nerve

Sphenopalatine foramen
Sphenopalatine artery
Nasal branches of pterygopalatine
    ganglion and maxillary nerve

Foramen rotundum
Maxillary nerve

Foramen ovale
Mandibular and lesser petrosal nerve

Foramen spinosum
Middle meningeal vessels

Carotid canal
Internal carotid artery and sympathetic
    plexus

Jugular foramen
Inferior petrosal sinus
Glossopharyngeal, vagus and accessory
    nerves
Internal jugular vein (emerging below) as
    continuation of sigmoid sinus

Internal acoustic meatus
Facial and vestibulocochlear nerves
Labyrinthine artery

Hypoglossal canal
Hypoglossal nerve

Stylomastoid foramen
Facial nerve

Foramen magnum
Medulla oblongata and meninges
Vertebral and anterior and posterior spinal
    arteries
Accessory nerves (spinal parts)

INSIDE THE SKULL

ANTERIOR CRANIAL FOSSA

**Foramina in the cribriform plate of the
    ethmoid**
Olfactory nerve filaments
Anterior ethmoidal nerve and vessels

Foramen caecum: between the frontal crest
    of the frontal bone and the ethmoid in
    front of the crista galli
Emissary vein (between nose and superior
    sagittal sinus)

MIDDLE CRANIAL FOSSA

Optic canal: in the sphenoid between the
    body and the two roots of the lesser wing
Optic nerve
Ophthalmic artery

Superior orbital fissure: in the sphenoid
    between the body and greater and lesser
    wings, with a fragment of the frontal bone
    at the lateral extremity
Oculomotor, trochlear and abducent nerves
Lacrimal, frontal and nasociliary nerves
Filaments from the internal carotid
    (sympathetic) plexus
Orbital branch of the middle meningeal artery
Recurrent branch of the lacrimal artery
Superior ophthalmic vein

Foramen rotundum: in the greater wing of
    the sphenoid
Maxillary nerve

Foramen ovale: in the greater wing of the
    sphenoid
Mandibular nerve
Lesser petrosal nerve (usually)
Accessory meningeal artery
Emissary veins (from cavernous sinus to
    pterygoid plexus)

Foramen spinosum: in the greater wing of
    the sphenoid
Middle meningeal vessels
Meningeal branch of the mandibular nerve

Venous (emissary sphenoidal) foramen: in
    40% of skulls, in the greater wing of the
    sphenoid medial to the foramen ovale
Emissary vein (from the cavernous sinus to the
    pterygoid plexus)

Petrosal (innominate) foramen: occasional, in
    the greater wing of the sphenoid, medial to
    the foramen spinosum
Lesser petrosal nerve (if not through foramen
    ovale)

Foramen lacerum: between the sphenoid,
    apex of the petrous temporal and the
    basilar part of the occipital
A meningeal branch of the ascending
    pharyngeal artery
Emissary veins (from the cavernous sinus to
    the pterygoid plexus)

Hiatus for the greater petrosal nerve: in the
    tegmen tympani of the petrous temporal,
    in front of the arcuate eminence

Greater petrosal nerve
Petrosal branch of the middle meningeal
    artery

Hiatus for the lesser petrosal nerve: in the
    tegmen tympani of the petrous temporal,
    about 3 mm in front of the hiatus for the
    greater petrosal nerve
Lesser petrosal nerve

POSTERIOR CRANIAL FOSSA

Internal acoustic meatus: in the posterior
    surface of the petrous temporal
Facial nerve
Vestibulocochlear nerve
Labyrinthine artery

Aqueduct of the vestibule: in the petrous
    temporal about 1 cm behind the internal
    acoustic meatus
Endolymphatic duct and sac
A branch from the meningeal branch of the
    occipital artery
A vein (from the labyrinth and vestibule to
    the sigmoid sinus)

Jugular foramen: between the jugular fossa
    of the petrous temporal and the occipital
    bone
Glossopharyngeal, vagus and accessory nerves
Meningeal branches of the vagus nerve
Inferior petrosal sinus
Internal jugular vein
A meningeal branch of the occipital artery

Hypoglossal canal: in the occipital bone
    above the anterior part of the condyle
Hypoglossal nerve and its (recurrent)
    meningeal branch
A meningeal branch of the ascending
    pharyngeal artery
Emissary vein (from the basilar plexus to the
    internal jugular vein)

Condylar canal: occasional, from the lower
    part of the sigmoid groove in the lateral
    part of the occipital bone to the condylar
    fossa on the external surface of the
    occipital bone behind the condyle
Emissary vein (from the sigmoid sinus to
    occipital veins)
A meningeal branch of the occipital artery

Mastoid foramen: in the petrous temporal
    near the posterior margin of the lower
    part of the sigmoid groove, passing
    backwards to open behind the mastoid
    process
Emissary vein (from the sigmoid sinus to
    occipital veins)
A meningeal branch of the occipital artery

Foramen magnum: in the occipital bone
Apical ligament of the dens of the axis
Tectorial membrane
Medulla oblongata and meninges (including
    first digitations of denticulate ligaments)
Spinal parts of the accessory nerves
Meningeal branches of the upper cervical
    nerves
Vertebral arteries
Anterior spinal artery
Posterior spinal arteries

IN THE BASE OF THE SKULL EXTERNALLY

Foramen lacerum
Foramen ovale
Foramen spinosum
Jugular foramen } see INSIDE THE SKULL
Hypoglossal canal
Condylar canal
Mastoid foramen
Foramen magnum

Inferior orbital fissure – see IN THE ORBIT

Lateral incisive foramen: opens into the incisive fossa, in the midline at the front of the hard palate
Nasopalatine nerve
Greater palatine vessels

Greater palatine foramen: between the maxilla and the palatine bone at the lateral border of the hard palate behind the palatomaxillary fissure
Greater palatine nerve and vessels

Lesser palatine foramina: two or three, in the inferior and medial aspects of the pyramidal process of the palatine bone
Lesser palatine nerves and vessels

Palatovaginal canal: between lower surface of the vaginal process of the root of the medial pterygoid plate and the upper surface of the sphenoidal process of the palatine bone
Pharyngeal branch of the pterygopalatine ganglion
Pharyngeal branch of the maxillary artery

Vomerovaginal canal: occasional, medial to the palatovaginal canal, between the upper surface of the vaginal process of the root of the medial pterygoid plate and the lower surface of the ala of the vomer
Pharyngeal branch of the sphenopalatine artery

Petrosquamous fissure: between the squamous temporal and the tegmen tympani
Petrosquamous vein

Petrotympanic fissure: between the tympanic part of the temporal bone and the tegmen tympani
Chorda tympani
Anterior ligament of the malleus
Anterior tympanic branch of the maxillary artery

Cochlear canaliculus: in the petrous temporal, at the apex of a notch in front of the medial part of the jugular fossa
Perilymphatic duct
Emissary vein (from the cochlea to the internal jugular vein or inferior petrosal sinus)

Carotid canal: in the inferior surface of the petrous temporal
Internal carotid artery
Internal carotid (sympathetic) plexus
Internal carotid venous plexus (from the cavernous sinus to the internal jugular vein)

Tympanic canaliculus: in the inferior surface of the petrous temporal, on the ridge of bone between the carotid canal and the jugular fossa
Tympanic branch of the glossopharyngeal nerve
Inferior tympanic branch of the ascending pharyngeal artery

Mastoid canaliculus: in the inferior surface of the petrous temporal, on the lateral wall of the jugular fossa
Auricular branch of the vagus nerve

Stylomastoid foramen: between the styloid and mastoid processes of the temporal bone
Facial nerve
Stylomastoid branch of the posterior auricular artery

IN THE ORBIT

Superior orbital fissure } see INSIDE THE SKULL
Optic canal

Frontal notch or foramen: in the supra-orbital margin of the frontal bone one finger's breadth from the midline
Supratrochlear nerve and vessels

Supra-orbital notch or foramen: in the supra-orbital margin of the frontal bone two fingers' breadths from the midline
Supra-orbital nerve and vessels

Anterior ethmoidal foramen: in the medial wall of the orbit between the orbital part of the frontal bone and the ethmoid labyrinth
Anterior ethmoidal nerve and vessels

Posterior ethmoidal foramen: occasional, 1 to 2 cm behind the anterior ethmoidal foramen
Posterior ethmoidal nerve and vessels

Zygomatico-orbital foramen: in the orbital surface of the zygomatic bone
Zygomatic branch of the maxillary nerve

Nasolacrimal canal: at the front, lower, medial corner of the orbit formed by the lacrimal bone and maxilla
Nasolacrimal duct

Inferior orbital fissure: towards the back of the orbit, between the maxilla and the greater wing of the sphenoid
Maxillary nerve
Zygomatic nerve
Orbital branches of the pterygopalatine ganglion
Infra-orbital vessels
Inferior ophthalmic veins

Infra-orbital canal: in the orbital surface of the maxilla
Infra-orbital nerve and vessels

MISCELLANEOUS

Infra-orbital foramen: the anterior opening of the infra-orbital canal, in the maxilla below the infra-orbital margin
Infra-orbital nerve and vessels

Mental foramen: on the outer surface of the body of the mandible below the second premolar tooth or slightly more anteriorly
Mental nerve and vessels

Mandibular foramen: on the inner surface of the ramus of the mandible, overlapped anteriorly and medially by the lingula
Inferior alveolar nerve and vessels

Foramina in the infratemporal (posterior) surface of the maxilla
Posterior superior alveolar nerves and vessels

Pterygomaxillary fissure: between the lateral pterygoid plate and the infratemporal (posterior) surface of the maxilla, and continuous above with the posterior end of the inferior orbital fissure
Maxillary artery (entering pterygopalatine fossa)
Maxillary nerve (entering inferior orbital fissure)
Sphenopalatine veins

Sphenopalatine foramen: at the upper end of the perpendicular plate of the palatine between its orbital and sphenoidal processes and (above) the body of the sphenoid, in the medial wall of the pterygopalatine fossa (viewed laterally through the pterygomaxillary fissure) and lateral wall of the nasal cavity (viewed medially)
Nasopalatine and posterior superior nasal nerves
Sphenopalatine vessels

Foramina in the perpendicular plate of the palatine
Posterior inferior nasal nerves

Pterygoid canal: at the root of the pterygoid process of the sphenoid in line with the medial pterygoid plate, leading from the anterior wall of the foramen lacerum to the posterior wall of the pterygopalatine fossa (and only clearly seen in a disarticulated sphenoid)
Nerve of the pterygoid canal
Artery of the pterygoid canal

Musculotubular canal: at the lateral side of the apex of the petrous temporal, at the junction of the petrous and squamous parts, and divided by a bony septum into upper and lower semicanals
Tensor tympani (upper semicanal)
Auditory tube (lower semicanal)

Parietal foramen: in the parietal bone near the posterosuperior (occipital) angle
Emissary vein (from the superior sagittal sinus to the scalp)

Appendix II   *Lymphatic system*

THORACIC DUCT AND CISTERNA CHYLI TRIBUTARIES

Thoracic duct
Left jugular trunk
Left subclavian trunk
Left bronchomediastinal trunk

Right lymphatic duct
Right jugular trunk
Right subclavian trunk
Right bronchomediastinal trunk

Cisterna chyli
Left lumbar trunk
Right lumbar trunk
Intestinal trunk

LYMPH NODES OF THE HEAD AND NECK

Deep cervical
Superior (including jugulodigastric)
Inferior (including jugulo-omohyoid)

Draining superficial tissues in the head
Occipital
Retro-auricular (mastoid)
Parotid
Buccal (facial)

Draining superficial tissues in the neck
Submandibular
Submental
Anterior cervical
Superficial cervical

Draining deep tissues in the neck
Retropharyngeal
Paratracheal
Lingual
Infrahyoid
Prelaryngeal
Pretracheal

LYMPH NODES OF THE UPPER LIMB AND MAMMARY GLAND

Draining the upper limb
Axillary
  Apical
  Central
  Lateral
  Pectoral (anterior)
  Subscapular (posterior)
Infraclavicular
Supratrochlear
Cubital

Draining the mammary gland
Pectoral
Subscapular
Apical
Parasternal
Intercostal

LYMPH NODES OF THE THORAX

Draining thoracic walls
Superficial
  Pectoral
  Subscapular
  Parasternal
  Inferior deep cervical
Deep
  Parasternal
  Intercostal
  Phrenic
  Diaphragmatic

Draining thoracic contents
Brachiocephalic
Posterior mediastinal
Tracheobronchial
  Paratracheal
  Superior tracheobronchial
  Inferior tracheobronchial
  Bronchopulmonary
  Pulmonary

LYMPH NODES OF THE ABDOMEN AND PELVIS

Lumbar
  Pre-aortic
    Coeliac
      Gastric
        Left gastric
        Right gastro-epiploic
        Pyloric
      Hepatic
      Pancreaticosplenic
    Superior mesenteric
    Inferior mesenteric
  Lateral aortic
    Common iliac
    External iliac
    Internal iliac
    Inferior epigastric
    Circumflex iliac
    Sacral
  Retro-aortic

LYMPH NODES OF THE LOWER LIMB

Superficial inguinal
  Upper
  Lower
Deep inguinal
Popliteal

Appendix III *Nerves*

CRANIAL NERVES AND BRANCHES

I Olfactory (from olfactory mucous membrane)

II Optic (from retina)

III Oculomotor
Superior ramus (to superior rectus and levator palpebrae superioris)
Inferior ramus (to medial rectus, inferior rectus, inferior oblique and ciliary ganglion)

IV Trochlear (to superior oblique)

V Trigeminal
Ophthalmic
  Lacrimal
  Frontal
    Supratrochlear
    Supra-orbital
  Nasociliary → anterior ethmoidal → external nasal
    Internal nasal (from anterior ethmoidal)
    Ciliary ganglion
    Long ciliary
    Infratrochlear
    Posterior ethmoidal
Maxillary → infra-orbital
  Meningeal
  Pterygopalatine
    Orbital
    Palatine
    Nasal
    Pharyngeal
  Zygomatic
    Zygomaticotemporal
    Zygomaticofacial
  Posterior superior alveolar
  Middle superior alveolar
  Anterior superior alveolar
  Palpebral ⎤
  Nasal ⎬ (from infra-orbital)
  Superior labial ⎦

Mandibular
  Meningeal
  Nerve to medial pterygoid (and tensor veli palatini and tensor tympani)
  Anterior trunk
    Buccal
    Masseteric
    Deep temporal
    Nerve to lateral pterygoid
  Posterior trunk
    Auriculotemporal
    Lingual
    Inferior alveolar
      Nerve to mylohyoid
      Mental

VI Abducent (to lateral rectus)

VII Facial
Greater petrosal
Nerve to stapedius
Chorda tympani
Posterior auricular (to occipitalis and auricular muscles)
Nerve to posterior belly of digastric
Nerve to stylohyoid
Temporal ⎤
Zygomatic ⎮ to frontalis and
Buccal ⎬ muscles of facial
Mandibular ⎮ expression
Cervical ⎦

VIII Vestibulocochlear
Cochlear (from coils of cochlea)
Vestibular (from utricle, saccule and ampullae of semicircular ducts)

IX Glossopharyngeal
Tympanic
  Lesser petrosal
Carotid sinus
Pharyngeal
Muscular (to stylopharyngeus)
Tonsillar
Lingual

X Vagus
Meningeal
Auricular
Pharyngeal (to muscles of pharynx and soft palate except stylopharyngeus and tensor veli palatini)
Carotid body
Superior laryngeal
  Internal laryngeal
  External laryngeal (to cricothyroid)
Right recurrent laryngeal (to muscles of larynx except cricothyroid)
Cardiac (cervical)
Cardiac (thoracic)
Left recurrent laryngeal (to muscles of larynx except cricothyroid)
Pulmonary
Oesophageal
Anterior trunk
  Gastric
  Hepatic
Posterior trunk
  Coeliac
  Gastric

XI Accessory
Cranial root (to muscles of palate and possibly larynx via vagus)
Spinal root (to sternocleidomastoid and trapezius)

XII Hypoglossal
Descending (upper root of ansa cervicalis, from C1 to superior belly of omohyoid, then forming ansa cervicalis – see cervical plexus)
Nerve to thyrohyoid (from C1)
Muscular (to geniohyoid from C1) and to muscles of tongue except palatoglossus

HEAD AND NECK NERVE SUPPLIES

All the muscles of	Supplied by	Except	Supplied by
Pharynx	Pharyngeal plexus	Stylo-pharyngeus	Glosso-pharyngeal nerve
Palate	Pharyngeal plexus	Tensor veli palatini	Nerve to medial pterygoid
Larynx	Recurrent laryngeal nerve	Cricothyroid	External laryngeal nerve
Tongue	Hypoglossal nerve	Palatoglossus	Pharyngeal plexus
Facial expression (including buccinator)	Facial nerve		
Mastication	Mandibular branch of trigeminal nerve		

Index